Question Bank for Dental Postgraduate Entrance Examination

(Including Syllabus and AIPGEE's Solved Question Paper)

Question Bank for Dental Postgraduate Entrance Examination

(A comprehensive and multidisciplinary review of basic and clinical science subjects with explanatory answers)

Pankaj Goel
Kanwarjit Singh
Sanjay Saraf
Rohit Chopra
Sujata Mohanty
Pankaj Datta

Foreword by

Dr Mahesh Verma
Principal
Maulana Azad Dental College and Hospital
New Delhi

PEEPEE
PUBLISHERS and DISTRIBUTORS (P) LTD.

Question Bank for Dental Postgraduate Entrance Examination

Published by
Pawaninder P. Vij

Peepee Publishers and Distributors (P) Ltd.
Head Office: 160, Shakti Vihar, Pitam Pura, Delhi 110 034 (India)

Corporate office: 7/31, Ansari Road, Daryaganj, Post Box-7243
New Delhi 110002 (India)

Ph: 55195868, 9811156083

e-mail: peepee160@yahoo.co.in

e-mail: peepee160@rediffmail.com

First Edition: **2005**

ISBN: 81-88867-44-6

Printed at
Lordson, C-5/19, Rana Pratap Bagh, Delhi-110 007

Foreword

It gives me immense pleasure in writing this foreword for the title *"Question Bank for Dental Postgraduate Entrance Examination"* that has been jointly authored by Dr(s) Pankaj Goel, Kanwarjit Singh, Sanjay Saraf, Rohit Chopra, Sujata Mohanty and Pankaj Datta. Most of the authors of this book have been working at Maulana Azad Dental College and Hospital, New Delhi, for many years and I have had a close association with all of them. They are brilliant teachers who have tremendous research potential. Their clinical and didactic skills have been especially noteworthy for undergraduate teaching and training activities. In fact it is the synergy of their combined efforts that has culminated in the form of this much-needed book for students of Dentistry.

In today's scenario where everybody is trying to outdo others, examinations based on multiple-choice questions have become a gold standard to gauge a student's ability. This book would surely prove to be a cutting edge tool for candidates who endeavor to gain entry to top Dental institutions in India and abroad. Authors have taken great care to frame model questions covering important aspects of syllabus as prescribed by Dental Council of India for both basic and clinical science subjects. Explanatory answers and cross-references have also been provided to facilitate learning.

Science is ever changing and is truly dynamic. What was dead right ten years back may be dead wrong today. I am sure that this bunch of young authors will keep on updating their text accordingly and incorporate newer topics as they emerge. Wishing many more editions to their efforts.

Maheshverma

Dr Mahesh Verma
Principal
Maulana Azad Dental College and Hospital
New Delhi

Foreword

It gives me immense pleasure in writing this foreword for the title "*Question Bank for Dental Postgraduate Entrance Examinations*" that has been jointly authored by Drs Pankaj Goel, Kanwarjit Singh Sandhu, Sarit Rohit Kapoor, Sujata Mohanty and Pankaj Datta. Most of the authors of this book have been working at Maulana Azad Dental College and Hospital, New Delhi, for many years and I have had a close association with all of them. They are brilliant teachers who have tremendous research potential. Their clinical and didactic skills have been especially noteworthy for undergraduate teaching and training endeavors. In fact it is the synergy of their combined efforts that has culminated in the form of this much-needed book for students of Dentistry.

In today's scenario where everybody is trying to outdo others, examinations based on multiple-choice questions have become a gold standard to gauge a student's ability. This book would surely prove to be a cutting edge tool for candidates who endeavor to gain entry to top Dental institutions in India and abroad. Authors have taken great care to frame model questions covering important aspects of syllabus as prescribed by [illegible]. Explanatory answers and cross-references have been provided to facilitate learning.

Science is ever changing and evolving. What one read ten years back may be dead wrong today. I am sure that this first attempt of authors will keep on getting better with [illegible] and the addition of newer topics in their next edition. Wishing many more editions to their efforts.

[illegible]

Dr Mahesh Verma
Director-Principal
Maulana Azad Dental College and Hospital
New Delhi

Contributors

PANKAJ GOEL
MDS (Community Dentistry)
Maulana Azad Dental College
and Hospital
New Delhi

KANWARJIT SINGH ASI
MDS (Periodontics)
Maulana Azad Dental College
and Hospital
New Delhi

SANJAY SARAF
MDS (Oral Pathology)
Maulana Azad Dental College
and Hospital
New Delhi

ROHIT CHOPRA
MDS (Orthodontics)
Maulana Azad Dental College
and Hospital
New Delhi

SUJATA MOHANTY
MDS (Oral-Maxillofacial Surgery)
Maulana Azad Dental College
and Hospital
New Delhi

PANKAJ DATTA
MDS (Prosthodontics)
Department of Prosthodontics
Institute of Dental Studies and Technology
Modi Nagar (U.P.)

RITU CHOPRA
MD (Paediatrics)
Aruna Asaf Ali (Civil) Hospital
Govt. of NCT Delhi
Delhi

POONAM SARAF
MD (Medicine)
St. Stephen's Hospital
Delhi

Preface

A phenomenal increase in the number of Dental Colleges over the last decade has created a challenging situation for the profession in contemporary India. Charles Darwin's theory of ***natural selection*** (of the fittest) is most applicable to the 7500 Dental graduates entering the professional mainstream every year with a zest of making a mark in their careers. A postgraduate qualification is an obvious choice for a majority of those who aspire for professional satisfaction and prestige. However limited number of seats for postgraduation makes success difficult and thus a thorough preparation is warranted. This book is an humble step in this direction and at the same time it is much more than a compendium of MCQs. It is a ready reckoner to guide aspirants through the maze of ambiguity that surrounds entrance examinations. A team of Dental and Medical specialists have put together their efforts and experiences to bring to you the essentials of preparing for such examinations, that includes:

- Complete syllabus
- Model questions
- Explanatory answers
- Relevant diagrams and references
- Solved paper of latest AIPGEE.

We suggest that an aspirant should not limit him/herself to remembering answers only but should also probe into the reasoning for the same as provided in this book. Care has been taken to cover most aspects of the syllabus and queries/suggestions from readers are most welcome as they will help us strengthen the book further. We thanks our students at Maulana Azad Dental College and Hospital for reviewing the manuscript and helping us in understanding *their* topics of concern. Last but not the least we are thankful to our publisher, Mr Pawaninder Vij, and his dedicated team for their efforts.

Dr Pankaj Goel
(on behalf of all the authors)

Contents

BASIC SCIENCE

CLINICAL SCIENCE

Syllabus

1. Introduction.
2. Detailed Anatomy and Osteology of Head and Neck.
3. Gross Anatomy of Thorax, Abdomen and Extremities.
4. Embryology of Head, Neck with emphasis on development of face, jaws, tongue, palate, salivary glands, pharyngeal arches and pouches. Lymphatic and blood vessel system, G.I. system.
5. Paranasal air sinuses.
6. a. Gross Anatomy of the brain.
   b. Study of Cranial nerves–in detail extra cranial course of 5th, 7th and 9th nerves and upper cervical nerves.
7. Genetics: Fundamentals of Genetics.
8. Anthropology: General Principles.

Chapter 1

General Human Anatomy including Embryology and Histology

1. **Which of the following arteries contain impure blood?**
   A. Pulmonary artery
   B. Coronary artery
   C. Common carotid artery
   D. Descending aorta

2. **Tunica externa, tunica adventitia and tunica intima are parts of**
   A. Arteries
   B. Nerves
   C. Veins
   D. A and C both

3. **Continuous types of capillaries**
   A. Have no pores in the wall
   B. Have interrupted endothelium
   C. Are found in endocrine glands and pancreas
   D. All of the above

4. **All the blood vessels are of ____ origin**
   A. Endodermal
   B. Ectodermal
   C. Mesodermal
   D. Teratomatous

5. **The opening of the superior vena cava is situated at**
   A. Lower and anterior part of left atrium
   B. Posterior part of left ventricle
   C. Upper and posterior part of right atrium
   D. Anterior and inferior part of right ventricle

6. **'The fibres of Purkinje'**
   A. Are remains of embryonic cardiac muscle fibres
   B. Are placed over the pericardium
   C. Arise from the sinu-arterial node
   D. A and B both

7. **'Pacemaker' of the heart is**
   A. Atrioventricular node
   B. Sinu-atrial node
   C. Tricuspid valve
   D. Purkinje fibres

8. **Lingual artery arises from the antero-medial part of ECA opposite the tip of greater cornu of hyoid in between**
   A. Superior thyroid and facial arteries
   B. Maxillary and superficial temporal arteries
   C. Superior thyroid and posterior auricular arteries
   D. Posterior auricular and occipital arteries

9. **The cubital fossa is an intermuscular space situated**
   A. At the wrist
   B. In front of the elbow
   C. At the back of the knee
   D. At the midsternum

10. All of the following are branches of internal carotid artery *except*
A. Superior hypophyseal artery
B. Anterior cerebral artery
C. Posterior auricular artery
D. Middle cerebral artery

11. Vagus nerve supplies
A. Liver and pancreas only
B. Upto rectum
C. Upto duodenojejunal junction
D. Upto middle 2/3rd of transverse colon

12. Inferior thyroid artery is a branch of
A. Thyrocervical trunk
B. Facial artery
C. Lingual artery
D. External carotid artery

13. The following structures pass through cavernous sinus *except*
A. Internal carotid artery
B. IVth cranial nerve
C. IInd cranial nerve
D. VIth cranial nerve

14. Sensory nerve supply to skin over the angle of mandible is by
A. Greater auricular
B. Transverse cervical
C. Lesser occipital
D. Mandibular

15. The two hemispheres of brain are connected by all *except*
A. Anterior commissure
B. Posterior commissure
C. Corpus striatum
D. Corpus callosum

16. Cerebellum is connected to mid brain by
A. Superior cerebellar peduncle
B. Middle cerebellar peduncle
C. Inferior cerebellar peduncle
D. All of the above

17. Posterior interosseous nerve supplies
A. Brachioradialis
B. Triceps
C. Supinator
D. Pronator teres

18. Which of the following is true about femoral nerve?
A. Nerve to pectinus arises from it
B. Arises from ventral divisions $L_{2,3,4}$ roots
C. Gives cutaneous supply to the lateral thigh
D. Supplies adductor longus

19. Choroid plexus is present in all *except*
A. Lateral ventricles
B. IIIrd ventricle
C. IVth ventricle
D. Cerebral aqueduct

20. All of the following are branches of vertebral artery *except*
A. Anterior spinal
B. Posterior spinal
C. Anterior choroid
D. Posterior inferior cerebellar

21. The palaține tonsil develops from
A. 2nd branchial cleft
B. 4th branchial cleft
C. 1st branchial arch
D. 2nd branchial arch

22. 'Oligodendroglia' forms ____ in the CNS
A. Axons B. Myelin sheath
C. Ganglion D. Nodes of Ranvier

23. Widest cross sectional area is of
A. Artery B. Vein
C. Capillary D. Venule

24. Biceps is attached to
A. Posterior surface of radial tuberosity
B. Anterior surface of radial tuberosity
C. Olecranon process
D. Ulnar tuberosity

25. Normal pleura is
A. 1 cm above 1st rib
B. 2 cm above 1st rib
C. At upper edge of 1st rib
D. At lower edge of 1st rib

26. Structures derived from the neural crest are
A. Adrenal medulla
B. Pia
C. Schwann cells
D. All of the above

27. Which nerve does not arise from the medulla?
A. Facial
B. Glossopharyngeal
C. Vagus
D. Hypoglossal

28. The oesophageal opening in the diaphragm is at the level of
A. T_8 B. T_9
C. T_{10} D. T_{11}

29. The shortest part of colon is
A. Descending colon
B. Ascending colon
C. Transverse colon
D. Sigmoid colon

30. The number of spinal nerve pairs are
A. 30 B. 31
C. 33 D. 40

31. 'Risorius' is known as the ____ muscle
A. Frowning
B. Laughing
C. Grinning
D. None of the above

32. Internal thoracic veins are Tributaries of
A. Brachiocephalic vein
B. Azygous vein
C. Subclavian vein
D. Internal jugular vein

33. The two lobes of liver are divided by
A. Inferior vena cava
B. Triangular ligament
C. Falciform ligament
D. Superior vena cava

34. Brunner's glands are seen in
A. Illeum
B. Rectum
C. Jejunum
D. Duodenum

35. 'Aurbach's plexus' supplies
A. Pancreas B. Liver
C. Jejunum D. Rectum

36. 'Ligament of Bigelow' is present in
A. Hip joint
B. Ankle joint
C. Shoulder joint
D. Knee joint

37. All of the following are anterior relations of cervical part of oesophagus *except*
A. Trachea throughout its course in the neck
B. Common carotid artery
C. Lobes of thyroid gland at the lower part of neck
D. Recurrent laryngeal nerve

38. 'Riedel's lobe' is a part of ____
A. Spleen B. Liver
C. Oesophagus D. Thyroid gland

39. Eustachian tube is
A. Totally bony
B. Supplied by glossopharyngeal nerve
C. Lined by cuboidal epithelium
D. A tube connecting oropharynx to middle ear

40. Deep circumflex iliac artery is a branch of
A. Internal iliac
B. Vaginal
C. External iliac
D. Common iliac

41. External jugular vein is formed by
A. Union of posterior auricular and posterior division of retromandibular veins
B. Direct continuation of sigmoid sinus
C. Union of maxillary and superficial temporal veins
D. Union of anterior retromandibular with facial veins

42. **Following are some peculiarities of emissary veins *except***
   A. Devoid of any valves
   B. Blood flow is in both directions
   C. There is no muscular coat in the endothelial wall
   D. Are not connected to any cerebral sinus

43. **Which of the following vessels are prone for varicosity**
   A. Superficial veins of lower limb
   B. Deep veins of lower limb
   C. Superficial and deep arteries of lower limb
   D. All of the above

44. **All of the following structures pass through the parotid gland *except***
   A. External carotid artery
   B. Internal carotid artery
   C. Maxillary vein
   D. Facial nerve

45. **Which of the following structures pass through inferior orbital fissure?**
   A. Lacrimal nerve
   B. Infraorbital nerve
   C. Abducent nerve
   D. Olfactory nerve

46. **The difference between the composition of the lymph of lymphatic capillaries and tissue fluids lies in their ____ content.**
   A. Carbohydrate
   B. Fat
   C. Protein
   D. No difference in composition

47. **The collecting lymph vessels which drain into the lymphnode by piercing it at its periphery are**
   A. Afferent lymph vessels
   B. Efferent lymph vessels
   C. Lymph trunk
   D. All of the above

48. **All are the branches of cervical plexus *except***
   A. Supra clavicular nerve
   B. Greater auricular nerve
   C. Suprascapular nerve
   D. Lesser occipital nerve

49. **Pain sensitive structure in brain is**
   A. Grey mater
   B. Venous sinuses and durameter
   C. Pia and arachnoid mater
   D. Cerebellum

50. **Structures present in Radial groove besides radial nerve is**
   A. Median nerve
   B. Anterior circumflex humeral artery
   C. Posterior circumflex humeral artery
   D. Profunda brachi artery

51. **Ciliary ganglion is situated**
   A. In between optic nerve and lateral rectus
   B. In between optic nerve and medial rectus
   C. Apex of orbit lateral to optic nerve
   D. In between lateral and medial rectus

52. **All of the following are superficial group of lymphnodes *except***
   A. Occipital nodes
   B. Sub-mandibular nodes
   C. Jugulo-digastric nodes
   D. Submental nodes

53. **Cisternachyli continues upwards as**
   A. Ends blindly
   B. Thoracic duct
   C. Intestinal lymph trunk
   D. Left lumbar lymph trunk

54. **Cranial nerve with largest intra-cranial course is**
   A. Occulomotor B. Hypoglossal
   C. Trochlear D. Abducent

55. **All of the following are hamstring muscles *except***
   A. Semimembranosus
   B. Sartorius
   C. Semitendinosus
   D. Biceps femoris

56. **Bed of stomach is formed by all *except***
A. Spleen
B. Left suprarenal gland
C. Tail of pancreas
D. Splenic artery

57. **All of the following organs have an end arterial blood supply *except***
A. Lung B. Liver
C. Kidney D. Spleen

58. **The action of musculus uvulae is to**
A. Elevate the pharynx
B. Depress and elongate the uvula
C. Draw the soft palate to the same side
D. Elevate and shorten the uvula

59. **Sinus of 'Morgagni' is**
A. Gap between the base of the skull and upper concave margin of superior pharyngeal constrictor
B. Gap between inferior border of parietal bone and upper end of frontal bone
C. Sinusoidal space present in base of skull
D. None of the above

60. **The salivary gland duct which contain secretary cells are known as**
A. Interlobar duct
B. Striated ducts
C. Intercalated duct
D. Serous demilunes

61. **The superior parathyroid glands are derived from**
A. IInd Endodermal pouch
B. IIIrd Endodermal pouch
C. IVth Endodermal pouch
D. Vth Endodermal pouch

62. **Which of the following structures is not derived from the 1st branchial arch?**
A. Incus B. Stapes
C. Malleus D. Mandible

63. **Which of the following structure lies between external and internal carotid artery?**
A. Superior laryngeal nerve
B. Stylohyoid muscle
C. Glossopharyngeal nerve
D. Styloglossus muscle

64. **Sphenoid air sinus**
A. Opens into middle meatus
B. Lined by stratified squamous epithelium
C. Present at birth
D. Occupies the greater wing of sphenoid

65. **The following nerves are related to the humerus *except***
A. Radial B. Ulnar
C. Axillary D. Median

66. **The innervation of muscles of lateral compartment of leg is by**
A. Tibial nerve
B. Sural nerve
C. Deep peroneal nerve
D. Superficial peroneal nerve

67. **'Bergman cells' are microglial cells present in**
A. Retina
B. Cerebellum
C. Pituitary
D. Ventricles of brain

68. **Lateral rotators of shoulder are all *except***
A. Supraspinatus
B. Infraspinatus
C. Teres minor
D. Posterior fibres of Deltoid

69. **'Winging of scapula' results from paralysis of**
A. Dorsal scapular nerve
B. Long thoracic nerve
C. Axillary nerve
D. Suprascapular nerve

70. **The following ganglion are functionally related to parasympathetic nervous system *except***
A. Submandibular
B. Otic
C. Ciliary
D. Geniculate

71. Muscles supplied by occulomotor nerve are all *except*
A. Superior rectus B. Inferior rectus
C. Superior oblique D. Inferior oblique

72. Taste buds are absent on
A. Vallate papillae
B. Soft palate
C. Foliate papillae
D. Posterior 1/3rd tongue

73. Splenic artery is a branch of
A. Coeliac artery
B. Hepatic artery
C. Oesophageal artery
D. Superior mesenteric artery

74. Following cranial nerves are purely sensory *except*
A. I B. II
C. V D. VIII

75. Abductor of the vocal cord is
A. Posterior crico-arytenoid
B. Lateral arytenoid
C. Interarytenoid
D. Cricothyroid

76. The first bone to ossify in the body is
A. Femur B. Clavicle
C. Humerus D. Radius

77. Structure passing between superior constrictor of pharynx and base of the skull is
A. Tensor tympany
B. Tensor palati
C. Tensor palati and auditory tube
D. Stylohyoid and styloglossus

78. The lacrimal gland is supplied by ____ nerves
A. Sensory B. Secretomotor
C. Sympathetic D. All of the above

79. Secretomotor fibres to the parotid is via
A. Auriculotemporal nerve
B. Trigeminal nerve
C. Maxillary nerve
D. Facial nerve

80. Meningocytes are usually found in
A. Arachnoidal villi
B. In CSF
C. Within tentorium cerebelli
D. A and B both

81. 'Arachnoid mater' in Greek means
A. 'Compartment'
B. 'Like a spider's web'
C. 'Tender'
D. 'Irregularities'

82. Carotid canal transmits
A. Internal carotid artery
B. External carotid artery
C. Common carotid artery
D. All of the above

83. The largest ear ossicle is
A. Incus
B. Malleus
C. Stapes
D. All are of the same size

84. Damage to internal laryngeal nerve leads to
A. Weakness of phonation
B. Paralysis of vocal cords
C. Anaesthesia of mucous membrane of supraglottic part of larynx
D. No abnormality is produced

85. Waldeyer's lymphatic ring is formed by
A. 2 palatine, 1 pharyngeal and 1 lingual tonsils
B. 1 palatine, 2 pharyngeal and 1 lingual tonsils
C. 4 palatine, 1 pharyngeal and 2 lingual tonsils
D. 2 palatine, 2 pharyngeal and 2 lingual tonsils

86. Nucleus ambiguous and nucleus of tractus solitarius are nuclei of
A. Facial nerve
B. Vagus nerve
C. Glossopharyngeal nerve
D. Trochlear nerve

87. The temporal, zygomatic, buccal, mandibular and cervical branches of facial nerve
- **A.** Run within the facial canal
- **B.** Arise at its exit from stylomastoid foramen
- **C.** Are terminal branches within the parotid gland
- **D.** Communicate with adjacent cranial and spinal nerves

88. The anterior tubercle of transverse process of 6th cervical vertebra is
- **A.** Carotid tubercle
- **B.** Aortic body
- **C.** Adam's apple
- **D.** Subhyoid bursa

89. The investing layer of deep cervical fascia splits to enclose all of the following *except*
- **A.** Trapezius and sternomastoid muscles
- **B.** Parotid and submandibular glands
- **C.** Suprasternal and supraclavicular spaces
- **D.** Sternomastoid and vertebral arteries

90. Infection from nose can spread directly into
- **A.** Anterior cranial fossa
- **B.** Lacrimal apparatus
- **C.** Middle cranial fossa
- **D.** A and B

91. The 'Vestibular' part of vestibulocochlear nerve deals with
- **A.** Balance
- **B.** Hearing
- **C.** Smell
- **D.** Touch

92. Middle cerebral artery is a branch of
- **A.** External carotid artery
- **B.** Internal carotid artery
- **C.** Basilar artery
- **D.** Vertebral artery

93. Vidian's nerve is formed by union of
- **A.** Greater petrosal and deep petrosal nerves
- **B.** Greater petrosal and lesser petrosal nerves
- **C.** Greater petrosal and 3rd petrosal nerves
- **D.** Lesser and deep petrosal nerves

94. The suture between the 2 parietal and occipital bones is
- **A.** Superior nuchal line
- **B.** Inferior nuchal line
- **C.** Lambdoid suture
- **D.** Occipitomastoid suture

95. 'Rhinion' is
- **A.** Part of the nasal bone near the median plane
- **B.** Lower part of internasal suture
- **C.** Part of anterior nasal spine
- **D.** Part of frontal process of maxilla

96. 'Levator palati'
- **A.** Elevates soft palate and closes pharyngeal isthmus
- **B.** Tightens soft palate
- **C.** Pulls up uvula
- **D.** Pulls up root of tongue

97. Anterior relations of 1st part of vertebral artery are
- **A.** Transverse process of C_7 and stellate ganglion
- **B.** Common carotid artery, vertebral vein
- **C.** Ventral rami of C_{2-6} nerves
- **D.** Lateral mass of atlas

98. Subclavian trunk drains lymph from
- **A.** Lung and half of mediastinum
- **B.** Half of the head and neck
- **C.** Upper limb
- **D.** Most of the body except right upper limb, right halves of head, neck, thorax and superior surface of liver

99. Lesser occipital, great auricular and supraclavicular nerves are ________ branches of cervical plexus
- **A.** Superficial (cutaneous)
- **B.** Deep (communicating)
- **C.** Muscular
- **D.** Above are not branches of cervical plexus

Answers

1 A

2 D All these layers are parts of vessels i.e. arteries and veins with the outermost layer being the tunica externa. The middle one is tunica media and the inner layer is called tunica intima.

3 A 'B' and 'C' are features of fenestrated capillaries.

4 C

5 C

6 A These form specialized fibres of the heart and are supposed to be terminal filaments of bundle of His. They are placed beneath the endocardium and intervene between it and the myocardium.

7 B SA node commands the whole heart to beat at a rate of 60-80/min in an adult which is called a sinus rhythm.

8 A

9 B

10 C Which is a branch of ECA.

11 D

12 A 'B' and 'C' are branches of ECA; 'D' is a branch of commoncarotid artery. Superior thyroid is a branch of ECA but not inferior thyroid.

13 C Passes through optic formen.

14 A 'B' supplies skin over neck, 'C' supplies skin covering the head behind the auricle and 'D' is sensory to skin and mucous membrane covering buccinator muscle, skin covering upper part of auricle, external auditory meatus, TMJ area, tympanic membrane and the skin over temporal region.

15 C

16 A

17 C

18 A

19 D

20 C Is a branch of internal carotid artery.

21 A

22 B

23 B

24 A

25 B

26 D

27 A Arises from the Pons.

28 C

29 B The length is 5 inches; where as the lengths of 'A', 'C' and 'D'are 10, 20 and 15 inches respectively.

30 B

31 C 'A' is by corrugator supercilli and procerus and 'B' is by zygomaticus major muscles.

32 A

33 C

34 D These are duodenal glands.

35 C The superior mesenteric plexus of sympathetics and the vagus nerves (parasympathetics) arrange themselves in ganglionated plexus form situated inbetween the two muscular coats of Jejunum and Illium known as the myenteric or Aurbach's plexus mainly made of motor neurones.

36 A This is the Illeo-femoral ligament.

37 B Lies lateral to oesophagus (cervical part).

38 B Occasionally, a tongue shaped process known as 'Riedel's lobe' projects downwards from the inferior border of right lobe of liver on the right side of gall bladder.

39 B

40 C Deep circemflex iliac artery arises from the lateral aspect of external iliac artery immediately above the inguinal ligament and passes upwards and laterally to reach anterior superior iliac spine.

41 A 'B' is internal jugular vein, 'C' forms retromandibular vein and 'D' is the common facial vein.

42 D Are connected to superior sagittal, transverse, and cavernous sinuses.

43 A

44 B

45 B

46 C Protein content of lymph is almost equal to blood plasma and varies from 4-6% while the protein content of tissue fluid is less than 0.2%.

47 A 'B' is lymph vessel which drain the node and emerge through its hilium, 'C' is formed by efferent lymph vessels from the most centrally placed lymph nodes of the different lymphatic chains.

48 C Is a branch of Bracheal plexus.

49 B

50 D

51 A

52 C These nodes are grouped under Deep cervical lymphnodes.

53 B Which in turn ends blindly inferiorly.

54 D

55 B

56 C

57 A

58 D 'A' Pharynx is elevated by palatopharyngeus, 'C' Tensor vali palatini draws the soft palate to the same side.

59 A

60 B Some segments of the interlobular ducts are lined by secretory cells and are known as striated duct; Interlobar ducts are lined by pseudostratified columnar epithelium whereas intercalated ducts are lined by low or flat epithelium. Some mucous alveoli are capped by serous demilunes which are formed by serous type of cells.

61 C Tonsils develop from the 2nd, and inferior parathyroid glands from 3rd endodermal pouches.

62 B Derived from 2nd branchial arch.

63 C

64 C It opens into sphenoethmoidal recess of the superior meatus of nose, is lined by ciliated pseudo stratified columnar epithelium and occupies the body of sphenoid and may extend into the basilar part of occipital bone.

65 D

66 D Tibial nerve branches supply the ankle joint, gastrocnemius, soleus, plantaris and popliteus muscles etc. Sural nerve is a branch of Tibial nerve which supplies the lateral margin of foot and lateral side of the little toe. Deep peroneal nerve supplies the muscle of anterior cural region.

67 B

68 A

69 B

70 D

71 C Supplied by Trochlear nerve.

72 B

73 A

74 C

75 A All others close the glottis, where as posterior crioarytenoids opens it.

76 B

77 C

78 D

79 A

80 D These are mesothelial cells found in different parts of CNS and function in a variety of ways for the defence of the body.

81 B

82 A Carotid canal runs in the petrous part of temporal bone and transmits the internal carotid artery and the venous and sympathetic plexuses around the ICA.

83 B Followed by 'A' and 'C' respectively.

84 C 'A' results from damage to external laryngeal nerve and 'B' results from damage to both recurrent lanyngeal nerves.

85 A The Waldeyer's lymphatic ring guards entry to the digestive and respiratory passages. The ring is formed by four main masses of lymphoid tissue i.e. 2 palatine, 1 pharyngeal and 1 lingual tonsils connected together by the scattered lymphoid tissue.

86 B These are nuclei of vagus nerve. Nucleus ambiguus is branchiomotor and nucleus of tractus solitarius is gustatory.

87 C

88 A It is the largest of all and is known as "Carotid tubercle of chassaignac" and is felt at the level of cricoid cartilage.

89 D

90 D Nose is connected to anterior cranial fossa via cribriform plate and to the lacrimal apparatus through nasolarymal duct.

91 A The cochlear part of the nerve deals with 'B', 'C' is related to olfactory nerve.

92 B It is the largest and direct branch of ICA.

93 A Vidian's nerve is also called nerve of pterygoid canal.

94 C

95 B

96 A 'B', 'C' and 'D' are the actions of tensor palati, musculus uvulae and palatoglossus respectively.

97 A 'B' is posterior relation of 1st part, 'C' and 'D' are related to 2nd and 3rd parts of the vertebral artery respectively.

98 C Bronchomediastinal trunk drains 'A', Jugular trunk drains 'B' and Thoracic duct drains 'D'.

99 A

Notes

Syllabus

1. Introduction to Physiology: The cell, the components of cell and their functions. Tissues of the body: Functions of epithelial tissues; glandular tissues, connective tissue and other tissues.
2. Blood: Fundamentals of muscle nerve physiology, composition and functions of RBC–variations in number in physiological and pathological states–life span and development of RBC. Blood volume, methods of measurement and variation.
   - Haemoglobin: Basic Chemistry and fate of Hb. Blood groups. WBC types, number, variations, functions, formation, circulation. Functions of lymph; Physiology of clotting.
3. Cardio-Vascular System: Basic haemodynamic principles, arterial blood pressure and factors affecting it. The structure and physiological properties of cardiac muscle. Origin and conduction of heart beat. Cardiac cycle, heart sounds, ECG. Regulation of heart's action Vasomotor system and its regulation–Physiology of shock.
4. Respiration: Mechanics of respiration. Sub-divisions of lung air. Transport of respiratory gases in blood. Anoxia-types and physiological changes in artificial respiration.
5. Excretion: Urine-volume, normal and abnormal constituents, Mechanism of urine formation.
6. Digestion: Digestion in the mouth, digestion in the stomach and intestines, enzymes of the gastro-intestinal tract and their functions. Movements of the gastro-intestinal tract. Physiology of liver, pancreas, absorption and assimilation of food.
7. Endocrines: Thyroid–Iodine metabolism–functions of thyroid gland, Hyper and hypofunctioning of thyroid.
   a. Adrenal Corte X—Secretion of the cortical cells. Actions of gluco and minerals corticoids, hyper and hypo functions of adrenal cortex adrenaline and non-adrenaline action on various systems.
   b. Pituitary gland—Hormones, actions, abnormal functions of pituitary gland. Physiology of posterior diabetes insipidus.
   c. Parathyroid—Actions of parathromone and calcium metabolism.
8. Reproduction: Ovary–Ovariam hormone –their actions, menstrual cycle, pregnancy, hormonal changes in pregnancy. Tests for pregnancy. Functions of testes, actions of testesterone. Physiological basis of Family Planning methods.
9. Central Nervous System: Reflex action, spinal cord, conditional reflix, ascending and descending tracts, cerebral cortex, various areas and functions of Cerebellum.
   - Carebellum: Physiology of thalamus, autonomic nervous system. Cerebrospinal fluid Fundamental knowledge of C.N.S. and special senses—Regulation of body temperature.
10. Special senses: Fundamental knowledge of vision, hearing, taste and smell.
11. Nutrition: General metabolism, principles of colorimetry. Basal Metabolic rate; Metabolism of proteins, fats and carbohydrates. Vitamins—Sources, requirement and actions. Basic principles of dietetics.

Chapter 2

General Human Physiology and Biochemistry

1. **The sympathetic reflex activity after blood loss basically aims at maintaining**
   A. Cardiac output
   B. Blood Pressure
   C. Renal Perfusion
   D. None of the above

2. **What happens to pH in Shock?**
   A. Acidosis
   B. Alkalosis
   C. No change
   D. None of the above

3. **In vasovagal syncope, the cardiac output falls due to all *except***
   A. Vasomotor failure
   B. Slowing of heart
   C. Dilatation of blood vessels
   D. None of the above

4. **Macula densa is located in**
   A. Proximal tube
   B. Distal Tube
   C. Ascending loop of Henle
   D. Collecting duct

5. **The net filtration pressure in kidneys is**
   A. 60 mm Hg B. 50 mm Hg
   C. 10 mm Hg D. 22 mm Hg

6. **Angiotensin converting enzyme inhibitors reduce GRF because they**
   A. Constrict afferent arteriole
   B. Constrict efferent arteriole
   C. Dilate efferent arteriole
   D. Dilate afferent arteriole

7. **Counter Transport mechanism helps in secretion of**
   A. H^+
   B. Cl^-
   C. Bicarbonate
   D. All of the above

8. **All the following are reabsorbed in distal tubule *except***
   A. Na^+ B. K^+
   C. Urea D. Cl^-

9. **Vasopressin (ADH) acts on**
   A. Proximal tubule
   B. Ascending limb
   C. Distal tubule
   D. Descending limb

10. **Which of the following is function of aldosterone?**
    A. NaCl absorption
    B. K^+ secretion
    C. H_2O absorption
    D. All of the above

11. **The threshold for drinking is (change in Na^+ concentration)**
    A. 10 mEq/Lit
    B. 07 mEq/Lit
    C. 05 mEq/Lit
    D. 2 mEq/Lit

12. **PTH regulates plasma concentration calcium through**
    A. Stimulates bone resorption
    B. Stimulation of renal hydroxylation of Vitamin D
    C. Direct stimulation of renal tubular calcium reabsorption
    D. All of the above

13. **The slowest acting body system to maintain pH is**
    A. Buffer of the body fluid
    B. Lungs
    C. Kidneys
    D. All of the above

14. **What will be the blood pH if alveolar ventilation is reduced to one forth of normal?**
    A. 7 B. 7.2
    C. 7.4 D. 7.8

15. **In chronic acidosis, the major mechanism of urinary H^+ excretion is**
    A. Ammonium ions
    B. Phosphate
    C. Urate ions
    D. None of the above

16. **Urine passes through ureter by**
    A. Gravity
    B. Parasympathetic tone
    C. Sympathetic tone
    D. All of the above

17. **Loop diuretics mainly act upon**
    A. Na^+K^+ ATPase
    B. Sodium-hydrogen counter transport
    C. 1 sodium, 2 chloride, -1 potassium contransport
    D. Carbonic anhydrase

18. **Bones become decalcified in chronic renal failure due to**
    A. Decreased calcium intake
    B. Increased urinary calcium loss
    C. Decreased Vit D production
    D. Decreased Vit D intake

19. **Renal Phosphaturia leads to**
    A. No Symptoms
    B. Rickets that promptly responds to Vitamin D
    C. Ricket refractory to Vitamin D
    D. None of the above

20. **In the macrocytic anaemia due to B_{12} folic acid deficiency there is failure of**
    A. Haemoglobin formation
    B. Haemoglobin incorporation
    C. Maturation
    D. All of the above

21. **In Sickle cell anaemia, the defect lies in**
    A. Alpha chain
    B. Beta chain
    C. Gamma chain
    D. Delta chain

22. **What is erythroblastosis Foetalis?**
    A. Destruction of RBCs of mother by the foetal antibodies
    B. Haemolysis in foetus due to maternal Rh antibodies
    C. Haemolysis in mother due to foetal ABO antibodies
    D. All of the above

23. **What is not true of polycythemia vera?**
    A. All the three cells lines proliferate
    B. Rise in blood viscosity
    C. Rapid blood flow in capillaries
    D. Ruddy complexion with bluish skin

24. **The half life of platelet is**
    A. 10 days B. 24 days
    C. 6 weeks D. 6 months

25. **Neutrophil invasion of inflamed areas is**
    A. First line of defence
    B. Second line of defence
    C. Third line of defence
    D. Fourth line of defence

26. **B-cell immunity refers to**
    A. Humoral immunity
    B. Cell mediated immunity
    C. Innate immunity
    D. None of the above

27. The number of proteins constituting complement system number
A. 8 B. 15
C. 20 D. 27

28. The most T-cell population consists of
A. Helper T cell
B. Memory T cells
C. Suppressor T cells
D. NK cells

29. Anaphylaxis results from liberation of all *except*
A. Histamine B. SRSA
C. Inter Leukins D. Leukotrienes

30. The least frequent blood group is
A. AB B. A
C. O D. B

31. The difference between plasma and serum is that latter does not contain
A. Platelets
B. RBC
C. Clotting Factors
D. All of the above

32. Which pathway of coagulation is very fast?
A. Intrinsic
B. Extrinsic
C. Both are equally fast

33. Lack of Vit K Causes defficency of all *except*
A. Prothrombin B. Fibriogen
C. Factor VII D. Factors IX and X

34. All the following muscles help in respiration *except*
A. Sterno cleidomostoid
B. Intercostals
C. Deltoid
D. Serratus anterior

35. Surfactant is secreted by
A. Type I pneumocytes
B. Type II pneumocytes
C. Both of the above
D. None of the above

36. When Vital Capacity is added to residual volume it gives to
A. Total lung capacity
B. Functional residual capacity
C. Inspiratory reserve volume
D. All of the above

37. One gram of Haemoglobin can approximately carry how much of oxygen?
A. 3.3 ml B. 2.3 ml
C. 1.3 ml D. 0. 3 ml

38. What is Bohr effect?
A. Rise in O_2 saturation of blood with rise in alveolar oxygen concentration
B. Fall in O_2 saturation of blood with rise in alveolar CO_2 concentration
C. Shift in oxygen-haemoglobin dissociation in response to hydrogen ion concentration
D. All of the above

39. All the following cause O_2 dissociation curve shift to right *except*
A. Alkalosis B. Raised PCO_2
C. Fever D. Increased DPG

40. What is chloride shift?
A. Exchange of chloride for sodium
B. Exchange of chloride for bicarbonates
C. Exchange of chloride for potassium
D. None of the above

41. What is Haldane effect?
A. Binding of CO_2 to Hb displaces O_2
B. Binding of O_2 to Hb displaces CO_2
C. Binding of CO to Hb displaces O_2

42. Respiratory exchange ratio for fat is
A. 1 B. 3
C. 0.7 D. 0.5

43. Rate and pattern of Breathing is controlled by
A. Dorsal respiration centre
B. Ventral respiration centre
C. Pneumotaxic centre
D. All of the above

44. What is Hering's nerve?
A. Nerves from aortic bodies to recurrent laryngeal
B. Nerve from carotid bodies to glossopharyngeal
C. Nerves from J.G. apparatus to renal sympathetic
D. None of the above

45. Pulmonary J receptors are responsible for
A. Inspiration B. Expiration
C. Breathlessness D. Apneusis

46. Total alveolar ventilation volume is ____ liters/ minute
A. 1.5 B. 3.5
C. 4.2 D. 5.0

47. During isovolumetric contraction phase
A. AV closed and semi lunar valve open
B. AV open and semi lunar valve closed
C. AV closed and semi lunar valve closed
D. Blood ejected in aortic and pulmonary vessels

48. Thromboplastenin is a
A. Coagulation protein
B. Contractile protein
C. Thrombosis protecting protein
D. Protein for regulating platlet production

49. Difference between adult RBC and fetal RBCs are all *except*
A. Fetal RBCs are bigger
B. More 2-3 DPG in fetal RBCs
C. Less carbonic anhydrase
D. Fetal RBC has shorter life span

50. Bile acids act as detergent due to
A. Amphipathic nature of bile acid
B. Formation of zwitter ion
C. Formation of soap
D. Formation of medium chain tryglyceride

51. Insensible daily water loss from body is
A. 1500 ml B. 700 ml
C. 100 ml D. 300 ml

52. The smallest fluid compartment of body is
A. Extra-cellular B. Intracellular
C. Interstitial D. Transcellular

53. Which statement describes Donnan effect the best?
A. Positively charged plasma proteins hold up sodium
B. Negatively charged plasma proteins hold up sodium
C. Negatively charged plasma proteins bind bicarbonates
D. None of the above

54. If the plasma volume is 3 liters and the hematocrit is 0.4, then the total blood volume is
A. 5 liters B. 4 liters
C. 1.2 liters D. 7.2 liters

55. The saline concentration isotonic to plasma is
A. 1% B. 0.9%
C. 1.9% D. 5%

56. The total safety factor against edema is
A. 17 mm Hg B. 7 mm Hg
C. 27 mm Hg D. 37 mm Hg

57. Water content of a cell excluding fat cells is
A. 50-60% B. 40-50%
C. 80-90% D. 70-80%

58. Carbohydrate is maximum in
A. Muscle cell
B. Hepatocyte
C. Red blood cell
D. Nerve cell

59. Maximum alcohol detoxification within cell is in
A. Lysosomes B. Micro tubules
C. Peroxisomes D. Mitochondria

60. The constituents of ATP are all *except*
A. Ribulose B. Adenine
C. Ribose D. Phosphate

61. **Which of the following is not a component of DNA?**
   A. Uracil B. Adenine
   C. Guanine D. Cytosine

62. **Which of the following statement is true regarding osmolality?**
   A. One osmoles is 1 gram molecular weight of dissociated solute
   B. One osmoles is 1 gram molecular weight of undissociated solute
   C. Normal osmolality of intra and extracellular fluids is 350 milliosmoles/kg
   D. All are true

63. **Glucose is transported into cell with**
   A. Sodium B. Potassium
   C. Calcium D. All of the above

64. **The resting membrane potential of a large nerve fiber is**
   A. –50 mV B. –90 mV
   C. 90 mV D. 60 mV

65. **The K^+ concentration within a nerve fiber is**
   A. 160 mEq/L B. 140 mEq/L
   C. 60 mEq/L D. 100 mEq/L

66. **The plateau of action potential is due to**
   A. Fast sodium channels
   B. Slow calcium channels
   C. Potassium channels
   D. All of the above

67. **The nerve conduction in myelinated nerve fiber is called**
   A. Continuous B. Interrupted
   C. Saltatory D. None of the above

68. **The light I bands in electron photo micrograph of the muscle fiber correspond to**
   A. Actin filaments
   B. Myosin filaments
   C. Actin myosin cross bridge
   D. None of the above

69. **Actin myosin interaction in resting stage is inhibited by**
   A. Calcium ions
   B. Troponin
   C. Troponin-tropomyosin
   D. ATP

70. **What is not true of rigor mortis?**
   A. Occurs after death
   B. Muscle is rigid and contracted
   C. Muscle action potential is high
   D. Depleted ATP store

71. **Smooth muscle does not contain**
   A. Actin B. Myosin
   C. Troponin D. Calmodulin

72. **The depolarization time in ventricular muscle is**
   A. 0.2 sec B. 0.3 sec
   C. 0.4 sec D. 0.4 sec

73. **With rise in heart rate which phase is shortened more**
   A. Systole
   B. Diastole
   C. Both of the above
   D. None of the above

74. **Blood ejected into pulmonary and systemic circulation during rapid ejection period is**
   A. 50% B. 60%
   C. 70% D. 90%

75. **The normal endsystolic volume is**
   A. 100 ml B. 75-85 ml
   C. 50-60 ml D. 40-50 ml

76. **The location of sinus node is**
   A. Lateral wall of RA at the entry of IVC
   B. Superior lateral wall of RA at the entry of SVC
   C. Superior lateral wall of RA at the entry of IVC
   D. Just above the interatrial septum

77. Which of the following is not recorded in ECG?
A. Atrial depolarization
B. Atrial repolarization
C. Ventricular repolarization
D. None of the above

78. The normal QRS duration is
A. 0.1 to 0.12 seconds
B. 0.08 to 0.12 seconds
C. 0.06 to 0.08 seconds
D. 0.02 to 0.04 seconds

79. The volume of blood in pulmonary circulation at any given time is
A. 20% B. 2%
C. 5% D. 9%

80. The functional pressure in most vascular bed is
A. 25 mm Hg
B. 30 mm Hg
C. 17 mm Hg
D. 20 mm Hg

81. 1 mm Hg pressure equals to
A. 1.46 cm of water
B. 1.56 cm of water
C. 1.36 cm of water
D. 1.16 cm of water

82. Because of good reservoir system, healthy man can tolerate safely acute blood loss of
A. 20% B. 80%
C. 40% D. 60%

83. Which of the molecules has the smallest diameter?
A. Na^+ B. H_2O
C. Ca^{++} D. Protein

84. Normal plasma colloid osmotic pressure is
A. 42 mm Hg
B. 50 mm Hg
C. 28 mm Hg
D. 21 mm Hg

85. The total quantity of lymph entering circulation daily is
A. 1 liter
B. 3 liter
C. 5 liter
D. ½ liter

86. Vasomotor center is located in
A. Medulla
B. Midbrain
C. Hypothalamus
D. Frontal cortex

87. What is brain bridge reflex?
A. Rise in heart rate with atrial dilatation
B. Decrease in BP with atrial dilatation
C. Slowing of heart rate with atrial dilatation
D. Increase in BP with atrial dilatation

88. Aortic and carotid body chemoreceptors are sensitive to
A. Decrease pH
B. CO_2 excess
C. Oxygen lack
D. All of the above

89. What is Goldblatt Hypertension?
A. Hypertension in response to renal vascular obstruction
B. Hypertension that occurred in Goldblatt
C. Hypertension occurring due to aldosterone excess
D. None of the above

90. Normal cardiac index for adult is
A. 3.5 lit/min/m^2
B. 3 lit/min/m^2
C. 3.75 lit/min/m^2
D. 4 lit/min/m^2

91. During exercise blood flow of muscles is increased
A. 7-10 folds
B. 3-5 folds
C. 10-15 folds
D. 15-25 folds

92. At resting conditions, cardiac energy is mainly derived from

A. Fatty acids
B. Carbohydrates
C. Proteins
D. None of the above

93. Cardiac pain is related to release of which of the following

A. Kinins
B. Lactic acid
C. Histamine
D. All of the above

94. The fourth heart sound originates from

A. Atria
B. Ventricles
C. Moderator band
D. None of the above

95. The murmur across a stenosed valve is due to

A. Turbulence
B. Vigorous cardiac contraction
C. Vibration of myocardium
D. All of the above

Answers

1 B The decrease in arterial pressure, as well as decreases in pressures in the low-pressure areas of the thorax after hemorrhage, initiates powerful sympathetic reflexes (initiated mainly by the baroreceptors and by the low-pressure vascular stretch receptors. The reflexes stimulate the sympathetic vasoconstrictor system throughout the body, resulting in three important effects: (1) The arterioles constrict in most parts of the body, thereby increasing the total peripheral resistance. (2) The veins and venous reservoirs constrict, thereby helping to maintain adequate venous return despite diminished blood volume. (3) Heart activity increases markedly, sometimes increasing the heart rate from the normal value of 72 beats/min to a high as 160 to 180 beats/min.

2 A Most of the metabolic derangements that occur in shocked tissue can lead to blood acidosis all through the body. This results from poor delivery of oxygen to the tissues, which greatly diminishes oxidative metabolism of the foodstuffs. When this occurs the cell obtain their energy by the anaerobic process of glycolysis, which leads to tremendous quantities of excess lactic acid in the blood. In addition, the poor blood flow through the tissues prevents normal removal of carbon dioxide; the carbon dioxide reacts locally in the cells with water to form high concentrations of intracellular carbonic acid; this in turn reacts with the various tissues buffers to form still other intracellular acidic substances.

Thus, deteriorative effect of shock is both generalized and local tissues acidosis, leading to still further progression of the shock itself.

3 A A particularly interesting vasodilatory reaction occurs in people who experience intense emotional disturbances that cause fainting. The muscle vasodilator system becomes powerfully activated, and at the same time, the vagal cardioinhibitory centre transmits strong signals to the heart to markedly slow the heart rate. The arterial pressure falls instantly, which also reduces blood flow to the brain and causes the person to lose consciousness. This overall effect is called vasovagal syncopy. Emotional fainting begins with disturbing thoughts in the cerebral cortex. The pathway probably then goes to the vasodilatory center of the anterior hypothalamus, to the vagal centers of the medulla, and also through the spinal cord to the sympathetic vasodilator nerves of the muscles.

4 B At the end of thick ascending limb is a short segment, which is actually a plaque in its wall, known as the macula densa. As we discuss later, the macula densa plays an important role in controlling nephron function. Beyond the macula densa, fluid enters the distal tubule that, like the proximal tubule, lies in the renal cortex. This is followed by connecting tubules and cortical collecting tubule which lead to corlical collecting duct.

5 C The net filtration pressure represents the sum of the hydrostatic and colloid osmotic forces that either favor or oppose filtration across the glomerular capillaries. These forces include (1) hydrostatic pressure inside the glomerular capillaries (glomerular hydrostatic pressure, which promotes filtration); (2) the hydrostatic pressure in Bowman's capsule outside the capillaries, which opposes filtration; (3) the colloid osmotic pressure of the glomerular capillary plasma proteins, which opposes filtration; (4) The colloid osmotic pressure of the proteins in Bowman's capsule, which promotes filtration (under normal conditions, the concentration of protein in the glomerular filtrate is so low that the colloid osmotic pressure of the Bowman's capsule fluid is considered to be Zero). The net filtration pressure is around 10 mm of Hg.

6 C A preferential constrictor action of Angiotensin II on efferent arterioles helps to prevent serious reductions in glomerular hydrostatic pressure and GFR when perfusion pressure falls below normal. The administration of drugs that block the formation of Angiotensin II (Angiotensin-converting enzyme inhibitors) or that block the action of Angiotensin II (Angiotensin II antagonists) causes greater reductions in GFR that usual when the renal arterial pressure falls below normal.

7 A A few substances are secreted into the tubules by secondary active transport. This often involves counter-transport of the substances with sodium ions. In counter-transport, the energy liberated from the downhill movement of one of the substances (for example sodium ions) enables uphill movement of a second substance in the opposite direction.

One example of counter transport, is the active secretion of hydrogen ions coupled to sodium reabsorption in the luminal membrane. As sodium is carried to the interior to the cell, hydrogen ions are forced outward in the opposite direction into the tubular lumen.

8 C The very first portion of the distal tube forms part of the juxtaglomerular complex that provides feedback control of GFR and blood flow in the same nephron. The next early part of the distal tubule is highly convoluted and has many of the same reabsorptive characteristics of the thick segment of the ascending limb of the loop of Henle. That is, it avidly reabsorbs most of the ions, including sodium, potassium, and chloride, but is virtually impermeable to water and urea. For this reason, it is referred to as the diluting segment because it also dilutes the tubular fluid.

9 C The permeability of the late distal tubule and cortical collecting duct to water is controlled by the concentration of ADH, which is also called vasopressin. With high levels of ADH, these tubular segments are permeable to water. This special characteristic provides and important mechanism for controlling the degree of dilution or concentration of the urine.

10 B Aldosterone, secreted by the zona glomeruloca cells of the adrenal cortex, is an important regulator of sodium reabsorption and potassium secretion by the renal tubules. *The primary site of aldosterone action is on the principal cells of the cortical collecting tubule.* The mechanism by which aldosterone increases sodium reabsorption while at the same sodium-potassium ATPase pump on the basolateral side of the cortical collecting tubule membrane. Aldosterone also increased the sodium permeability of the luminal side of the membrane.

11 D The kidney must continually excrete at least some fluid, even in a dehydrated person, to rid the body of excess solutes that are ingested or reduced by metabolism. Water is also lost by evaporation from the lungs and the gastrointestinal tract and by evaporation and sweating from the skin. Therefore, there is always a tendency for dehydration, with resultant increased extra-cellular fluid sodium concentration and osmolarity. When the sodium concentration increases only about 2 mEq/L above normal, the thirst mechanism is activated, causing a desire to drink water. This is called the Threshold for drinking.

12 D PTH regulates plasma calcium concentration through three main effects: (1) by stimulating bone reabsorption; (2) by stimulation activation of vitamin D, which then increases intestinal reabsorption of calcium; and (3) by directly increasing renal tubular calcium reabsorption.

13 C There are three primary systems that regulate the hydrogen ion concentration in the body fluids to prevent acidosis or alkalosis: (1) *the chemical acid-base buffer systems of the body fluids,* which immediately combine with acid or base to prevent excessive changes in hydrogen ion concentration; (2) *the respiratory centre,* which regulates the removal of CO_2 (and, therefore, H_2CO_3) from the extracellular fluid; and (3) the kidneys, which can excrete either acid or alkaline urine, thereby readjusting the extracellular fluid hydrogen ion concentration toward normal during acidosis or alkalosis.

When there is a change in hydrogen ion concentration, the buffer systems of the body fluids react within a fraction of a second to minimize these changes. Buffer system do not estimate hydrogen from the body or add them to the body but only keep them tied up until balance can re-established. The second line of defense, the respiratory system, also reacts within few minutes to eliminate CO_2 and, therefore, H_2CO_3 from the body. These first two line of defense keep the hydrogen ion concentration from changing too much until the more slowly responding third line of defense, the kidneys, can eliminate the excess acid or base from the body. Although the kidneys are relatively slow to respond, compared with the other defenses, they are over a period of hours to several days by far the most powerful of the acid-base regulatory systems.

14 A A decrease in alveolar ventilation to one-fourth normal reduces the pH by 0.45. That is, if at a normal alveolar ventilation the pH is 7.4, reducing the alveolar ventilation to one fourth normal values the pH to 6.95.

15 A One of the most important features of the renal ammonium-ammonia buffer system is that it is subject to physiological control. An increase in extracellular fluid hydrogen ion concentration stimulates renal glutamine metabolism and, therefore, increases the formation of NH_4^+ and new bicarbonate to be used in hydrogen ion buffering; a decease in hydrogen ion concentration has the opposite effect.

16 B The walls of the ureters contain smooth muscle and are innervated by both sympathetic and parasympathetic nerves as well as by an intramural plexus of neurons and nerves fibers that extends along the entire length of the ureters. As with other visceral smooth muscle, peristaltic concentrations in the ureter are enhanced by parasympathetic stimulation and inhibited by sympathetic stimulation.

17 C See following Table:

Class of diuretric	*Mechanism of action*	*Tubular site of action*
Loop diuretics	Inhibits Na-K-Cl co-transport in luminal membrane.	Thick ascending loop of Henle.

18 C Prolonged renal failure also causes osteomalacia, a condition in which the bones are partially absorbed and, therefore, become greatly weakened. An important cause of this condition is the following: vitamin D must be converted by a two stage process, first in the liver and then in the kidneys, into 1,25-dihydroxycholecalciferoi before it is able to promote calcium absorption from the intestine. Therefore, serious damage to the kidney greatly reduces the blood concentration of active vitamin D, which in turn decreases intestinal absorption of calcium and the availability of calcium to the bones.

Another important cause of demineralization of the skeleton in chronic renal failure is the rise in serum phosphate concentration that occurs as a result of decreased GFR. This rise in serum phosphate causes increased binding of phosphate with calcium in the plasma, thus decreasing the plasma serum ionized calcium concentration, which in turn stimulates parathyroid hormone secretion. This secondary hyperparathyroidism then stimulates release to calcium from bones, causing further demineralization of the bones.

19 C In renal hypophosphatemia, the renal tubules fail to reabsorb large enough quantities of phosphate ions when the phosphate concentration of the body fluids falls very low. This condition usually does not cause serious immediate abnormalities because phosphate concentration of the extracellular fluids can vary widely without causing major cellular dysfunction. Over a long period, a low phosphate level causes diminished calcification of the bones, thus causing the person to develop rickets, which is refractory to vitamin D therapy.

20 C Important for final maturation of the red blood cells are two vitamins, Vitamin B_{12} and folic acid. Both of these are essential for the synthesis of DNA because each in a different way is required for the formation of thymidine triphosphate, one of the essential building blocks of DNA. Therefore lack of either vitamin B_{12} or folic acid causes diminished DNA and, consequently, failure of nuclear maturation and division. Furthermore, the erythroblastic cells of the bone marrow, in addition to failing to proliferate rapidly, produce mainly larger than normal red cells called macrocytes, and the cell has a flimsy membrane and is often irregular, large and oval instead of usual biconcave disc. These poorly formed cells, after entering the circulating blood, are capable of carrying oxygen normally, but their fragility causes them to have a short life, one-half to one-third normal. Therefore, it is said that either vitamin B_{12} or folic acid deficiency causes maturation failure in the process of erythropoiesis.

21 B In sickle cell anaemia, which is present in 0.3 to 1.0 percent of West African and American Blacks, the cells contain an abnormal type of hemoglobin called hemoglobin S, caused by abnormal beta chains of the hemoglobin molecule, as explained earlier in the chapter. When this hemoglobin is exposed to low concentrations of oxygen. It precipitates into long crystals inside the red blood cell. These crystals elongate the cells and give it the appearance of being a sickle, rather than biconcave disc.

22 B In *erythroblastosis fetalis,* Rh-positive red blood cells in the fetus are attacked by antibodies from an Rh-negative mother, these antibodies make the Rh-positive cells fragile, leading to rapid rupture and causing child to be born with serious anemia. The extremely rapid formation of the of a new red cells to make up for the destroyed cells in erythroblastosis fetalis causes a large number of early blast forms of red cells to be released into the blood.

23 C People who have physiological polycythemia, other have pathological condition known as polycythemia vera, in which the red blood cells count maybe 7 to 8 millions/mm^3 and the hematocrit 60 to 70 per cent. Polycythemia vera is caused by a genetic aberration that occurs in the hemocytoblastic cell line that produces the blood cells. The blast cells no longer stop producing red cells when too many cells are already present. This causes excess production of red blood cells in the same manner that a tumor to breast causes excess of production of a specific type of breast cell. It usually causes excess production of white blood cells and platelets as well.

24 A The platelets in the blood are replaced once about every 10 days; in other words, about 30,000 platelets are formed each day for each microliter of blood.

25 B 1. The Tissues Macrophage is a first line of defence against infection.
2. Neutrophil invasion of the inflamed area is second line of defence.
3. A second Macrophage invasion into the inflamed tissue is a third line of defence.

26 A The B lymphocytes that are destined to form antibodies–are preprocessed in the liver during midfetal life and in the bone marrow in late fetal life and after birth. This population of cells was first discovered in birds in which the preprocessing occurs in the bursa of fabricius, a structure not found in mammals. For this reason, these lymphocytes are called "B" lymphocytes to designate the role of the bursa, and they are responsible for humoral immunity.

27 C "Complement" is a collective term that describes a system of about 20 proteins, many of which are enzyme precursors. The principal actors in this system are 11 proteins designated CI through C9, B and D. All these are present normally among the plasma proteins in the blood cells as well as among the proteins that leak out the capillaries into the tissue spaces. The enzyme precursors are normally inactive, but they can be activated mainly by the so-called classic pathway.

28 A It has become clear that there are multiple types of T cells. They are classified into three major groups: *(1) helper T cells, (2) cytotoxic T cells (3) and the Suppressor T cells.* The function of each of these are distinct.

Helper T cells–Their role in overall regulation of immunity.

The helper T cells are by far the most numerous of the T cells, usually constituting more than three quarter of all of them. As their name implies, they help in the function of the immune system.

29 C When a widespread allergic reaction occurs throughout the vascular system and closely associated tissues, it is called anaphylaxis. Histamine is released into the circulation and causes body-wide vasodilatation as well as increased permeability of the capillaries with resultant marked loss of plasma from the circulation. An occasional person who experiences this reaction dies of circulatory shock within a few minutes unless treated with epinephrine to oppose the effects of the histamine. But also released from the cells is a mixture of leukotrienes called slow reacting substance of anaphylaxis. These leukotrienes can cause spasm of the smooth muscle of the bronchioles, creating an asthma-like attack and sometimes causes death by suffocation.

30 A Relative Frequencies of the blood group types. The prevalence of the different blood types among white people is approximately as follows:

O	47%
A	41%
B	9%
AB	3%

It is obvious from these percentages that the O and A genes occur frequently, whereas the B gene is infrequent.

31 C **Clot Retraction Serum.** With in a few minutes after a clot is formed, it begins to contract and usually express most of the fluid from the clot within 20 to 60 minutes. The fluid expressed is called serum because all its fibrogen and most of the other clotting factors have been removed; in this way, serum differs from plasma. Serum cannot clot because it lacks these factors.

32 B An especially important difference between the extrinsic and intrinsic pathways is that the extrinsic pathway can be explosive; once initiated, its speed of occurrence is limited only by the amount of tissue factor released from the traumatized tissues and by the quantities of factors X, IV and V in the blood. With severe tissue trauma, clotting can occur in as little as 15 seconds. The intrinsic pathway is much slower to proceed, usually requiring 1 to 6 minutes to cause clotting.

33 B One of the causes of depressed formation of clotting factors by the liver is vitamin K deficiency. Vitamin K is necessary for liver formation of five of the important clotting factors, prothrombin, factor VII, factor IX, factor X, and protein C. In the absence of vitamin K, subsequent insufficiency of these coagulation factors in the blood can lead to serious bleeding tendencies.

34 C The most important muscles that raise the rib cage are the external intercostals but others that help are (1) the sternocleidomastiod muscles, which lift upward on the sternum; (2) the anterior serrati, which lift many of the ribs; and (3) the scaleni, which lift the first two ribs.

The muscles that pull the rib cage downward during expiration are (1) the abdominal recti, which have the powerful effect of pulling downward on the lower ribs at the same time that they and the other abdominal muscles compress the abdominal contents upward toward the diaphragm, and (2) the internal intercostals.

35 B Surfactant is a surface active agent in water, which means that it greatly reduces the surface tension of the water. It is secreted by special surfactant-secreting epithelial cells that constitute about 10 per cent of the surface area of the alveoli. These cells are granular containing lipid inclusions; they are called type II alveolar epithelial cells.

36 A The total lung capacity is the volume, which the lungs can be expanded with greatest possible effort (about 5800 milliliters) it is equal to vital capacity plus residual volume.

37 C The blood of a normal person contains about 15 grams of hemoglobin in each 100 milliliters of blood, and each gram of hemoglobin can bind with a maximum of 1.34 milliliters of oxygen (1.29 milliliters when the hemoglobin is chemically pure but the purity is reduced by impurities such as methemoglobin).

38 C A shift of the oxygen-hemoglobin dissociation curve in response to changes in the blood carbon dioxide and hydrogen ions has a significant effect in enhancing oxygenation of the blood in the lungs and then again in enhancing release of oxygen from the blood in the tissues. This is called Bhor's effect.

39 A In addition to pH changes, several other factors are known to shift the curve. Three of these, all of which shift the curve to right are:

1. Increased carbon dioxide concentration,
2. Increased blood temperature, and
3. Increased 2,3-diphosphoglycerate (DPG) a metabolic important phosphate compound present in the blood but in different concentration under different metabolic conditions.

40 B Most of the hydrogen ions when combine with the hemoglobin in the red blood cells because the hemoglobin protein is a powerful acid-base buffer. In turn many of the bicarbonate ions diffuse from the red cells into the plasma while chloride ions diffuse into the red cells to take their place. This is made possible by the presence of a special bicarbonate chloride carrier protein in the red cell membrane that shuttles these two ions in opposite direction in rapid velocities. Thus, the chloride content of venous red blood cells is greater that of the arterial red cells, a phenomenon called the chloride shift.

41 B Binding of oxygen with hemoglobin tends to displace carbon dioxide from the blood. Indeed, this effect, called the Haldane effect, is quantitatively far more important in promoting carbon dioxide transport than is the Bhor effect in promoting oxygen transport.

42 C The ratio of the carbon dioxide output to oxygen uptake is called the respiratory ratio (R). That is,

$$R = \frac{\text{Rate of Carbon dioxide output}}{\text{Rate of Oxygen uptake}}$$

The value for R changes under different metabolic conditions. When a person is using exclusively carbohydrates for bodily metabolism, R rises to 1.00. Conversely, when a person is using exclusively fats for metabolic energy, the R level falls to as low as 0.7. The reason for this difference is that when oxygen is metabolized with carbohydrates, one molecule of carbon dioxide is formed for each molecule of oxygen consumed. Whereas when oxygen reacts with fats, a large share of oxygen combines with hydrogen from the fat to form water instead of carbon dioxide. In other words the respiratory quotient of the chemical reactions in the tissues when fats are metabolized is about 0.70 instead of 1.00.

43 C The pneumotaxic centre, located dorsally in the nucleus parabrachialis of the upper pons, transmits signals to the inspiratory area. The primary effect of this centre is to control the "Switch off" point of the inspiratory ramp, thus controlling the duration of the filling phase of the lung cycle.

44 B The carotid bodies are located bilaterally in the bifurcations of the common carotid arteries, and their afferent nerves fibers pass through Hering's nerves to the glossopharyngeal nerves and then to dorsal respiratory area of the medulla. The aortic bodies are located along the arch of the aorta; their afferent nerve fibers pass through the vagi also to the dorsal respiratory area.

45 C A few sensory nerve endings occur in the alveolar walls in juxtaposition to the pulmonary capillaries from where comes the name "J receptors". They are stimulated specially when the pulmonary capillaries become engorged with blood or when pulmonary edema occurs in such conditions as congestive heart failure. Although the functional role of the J receptors is not clear, their excitation perhaps gives the person a feeling of dyspnea.

46 C Alveolar ventilation is the amount of air reaching the alveoli per minute. Thus a man weighing 68 kg only the first 350 ml of the 500 ml inspired with each breath at rest mixes with the air in the alveoli, the remaining 150 ml remains in the dead space. Therefore total ventilation volume = alveolar ventilation × respiratory rate/minute (350 × 12 = 4200).

47 C At the start of ventricular systole the mitral and tricuspid valves close. Ventricular muscle initially shortens relatively little, but intraventricular pressure rises sharply as the myocardium presses on the blood in the ventricles. This period of isovolumetric contraction lasts about 0.05s, until the pressure in the ventricles exceed the pressures in the aorta (80 mm hg) and pulmonary artery (10 mm Hg) and aortic and pulmonary valve open. During this isovolumetric contraction, the AV valve bulge into the atria causing a small but sharp rise in atrial pressure.

48 B The extrinsic system is triggered by the release of tissue thromboplastenin, a protein-phospholipid mixture that activates factor VII. It is a contractile protein.

49 B Fetal hemoglobin is similar to adult hemoglobin except γ chains replace β chains IO. It is not the amount of 2,3 DPG in fetal RBC that is different but it binds less avidly to oxygen that is why it delivers more oxygen at a given PO_2.

50 A Bile salts have a number of important functions, they reduce the surface tension and, in conjunction with phospholipids and monoglycerides. They are amphipathic; they have both hydrophilic and hydrophobic domains. One surface of the molecule is hydrophilic because the polar peptide bond and the carboxyl and hydroxyl groups are on that surface whereas the other surface is hydrophobic. Therefore bile salts tend to form cylindrical disks called as micelles.

51 B Some water loss cannot be regulated, such as continuous loss of water by evaporation from the respiratory tract and diffusion through the skin, which together accounts for about 700 ml of water loss under normal circumstances. This is termed as insensible water loss because we are not consciously aware of it.

52 D The total body fluid is mainly distributed between two compartments, extracellular and intracellular fluid. The extracellular fluid in turn is divided into the interstitial fluid and the blood plasma. There is another small compartment of fluid that is referred to as transcellular fluid. This compartment includes fluid in the synovial, peritoneal, pericardial and intraocular spaces, as well as cerebrospinal fluid. It is considered to be specialized type of extracellular fluid. All the transcellular fluids together constitute about 1 to 2 liters, which is the smallest compartment.

53 B Because the plasma and interstitial fluids are separated only by highly permeable capillary membranes, their ionic compositions are similar except the concentration of the protein in the plasma is higher than the interstitial fluid. Because of Donnan effect the concentration of positively charged ions (cations) is slightly greater (about 2 %) in the plasma than in the interstitial fluid. This is because the plasma proteins have a net negative charge and therefore tend to bind cations, such as sodium or potassium ions thus holding extra amount of cations in the plasma along with plasma proteins. Similarly the negatively charged ions tend to have slightly higher concentration in the interstitial fluid.

54 A Blood volume can also be measured if one knows the hematocrit (the fraction of total blood volume composed of cells) using the following equation:

$$\text{Total blood volume} = \frac{\text{Plasma volume}}{(1\text{-hematocrit})}$$

Therefore, if the total plasma volume is 3 liters and the hematocrit is 0.4.

$$\text{Total blood volume} = \frac{3 \text{ liters}}{(1\text{-}0.4)} = 5 \text{ liters.}$$

55 B Using van't Hoff's law one can calculate the potential osmotic pressure of a solution. The osmotic pressure of 0.9% sodium chloride solution is calculated as follows: a 0.9% solution means 0.9 grams of sodium chloride in 100 ml of solution or 9 grams/liter. Because the molecular weight of sodium chloride is 58.5 g/mol, the molarity of the solution is 9 g/l divided by 58.5 g/mol or about 0.154 mol/l. because each molecule of sodium chloride is equal to 2 osmoles the osmolarity of the solution is 0.154 × 2 or 0.308 osm/l. Therefore the osmolarity of the solution is 308 mosm/l. The correct osmolarity of the solution is determined by applying the osmotic coefficient. For sodium chloride the osmotic coefficient is about 0.93, therefore the actual osmolarity of a 0.9 % sodium chloride is 308 × 0.93 = 286 m osm/l.

56 A If we look at all the safety factors together, we find the following:

Safety factor caused by low tissue compliance in the negative pressure range is about 3 mmHg.

The safety factor caused by increased lymph flow is about 7 mmHG.

The safety factor caused by wash down of proteins from the interstitial spaces is about 7 mmHg. Therefore the total safety factor against edema is about 17 mmHg. This means that the capillary pressure in a peripheral tissue could theoretically rise by 17 mmHg, or approximately double the normal value before significant edema would occur.

57 D The principal fluid medium of the cell is water, which is present in most cells (except fat cells) in a concentration of 70–85%. Many cellular chemicals are dissolved in the water. Others are suspended in the water as solid particulate. Chemical reactions take place among the dissolved chemicals or at the surface boundaries between the suspended particles or membranes and the water.

58 B Carbohydrates have little structural function in the cell except as parts of glycoprotein molecules, but they play a major role in nutrition of the cell. Most human cells do not maintain large stores of carbohydrates; the amount usually averages about 1% of their total mass but increases to as much as 3% in muscle cells and, occasionally 6% in liver cells. Carbohydrates in the form of dissolved glucose are always present in the surrounding extracellular fluid so that it is readily available to the cell.

59 C Peroxisomes are similar physically to lysosomes, but they are different in two important ways, first they are formed by self replication, second they contain oxidases rather than hydrolases. Several of the oxidases are capable of combining oxygen with hydrogen ions from different intracellular chemicals to form hydrogen peroxide. The hydrogen peroxide is in turn is itself a highly oxidizing substance and this is used in association with catalase (present in peroxisomes) may oxidize many substances that might otherwise be poisonous to the cell. About half of alcohol a person drinks is detoxified by peroxisomes of the liver cells in this manner.

60 A ATP is a nucleotide composed of the nitrogenous base adenine, the pentose sugar ribose, and three phosphate radicals. The last two phosphate radicals are connected with the reminder of the molecule by socalled high energy phosphate bonds.

61 A The basic chemical compounds involved in the formation of DNA are phosphoric acid, a sugar called deoxyribose and four nitrogenous bases. These bases are two purines (adenine and guanine) and two pyrimidines (thymine and cytosine). The phosphoric acid and deoxyribose form the two helical strands that are the backbone of the DNA molecule, and the bases lie between the two strands and connect them.

62 B A solution that has 1 osmole of solute dissolved in each kilogram of water is said to have an osmolality of 1 osmole per kilogram, and a solution that has 1/1000 osmole dissolved per kilogram has an osmolality of 1 milliosmoles per kilogram. The normal osmolality of the extracellular fluid is about 300 milliosmoles per kilogram of water.

63 A Glucose and many amino acids are transported into most cells against large concentration gradient; the mechanism of this is entirely by a co-transport mechanism. The transport carrier protein has two binding sites on its exterior side, one for the sodium and one for the glucose. Also the concentration of sodium ions is very high on the outside and very low inside which provides the energy for the transport. The sodium and glucose both are transported at the same time.

64 B The resting membrane potential of large nerve fibers when they are not transmitting nerve signals is about -90 mV. That is the potential inside the fiber is 90 mV more negative than the potential in the extracellular fluid on the outside of the fiber.

65 B The concentration of:

Sodium (outside) is	:	142 mEq/L
Sodium (inside) is	:	14 mEq/L
Potassium (outside) is	:	4 mEq/L
Potassium (inside) is	:	140 mEq/L

The sodium potassium pump causes large concentration gradient for sodium and potassium across the resting nerve membrane.

66 B The cause of plateau is a combination of several factors, in the heart muscle, two types of channel enter into depolarization process: (1) the usual voltage activated sodium channels called fast channels and (2) voltage activated calcium sodium channels, which are slow to open and therefore are called as slow channels. These slow channels allow diffusion mainly of calcium ions but of some sodium ions as well. It is this opening of slow channels is mainly responsible for the plateau portion of action potential.

67 C Even though no ions can flow through the thick myelin sheaths of myelinated nerves, they can flow through the nodes of Raniver. Therefore, action potential occurs only at the nodes. The action potential is conducted from node to node. This type of conduction is called saltatory conduction. The electrical current flows through the extracellular fluid outside the myelin sheath as well as through the axoplasm inside the axon from node to node.

68 A Myosin and actin filaments partially interdigitate and thus cause the myofibrils to have alternate

light and dark bands. The light bands contain only actin filaments and are called as I bands because they are isotropic to polarized light. The dark bands contain the myosin filaments as well as the ends of the actin filaments where they overlap the myosin and are called A bands because they are anisotropic to polarized light.

69 C A pure actin filaments without the presence of the troponin-tropomyosin complex binds instantly and strongly with the heads of the myosin molecules in the presence of magnesium ions and ATP, both of which are abundant in the myofibril. If the troponin-tropomyosin complex is added to the actin filament, this binding does not take place. Therefore it is believed that the active sites on the normal actin filament of the relaxed muscle are inhibited or physically covered by troponin-tropomyosin complex.

70 C Several hours after death, all the muscles of the body go into a state of contracture called rigor mortis that is the muscles contract and become rigid even without action potentials. This rigidity is caused by loss of all ATP, which is required to cause separation of the cross-bridges from the actin filaments during the relaxation process. The muscles remain in rigor mortis until the muscle proteins are destroyed which usually results from the autolysis cause by enzymes released from the lysosomes some 15 to 25 hours later.

71 C In place of troponin, smooth muscle cells contain a large amount of another regulatory protein called calmodulin. Although this protein is similar to troponin in that it reacts with four calcium ions, it is different in the manner in which it initiates contraction. Calmodulin does this by activating the myosin cross bridges.

72 B The action potential recorded in ventricular muscle averages around 105 millivolts that means that the membrane potential rises from its very negative value of about -85 millivolts between beats to a slightly positive value of about +20 millivolts during each beat. After the initial spike, the membrane remains depolarized for about 0.2 seconds in atrial muscle and about 0.3 seconds in ventricular muscle, exhibiting a plateau which is followed by abrupt repolarization. The presence of this plateau cause the cardiac muscle contraction to last upto 15 times as long as skeletal muscle.

73 B When the heart rate increases, the duration of each cycle of the heart, including both the contraction phase and the relaxation phase, decreases. The duration of action potential and the period of contraction also decrease but not by as great a percentage as does the relaxation phase. At a normal heart rate of 72 beats per minute the period of contraction is about 0.40 of the entire cycle. At three time normal heart rate this period is about 0.65 of the entire cycle, which means that a heart beating at a very fast rate sometimes does not remain relaxed long enough to allow complete filling of the cardiac chambers before the next contraction.

74 C When the left ventricular pressure rises slightly above 80 mm Hg (and right ventricular pressure slightly above 8 mm Hg), the ventricular pressure push the semi lunar valve open. Immediately the blood begins to pour out of the ventricles, with about 70% of the emptying occurring during the first third of the period of ejection and the remaining 30% during the next two thirds. Therefore the first third is called the period of rapid ejection and the last two thirds the period of slow ejection.

75 D During diastole filling of ventricles normally increases the volume of each ventricle to about 110 to 120 ml. This volume is known as the end-diastolic volume. Then as the ventricle empty during systole the volume decreases about 70 ml, which is called stroke volume output. The remaining volume in each ventricle about 40 to 50 ml is called endsystolic volume. The fraction of the end diastolic volume that is ejected is called the ejection fraction.

76 B The sinus node is a small strip of specialized muscle about 3 mm wide, 15 mm long and 1 mm thick, it is located in the superior posterolateral wall of right atrium immediately below and slightly lateral to the opening of the superior vena cava.

77 B Spread of the depolarization wave through the atrial muscle is much slower than in ventricles. Therefore the musculature around the sinus node becomes depolarized a long time before around the musculature in the distal part of the atria. Because of this the area in the atria that also becomes repolarized first is also the sinus nodal region, the area that had originally become depolarized first. Thus when repolarization begins the region around the sinus node becomes positive with respect to the rest of atria. Therefore the atrial repolarization vector is backward to the vector of depolarization. Therefore the atrial T wave follows about 0.15 second after the atrial P wave, but this T wave is on the opposite side of the zero reference line from the P wave. The atrial T wave

appears at about the same time that the QRS complex of the ventricles appears. Therefore it is almost always totally obscured by the large ventricular QRS complex.

78 C In general QRS complex lasts as long as depolarization continues to spread through the ventricles, that is as long as part of the ventricles is depolarized and part still is polarized. Therefore the cause of a prolonged QRS complex is always prolonged conduction of the impulse through the ventricles. The normal QRS complex lasts 0.06 to 0.08 seconds, whereas in hypertrophy or dilatation of the right/left ventricles, the QRS complex may be prolonged to 0.09 to 0.12 seconds.

79 D The percentage of the total blood in the different segments of circulation is as follows:

Systemic circulation	84%
Veins	64%
Arteries	13%
Systemic arterioles	7%
Heart	7%
Pulmonary vessels	9%

80 C The pressure in the systemic capillaries varies from as high as 35 mm of Hg near the arteriolar end to as slow as 10 mmHg near the venous ends, but their average functional pressure in most vascular beds is about 17 mmHg, a pressure low enough that little of plasma flows out of the porous capillaries even though nutrients can diffuse easily to the tissue cells.

81 C Occasionally pressure is measured in centimeters of water. A pressure of 10 cm H_2O means a pressure sufficient to raise a column of water against gravity to a height of 10 centimeters. One millimeter of mercury pressure equals 1.36 cm H_2O pressure because the specific gravity of mercury is 13.6 times that of water, and 1 centimeter is 10 times as great as 1 millimeter.

82 A When blood is lost from the body and the arterial pressure begins to fall, nervous reflexes are elicited from the carotid sinuses and other pressure sensitive areas of the circulation. These in turn send nerve signals from the brain and spinal cord mainly through the sympathetic nerves, to the veins causing them to constrict. This takes up much of the slack in the circulatory system caused by the lost blood. Even after 20% of the total blood volume has been lost, the circulatory system often functions almost normally because of variable reservoir function of the veins.

83 B The width of the capillary intercellular cleft pores, 6 to 7 nanometers, is about 20 times the diameter of the water molecule, which is the smallest molecule that normally passes through the capillary pores. The diameters of plasma protein molecules are slightly grater than the width of the pores. Other substances such as sodium ions, chloride ions, glucose and urea have intermediate diameters.

84 C The colloid osmotic pressure of normal human plasma averages about 28 mmHg, 19 mm of this is caused by molecular effects of the dissolved protein and 9 mm by the cations held in the plasma by the proteins, which is called the Donnan effect.

85 B About 100 ml per hour of lymph flows through the thoracic duct of a resting human, and approximately another 20 ml flows into the circulation each hour through other channels, making a total of 120 ml/hr that is between 2 to 3 liters per day.

86 A Vasomotor center is located bilaterally in the reticular substance of the medulla and of the lower third of the pons. This centre transmits parasympathetic impulses through the vagus nerves to the heart and transmits sympathetic impulses through the cord and peripheral sympathetic nerves to all or almost all of the blood vessels of the body.

87 A An increase in atrial pressure also causes an increase in heart rate, sometimes increasing the heart rate as much as 75%. A small part of this increase is caused by a direct effect of the increased atrial volume to stretch the sinus node. Such direct stretch can increase the heart rate as much as 15%. An additional 40 to 60% increase in heart rate is caused by a nervous reflex called the brain bridge reflex. The stretch receptors of atria that elicit the Bainbridge reflex transmit their afferent signals through the vagus nerve to the medulla of the brain. Then the efferent signals are transmitted back through both the vagal and sympathetic nerves to increase the heart rate and strengthen the heart contraction.

88 D Closely associated with the baroreceptor pressure control system is a chemoreceptor reflex that operates in much the same way as the baroreceptor reflex except that chemoreceptors, instead of stretch receptors, initiate the response. They are located in several small organs, 1 to 2 mm in size. The chemo receptors are chemosensitive cells sensitive to oxygen lack, carbon dioxide excess or hydrogen ion excess.

89 A Often patchy areas of one or both kidneys are diseased and become ischemic because of local vascular constriction, whereas other areas of the kidneys are normal. When this occurs almost identical effects occur as in two-kidney type of Goldblatt hypertension. That is the patchy ischemic kidney tissue secretes rennin, and this in turn, acting through the formation of angiotensin II, cause the remaining kidney mass also to retain the salt and water. Indeed one of the most common causes of renal hypertension, especially in older patients.

90 B Because the cardiac output changes markedly with body size, it has been important to find some means by which the cardiac output of different sized people can be compared with one another. Therefore cardiac output is frequently stated in terms of cardiac index, which is the cardiac output per square meter of body surface area. The normal human being weighing 70 kilograms has a body surface area of about 1.7 square meters, which means that the normal average cardiac index for adults is about 3 L/min/m^2 of body surface area.

91 D During rest, blood flow through skeletal muscle averages 3 to 4 ml/min/100 g of muscle. During exercise in a well conditioned athlete, this rate can increase 15-25 folds rising to 50 to 80 ml/min/100 g of muscle.

92 A Under resting conditions, cardiac muscle normally uses mainly fatty acids for its energy instead of carbohydrates, with about 70% of the energy being derived from fatty acids. However as is true with other tissues under anaerobic conditions cardiac metabolism must call on the anaerobic glycolysis mechanism for energy. The glycolysis uses tremendous quantities of the blood glucose and at the same time forms large amounts of lactic acid in the cardiac tissue, which is probably one of the causes of the cardiac pain in cardiac ischemic conditions.

93 D Normally a person cannot feel his or her heart but ischemic cardiac muscle often does not exhibit pain sensation. Under ischemic conditions heart muscle releases acidic substances such as lactic acid or other pain promoting substances such as histamine, kinins and cellular proteolytic enzymes that are not removed rapidly by the slowly moving coronary blood. The high concentration of these abnormal products then stimulate the pain endings in the cardiac muscle and pain impulses are transmitted through the sympathetic sensory afferent nerve fibers into the central nervous system.

94 A An atrial heart sound can be recorded in some people in the phonocardiogram, but it can almost never be heard with a stethoscope because of its low frequency–usually 20 cycles/sec or less. This sound occurs when the atria contracts, and presumably, it is caused by the inrush of blood into ventricles, which initiates vibrations similar to those of the third heart sound.

95 A In stenosis, the blood is ejected from the chamber through only a small opening of the valve. Because of the resistance to ejection, the blood pressure in the chamber rises as high as 300 mm Hg, whereas the pressure in the vessel is still normal. Thus a nozzle effect is created during systole, with blood jetting at tremendous velocity through a small opening of the valve. This cause severe turbulence of the blood in the root of the vessel. The turbulent blood impinging against the blood vessel causes intense vibration, and a loud murmur.

Notes

Syllabus

1. Introduction
   - Aims and scope of the science of dental materials.
2. Structure and behaviour of Matter.
3. Important physical properties applicable to Dental Materials including their biological considerations.
4. Gypsum products used in dentistry including casting investment materials with or without gypsum binder.
5. Impressions materials used in dentistry including duplicating materials.
6. Synthetic resins used in dentistry
   a. General properties and physical characteristics.
   b. Resins as denture base materials, repair and reline materials, soft liners, tissue conditioners.
   c. Resins as restorative materials: Unfilled and filled resin restorative materials, tissue sealant.
   d. Direct-bonding cement materials.
7. Metals and alloys: Their structure and behaviour, some important physical properties:
   a. Dental amalgam alloys.
   b. Gold foil.
   c. Dental casting gold alloys.
   d. Stainless steel, chrome–cobalt alloys.
8. Dental waxes including inlay casting wax.
9. Gold inlay casting procedures:
   - Preparation of the die-wax pattern, spruing, investing-control of shrinkage compensation. Wax elimination–casting machines, casting, defects in castings.
10. Welding and soldering–Materials used.
11. Dental Cements: Classification, composition, manipulation, properties and uses:
    - Zinc Cements, Copper cements, Zincoxide eugenol cements, Silicate cements, Cavity liners, cavity varnishers, resin cements.
12. Dental porcelain including porelain fused to metal. Porcelain furnace and fusing.
13. Mechanics of tooth cutting. Burs and points.
14. Abrasives and polishing agents.
15. Die and counter die materials including electroforming and electro-polishing. Practicals and Demonstrations to be arranged in the manipulation of the more common materials.

Chapter 3

Dental Materials

1. Which of the metal is not used as an implant material?

A. Stainless steel B. Nickel–chromium

C. Pure titanium D. Cobalt–chromium

2. Tissue conditioners are temporary materials because they

A. Are too expensive for permanent use

B. Are not color stable over time

C. Harden over time in the mouth

D. Are always irritating to the gums

3. Which of the following statements applies best to the poly vinyl siloxane impression materials?

A. Stiffest elastomeric impression material

B. Most dimensionally stable elastomeric impression material

C. Could not be used for edentulous arches

D. Pouring within 1 hour is most critical

4. It is common to use more than one type of direct gold material to fill a cavity because

A. Some are manufactured with less density as bulk-filling materials only

B. Roughness is enhanced when dense foils are used on the surface

C. Only alloys with calcium can be used in the final layer for optimal hardness

D. It is nor possible to truly condense certain materials in the base of cavities

5. Which of the following is recommended as an appropriate disinfection procedure for an alginate impression?

A. Complete immersion in bleach in a plastic bag for 1 hour

B. Spraying for 30 seconds with an iodophor and then wiping dry

C. Placing in an autoclave on low temperature for 3 minutes

D. Spraying with glutaraldehyde and sealing in a bag for 10 minutes

6. Which of the following is *not* one of the major components of dental porcelain?

A. Clay B. Feldspar

C. Cerium oxide D. Quartz

7. Gaps at the margins of composite restorations and teeth may be opened during the ingestion of foods and beverages as a result of

A. Differences in thermal conductivity

B. The presence of pulpal pressure

C. Differences in thermal expansion coefficients

D. Inadequate strength of composite

8. Which impression material(s) could theoretically be disinfected and used to make another impression?

A. Polyether B. ZnOE

C. Alginate D. Compound

9. A patient returns to the clinic complaining that the class II composite placed in a lower first molar 3 months ago remains very sensitive to hot and cold stimuli. It is determined that the restoration is leaking along the gingival margin, possibly as a result of all of the above *except*

A. Light-curing of the proximal box from the occlusal direction only
B. Due to delayed acid–base reaction in composite
C. Moisture contamination of the cavity preparation before placement
D. Placing the light-cured restoration as a single increment

10. Benefits directly derived from the use of a slightly higher Hg/alloy ratio than is necessary for an amalgam include all of the following, *except*

A. Enhanced plasticity of the mix
B. Better condensability
C. Longer working time
D. Greater strength

11. Flux is added to the casting metal during melting to

A. Minimize oxidation of the metal
B. Enhance the esthetics of the metal
C. Increase the stiffness of the metal
D. Reduce the fluidity of the metal

12. The large working range of orthodontic wires made from which alloy allows the most tooth movement with the fewest adjustments

A. Nickel-titanium
B. Stainless steel
C. β-Titanium
D. Cobalt-chromium

13. Agar hydrocolloid can be used for accurate crown and bridge impression taking, whereas alginate cannot because

A. Alginate is less stable
B. Alginate is less accurate
C. Agar is faster setting
D. Agar is more flexible

14. Which of the following does not represent a mode of activation commonly used to cause polymerization of dental polymers within the oral cavity?

A. Heat
B. Light
C. Chemical
D. Microwave

15. Which of the following is *not* a correct step during the preparation of an alginate impression?

A. Wiping the mix against the side of the bowl to remove air bubbles
B. Mixing for 60 seconds to provide ample working time
C. Loading a water-cooled tray from the posterior to eliminate trapped air
D. Holding the tray in the mouth for several minutes to ensure accuracy

16. Which of the following is least likely to have a significant effect on the setting rate of zinc phosphate cement?

A. Powder-to-liquid ratio
B. Size of the powder particles
C. Stiffness of the mixing spatula
D. Size of the mixing area

17. Why would it be inappropriate for a prophylaxis paste to contain diamond particles?

A. It would be too expensive
B. It would remove enamel
C. It would not remove plaque
D. It would not remove calculus

18. Compomers differ from resin-modified glass ionomers in that compomers

A. Do not contain water
B. Have a delayed acid-base reaction
C. Have properties similar to composites
D. All of the above

19. Compared with any of the resin-based sealants, glass ionomers

A. Have been shown to have greater retention rates in clinical studies
B. Release fluoride at a greater rate and to a greater extent
C. Have similar long-term preventive capabilities
D. Are more resistant to chipping

20. Which of the following is (are) *not* a part(s) of the direct gold restoration procedure?

A. Dipping each piece of gold in alcohol to improve cohesion
B. Condensing each piece of foil with 10 to 15 pounds of force
C. Using incremental method of placing gold in the cavity
D. Isolating the tooth with a rubber dam

21. What would be the rationale for placing a liner of glass ionomer under a large and deep composite restoration in a molar?

A. Provide thermal insulation for the tooth
B. Seal the dentinal surfaces under the composite
C. Improve the strength of the restoration
D. Minimize chances of corrosion on the surface

22. Dimensional changes that affect the accuracy of a cast dental crown include

A. Setting contraction of the investment material
B. Shrinkage of the wax pattern during cooling
C. Shrinkage of the metal during burnout
D. Expansion of the impression material during setting

23. Compared with conventional posterior composites, packable composites developed for posterior applications have improved

A. Wear resistance
B. Handling characteristics
C. Esthetics
D. Marginal adaptation

24. Which of the following is *not* recommended in the technique for curing light-cured composites?

A. Holding the light tip 1 cm from the tooth
B. Wearing special glasses with orange filters
C. Using an exposure duration of 40 to 60 seconds
D. Placing the composite in increments of 1 to 2 mm

25. A patient is allergic to earrings, which alloy would not be a good choice for her PFM crown?

A. 70% palladium, 30% silver
B. 80% nickle, 20% chromium
C. 90% gold, 10% palladium
D. 50% gold, 50% platinum

26. Which of the following produces the smoothest surface on dental porcelain?

A. Aluminum oxide
B. Tin oxide
C. Rubber wheels
D. Glazing

27. The hue of natural teeth is generally

A. 6-8
B. Yellow
C. 2-3
D. White

28. An ideal base for a deep amalgam restoration should be mixed to heavy consistency and placed to a thickness of approximately

A. 0.5 mm
B. 2.0 mm
C. 1.0 mm
D. 3.0 mm

29. You inspect a denture that has been returned from the laboratory for presentation to a patient that afternoon and notice a large number of bubbles, but only in the thickest areas. You suspect that the bubbles were caused by
- **A.** Heating the denture to less than 75°C during processing
- **B.** Heating the denture rapidly during the early stage of processing
- **C.** An inadequate application of pressure during packing
- **D.** Mixing with too low of a monomer-to-powder ratio

30. An abrasive material that would most efficiently abrade a surface with a hardness of 5 on the Moh's scale might be one with
- **A.** Irregular particles of hardness 6
- **B.** Spherical particles of hardness 6
- **C.** Irregular particles of hardness 3
- **D.** Spherical particles of hardness 3

31. After drinking cold beverages, a patient experiences severe pain in tooth 21, which has had a PFM crown for several years. A likely cause for this pain is
- **A.** Overextended margin of the crown
- **B.** Dissolution of the cement, producing a gap at the margin
- **C.** A gap between tooth and cement at the interior, away from the margins
- **D.** An inflammatory response to the cement

32. Failure to place a tray filled with agar impression material into the last bath before seating in the patient could cause
- **A.** A significant loss of accuracy
- **B.** Burning of the patient's tissues
- **C.** The material to remain unset
- **D.** A reduction in working time

33. The hardness of denture base acrylic plastic is
- **A.** Greater than that of glass
- **B.** Greater than that of enamel
- **C.** Less than that of metals
- **D.** Less than that of gingival tissue

34. In contrast to low-heat investments, high-heat investments
- **A.** Cannot be heated beyond 750°C
- **B.** Are used for PFM alloys
- **C.** Undergo lesser expansion
- **D.** Are made with gypsum

35. The excellent corrosion resistance of the base metal alloys used in restorations can be attributed to which of the following
- **A.** The formation of a protective oxide film
- **B.** Painting the surface with varnish as a final step
- **C.** The absence of sufficient chromium within the metal
- **D.** Their extremely smooth surfaces

36. Complete mixing of an addition silicone impression material is achieved when the material
- **A.** Begins to feel rubbery
- **B.** Can be poured into a syringe
- **C.** Has a uniform color
- **D.** No longer sticks to the pad or spatula

37. Which of the following waxes is hardest at room temperature?
- **A.** Base plate **B.** Boxing
- **C.** Inlay pattern **D.** Impression

38. Compare with pure gold, dental gold alloys are
- **A.** More expensive
- **B.** Harder
- **C.** More corrosion resistant
- **D.** More malleable

39. A significant weight gain in a denture base would be associated with all of the following *except*
- **A.** Swelling
- **B.** Water sorption
- **C.** Leaching of unreacted molecules
- **D.** Change in the fit

40. Which of the following would be least likely to scratch the surface of an acrylic denture?

A. Quartz dust B. Talc powder
C. Ground glass D. Pumice stone

41. Which of the following is *not* a step normally recommended for the intraoral repair of a chipped anterior PFM restoration?

A. Etch the porcelain surface with hydrofluoric acid
B. Place a glass ionomer liner over any exposed metal
C. Roughen the surfaces with an intraoral sandblaster
D. Make the repair with a light-cured composite

42. Replacement of the enamel portion of a tooth is optimally done with a composite having

A. Opacity
B. Low translucency
C. High Translucency
D. Chroma

43. When an amalgam is in contact with a gold onlay, a galvanic cell is established in which the amalgam Pick the odd one out

A. Oxidizes
B. Releases metallic ions
C. Serves as the cathode
D. Degrades more quickly

44. The smoothest surface on amalgam is achieved with a final polish using

A. Pumice B. Brown stones
C. Tin oxide D. Green points

45. A bioactive implant has all of the following characteristics, *except*

A. Stronger than steel
B. Ceramic
C. Chemically bonds to bone
D. Similar stiffness as bone

46. Which element is most responsible for reacting with mercury to cause the hardening of dental amalgam?

A. Copper
B. Silver
C. Tin
D. Zinc

47. The elastic modulus of a material is a measure of its

A. Hardness
B. Toughness
C. Percent elongation
D. Stiffness

48. An epoxy die has the following characteristics, compared with a stone die

A. Lower strength
B. Greater setting expansion
C. Lower abrasion resistance
D. Less brittleness

49. A patient requests a posterior composite in a lower second molar, even though it will be in direct contact with the opposing cusp during biting. What are your expectations for this restoration?

A. Wear will be greater in the contact site than in the noncontact sites
B. Wear in the contact site will be less than it would be for an amalgam
C. The opposing tooth may show an increased rate of wear
D. The composite cannot be placed with sealed margins

50. Which of the following is *not* a true statement about dental composites?

A. They contain monomers that chemically react to transform a paste into a rigid restorative
B. Glass particles are coated with coupling agents to enhance bonding to polymers
C. They contain spherical fillers that are generally 100 to 200 μm in diameter
D. Their strength depends on how much filler they contain

51. An acid-etched composite would *not* make a good provisional restorative because it would
- **A.** Have a poor marginal seal
- **B.** Not be strong enough
- **C.** Be too difficult to remove
- **D.** Set too slowly

52. Which type of composite would be expected to have the shiniest surface after polishing with prophylaxis paste?
- **A.** Small-sized hybrid
- **B.** Microfill
- **C.** Midsized hybrid
- **D.** All would be the same

53. Denture acrylics contain cross-linking agents, mainly to improve their
- **A.** Internal color
- **B.** Tissue compatibility
- **C.** Surface hardness
- **D.** Craze resistance

54. An image-conscious patient returns with a fractured class IV composite restoration that must be replaced. The chart shows the original restoration was a microfill composite placed 6 months ago. What treatment might be suggested to replace the restoration?
- **A.** Glass ionomer to prevent further decay
- **B.** A midsized hybrid because of its greater strength
- **C.** A microfill composite to maintain maximum esthetics
- **D.** A small-sized hybrid combining strength and esthetics

55. In explaining to a patient the benefits of polishing a recently placed occlusal amalgam restoration, one would be correct to say all of the following *except*
- **A.** A polished surface is better for oral hygiene
- **B.** Amalgam may show less tarnish and corrosion during aging
- **C.** A polished restoration will feel more natural to the tongue
- **D.** Amalgam will be less likely to wear down the opposing teeth

56. Glass ionomers should be mixed for approximately 30 to 40 seconds because
- **A.** Longer mixing times delay the setting reaction
- **B.** Shorter mixing times do not allow the powder to be entirely dissolved
- **C.** Longer mixing times increases the working time
- **D.** Shorter mixing times can compromise the material's strength

57. Which of the following is *not* one of the three basic components in most dentin-bonding agents?
- **A.** Antimicrobial agent
- **B.** Surface etchant
- **C.** Wetting primer
- **D.** Resin adhesive

58. Compared with multicomponent adhesives, one-component adhesives
- **A.** Can be applied in only a fraction of the time
- **B.** Have higher bond strengths to dentin
- **C.** Require fewer steps
- **D.** Are much less expensive

59. A base is placed on the floor of a deep cavity under a gold restoration to
- **A.** Provide thermal protection for the pulp
- **B.** Seal the dentin from toxic gold particles
- **C.** Prevent gold atoms from penetrating into the tooth
- **D.** Improve the stiffness of the restoration

60. **During the warm part of the year, the office air-conditioning system experiences problems, causing the operatory temperature to be noticeably warmer than usual. How will this affect the way you mix zinc phosphate cement for a bridge?**
   - **A.** Mix the powder into the liquid faster to leave enough working time
   - **B.** Chill the slab in the refrigerator before mixing to prolong the working time
   - **C.** Mix only one half of the recommended powder to slow setting
   - **D.** Dispense the liquid first to allow time for water to evaporate to slow setting

61. **A patient complains that tooth 3, which contains a crown, is sensitive to hot and cold, and the dentist notices that there has been a substantial loss of cement at the margins and suspects that it is leaking. Which of the following characteristics of the cement best explains the reason for the cement loss?**
   - **A.** Low compressive strength
   - **B.** Solubility in oral fluids
   - **C.** High thermal conductivity
   - **D.** Low elastic limit

62. **Which of the following materials is most often placed into a deep cavity with the intent of protecting the pulp and promoting reparative dentin formation?**
   - **A.** Zinc oxide eugenol
   - **B.** Glass ionomer
   - **C.** Calcium hydroxide
   - **D.** Zinc phosphate

63. **Glass ionomers are considered by some to be the material of choice for applying a base under an amalgam restoration because they**
   - **A.** Chemically adhere to enamel but not dentin
   - **B.** Are twice as strong as all other bases
   - **C.** Are completely insoluble in oral fluids
   - **D.** Provide fluoride protection under leaky fillings

64. **A patient with a history of very sensitive teeth requires an amalgam restoration of a maxillary molar. Which base material may be the best choice for this patient, and why?**
   - **A.** Glass ionomer, because it will never dissolve
   - **B.** Zinc phosphate, because it is very stiff
   - **C.** Zinc oxide eugenol, because it has a neutral pH
   - **D.** Light-cured calcium hydroxide, because it is so strong

65. **Good hand condensation of spherical amalgams requires**
   - **A.** Greater force than that used for admixed amalgams
   - **B.** Approximately 2 to 3 pounds of force
   - **C.** More force than that used for lathe-cut amalgams
   - **D.** The smallest-tipped condensers available

66. **Which of the following is *not* present in glass ionomer cements?**
   - **A.** Eugenol
   - **B.** Polyacrylic acid
   - **C.** Silicate glass
   - **D.** Tartaric acid

67. **Which of the following is (are) *not* a common component(s) of resin-based pit and fissure sealants?**
   - **A.** Silane coupling agent
   - **B.** Small glass filler particles
   - **C.** Bis-GMA monomers
   - **D.** Phosphoric acid

68. **Which of the following is *not* used in the procedure for preparing an indirect acrylic provisional restoration?**
   - **A.** A plaster model of the unprepared teeth
   - **B.** An impression of the prepared teeth
   - **C.** A plaster model of the prepared teeth
   - **D.** An impression of the restored teeth

69. A polyvinyl siloxane impression is taken of a tooth prepared for a crown. On removal from the mouth, the impression is inspected, and it is noted that the tooth surface and gingival areas around the tooth have a wrinkled appearance and seem moist. The most likely reason for this defect is the
- **A.** Impression material was not mixed properly
- **B.** Manufacturers packaged base pastes in both tubes of the cartridge
- **C.** Impression was removed from the mouth too soon
- **D.** Impression area was contacted by gloved fingers prior to taking the impression

70. Polymerization in which water or alcohol by-products are produced during the reaction is called
- **A.** Addition
- **B.** Condensation
- **C.** Ring-opening
- **D.** Cross-linking

71. Which of the following is (are) a practical way(s) to speed the setting rate of the pre encapsulated amalgam used in your office?
- **A.** Triturate the capsule at a slower speed
- **B.** Chill the capsule before trituration
- **C.** Open the capsule and remove some of the mercury
- **D.** Triturate the capsule for a longer time

72. A preventive resin restoration might be indicated for a patient with
- **A.** Extensive caries of both lower first molars
- **B.** An incipient lesion in an upper premolar
- **C.** A deep groove in a caries-free second molar
- **D.** Recurrent decay around an existing amalgam in a first molar

73. Which of the following is *not* a rationale for the wax burnout procedure?
- **A.** Increase the density of the investment material
- **B.** Expand the investment material
- **C.** Vaporize the wax pattern from the mold
- **D.** Increase the temperature of the investment

74. Mouth protectors are commonly made
- **A.** From hard plastics formed on metal frameworks for reinforcement
- **B.** By softening a plastic in boiling water and then forming on the teeth
- **C.** By a ready-made technique to improve fit and comfort
- **D.** From polyacrylic acid liquid and glass particles

75. Which type of bonding in a material is most associated with high electrical and thermal conductivity?
- **A.** Ionic
- **B.** Metallic
- **C.** Covalent
- **D.** Van der Waals

76. You did not have time to clean out the plaster bowl after making a mix, and the material has hardened. The easiest way to remove the gypsum is to
- **A.** Soak the rubber bowl in water for a period of 24 hours
- **B.** Soak the rubber bowl in a detergent solution for 10 minutes
- **C.** Place the bowl on a vibrator to break up the gypsum
- **D.** Flex the bowl several times to break up the gypsum

77. Tarnish differs from corrosion in that tarnish
- **A.** Is much more harmful to a metal
- **B.** Discolors metals and can easily be polished out
- **C.** Does cause metal ion release
- **D.** Involves an electrochemical reaction

78. Which of the following would not increase the rate of abrasion?
- **A.** Use of lubricant
- **B.** Increased pressure
- **C.** Smaller particles
- **D.** Increased speed

79. Which property describes the capability of an impression to be removed from around the teeth without permanently deforming?
A. Maximum flexibility
B. Percent elongation
C. Elastic modulus
D. Ductility

80. Fluoride gels differ from fluoride varnishes in that
A. Gels are for home use only
B. Varnishes are more acidic and more dangerous
C. Varnishes can cause surface deterioration of restorations
D. Gels are held in the mouth in trays

81. For light activated composite which of the following initiator-activator system is used?
A. Inorganic acid-peroxide
B. Diketone-amine
C. Peroxide-amine
D. Organic acid-amine

82. What is the maximum safe concentration of mercury vapor in the breathing zone for a 40-hour workweek?
A. 0.5 mg of Hg/m^3 of air
B. 0.05 mg of Hg/m^3 of air
C. 0.05 ng of Hg/m^3 of air
D. 5 mg of Hg/m^3 of air

83. Final polishing of amalgam should be done with
A. Burnishing
B. Silicone carbide
C. Carving
D. Tin oxide

84. To achieve the best surface of microfilled composite which is ideal method?
A. Use of greenstone
B. Use of white stone
C. Use of silicone carbide
D. Use of Mylar strip

85. Which of the following material is used over pulp?
A. Glass ionomer
B. Composite
C. Calcium hydroxide
D. Zinc phosphate

86. Which of the cement has the highest elastic modulus?
A. Glass ionomer
B. Zinc polycarboxylate
C. Zinc phosphate
D. Hybrid ionomer

87. Which of the following is not a component of dental porcelain?
A. Alkali metal carbonates
B. Quartz
C. Zinc oxide
D. Feldspar

88. All of the following are advantages of heat pressed, all ceramic material *except*
A. Increased aesthetic
B. Reduced processing time
C. Reduced cost of equipment
D. Increased marginal accuracy

89. Which of the metallic pigment gives blue hue to ceramic?
A. Tin oxide
B. Magnesium oxide
C. Cobalt oxide
D. Iron oxide

90. Cavity varnishes are contraindicated under
A. Amalgam B. Glass ionomer
C. Composite D. Silicate

91. Materials used in endodontics to seal the root space are covered under ADA specification No.
A. 1 B. 6
C. 57 D. 3

92. Density of dental ceramic is around
A. 1-1.5 g/cm^3 B. 2-2.5 g/cm^3
C. 3-3.5 g/cm^3 D. 4-4.5 g/cm^3

93. Minimum what percentage of chromium is required to produce corrosion resistant iron is

A. 5% B. 44%
C. 8% D. 11-13%

94. Which of them has the highest melting temperature?

A. Osmium B. Iridium
C. Gold D. Platinum

95. Which of the following wax has the maximum coefficient of thermal expansion?

A. Ceresin B. Paraffin
C. Beeswax D. Inlay wax

96. Which of them is not obtained from plant kingdom?

A. Carnauba B. Candelilla
C. Ceresin D. Beeswax

97. What is the maximum allowable level of Hg in the blood?

A. 8 µg/l B. 3 µg/l
C. 12 µg/l D. 22 µg/l

Answers

1 B The first metals used as dental implants were surgical stainless steel. Stainless steel is an alloy of iron and carbon (0.05%), it has the minimal amount of carbon thus it is designated as the low carbon, with 18% chromium to provide corrosion resistance and 8% nickel to stabilize the particular steel structure.

Another alloy commonly used for dental implant was based on an alloy of cobalt (65%) and chromium (30%), which also contains a small amount of carbon. Both these alloys are very strong, hard, and stiff and have excellent corrosion resistance. Titanium is also used as implant metal either in pure form (commercially pure titanium) or as an alloy with aluminum (6%) and vanadium (4%). Other titanium alloys containing zirconium and niobium are also being used to a lesser extent. Titanium is strong, corrosion resistant metal, with lightweight.

Nickel chromium is not used as an implant material.

2 C A more temporary form of liner is available for patients whose mucosa is so irritated that they cannot wear their dentures. A tissue conditioner is the appropriate material in cases where tissue is damaged and needs time to heal. These materials are based on poly-methylmethacrylate polymers loaded with plasticizers such as alcohol to increase the softness. They are mixed as powder - liquid system, but no polymerization reaction occurs. Instead they are poured onto the tissue surface of a denture and pressed against the tissue to form an impression by a physical gelation between the polymer in the powder and the plasticizer in the liquid. Because of the alcohol the patient may experience a slight burning or stinging sensation with application, but not lasting adverse affects are noted. There also is no concern over heat generation because these materials do not polymerize. The soft conditioner occupies the space between the irritated tissue and the hard denture base, acting as shock absorber. The material is temporary lasting only a few weeks because the plasticizers leach out and cause the conditioner to harden in the mouth.

3 B Certain elastomeric impression materials should be poured as soon as possible; this is not a concern for the polyethers and addition silicones. Infact it is ideal to delay pouring of addition silicones for at least 45 minutes to 1 hour after taking the impression. Many of these materials release hydrogen gas during the setting reaction. If the impression is poured too soon this out gassing will produce tiny bubbles on the surface of the model or die material. The delay in pouring has no effect on the dimensional stability of silicones they can be poured even after a delay of many days.

Setting shrinkage in percentage of all elastomeric impression material is like:

Polysulfide	0.25
Condensation silicone	0.6
Polyether	0.1
Addition polysilicone	0.05

Impression materials, which are elastic, can be used for both dentulous and edentulous arches.

Polymers have much greater tear resistance than the hydrocolloids; therefore removal is not much of a concern. The one exception might be the polyether material that is very rigid but has very poor tear resistance.

4 A More than one type of direct gold is used for a single cavity even when one considers that the ultimate goal is to fill the cavity completely in a timely fashion, while producing a well-adapted restoration with excellent surface smoothness. Filling of the cavity preparation is most easily achieved by using the bulk forms of the material. Therefore it is common to use mat foil or chunks of mat or powdered gold. The surface must be smooth, however so the clinician uses a thinner and smoother foil or mat foil to fill the last portion or the outer surface of the preparation. 'The key parameters of a good gold restoration are to achieve excellent adaptation to the walls of the cavity and elimination of porosity, producing a dense hard restoration.

5 D ADA has developed general recommendations for the infection control in dental office that include specific recommendations for impression materials. Alginate impression materials can be immersed or sprayed with a disinfectant, but the resultant casts may be optimal when a spray technique is used. Therefore a typical procedure is to spray the alginate impression with an iodophor or hypochlorite compound and then place it into a sealed plastic bag for approximately 10 minutes. This recommendation is based on studies showing no significant loss of accuracy as result of an effective disinfection procedure. Before disinfecting the impression should be rinsed first to remove blood, debris and saliva.

6 C Porcelain contain three main components: quartz or flint (silica), feldspar (a potassium – aluminum silicate) and kaolin clay (aluminum silicate) in dental feldspathic porcelain, feldspar makes up 75 to 85% of the porcelain and serves as the amorphous glass phase that holds the silica mineral crystal together. Kaolin added at only 3 to 5% serves as an Opaquing agent and enhances the workability of the porcelain. Cerium oxide is not a component that is used in the dental porcelain.

7 C Temperature can have a profound effect on the dimensional accuracy of dental materials. A change in temperature can produce an immediate or delayed change in dimension. The magnitude of the change is determined by a thermal property called linear coefficient of thermal expansion. This property describes the change in length of an object produced by a certain increase or decrease in its temperature. The application or removal of heat causes any object to expand or contract respectively. The rate at which this occurs depends on the composition of the material. In a composite restoration the seal between the composite and the tooth may be compromised over time by the repeated temperature changes in the mouth, which cause different amounts of expansions and contraction of the composite and the tooth. This difference may create gaps between the two, which leads to leakage of salivary components into the tooth towards the pulp.
COTE of tooth — 8-11 × 10^{-6}/°C
COTE of composite — 20-50 × 10^{-6}/°C
COTE = Coefficient of Thermal expansion.

8 D Polyether, ZnOE and alginate all three are chemical setting and irreversible type of impression materials. Impression compound is the only material amongst the mentioned materials that is physical setting (thermoplastic), hence a reversible kind of material, which can be disinfected before making another impression.

9 B Micro leakage is very common in composite restoration. One of the causes is polymerization shrinkage that occurs when the bulk of the material is placed in the cavity and cured from occlusal direction, the resin shrinks towards the source of light thereby producing a gap gingivally. Therefore it is always recommended to place and cure the resin incrementally. For an optimum bonding, bond is placed on the etched enamel but boding may not take place if the enamel or dentin is contaminated with saliva. There is no acid–base reaction in the setting mechanism of composite, acid-base reaction takes place in GIC.

10 D The original alloy particles are the strongest and stiffest portion of the amalgam; anything that minimizes their content will decrease mechanical properties. Therefore higher Hg/alloy ratios, which result in more γ_1 matrix formation, produce a weaker amalgam. Although handling characteristics are improved when more mercury is used in the mix, using too much produces an amalgam with poorer properties.

11 A During melting of an alloy flux are added. Metals oxidize and form a skin or thickened outer surface; this is apparent in a melting metal because the oxide skin keeps the surface together and inhibits the metal from flowing. This obviously would be detrimental to the casting process. The flux is composed of borax and boric acid reacts with oxygen at the surface of the melting metal and removes the oxide skin thus reducing the surface tension and allowing the metal to become very fluid. At this stage the metal takes on a shiny mirror like appearance.

12 A The working range of an orthodontic wire is essentially equivalent to its maximum flexibility. A wire with a greater working range can move teeth greater distance than one with a lower working range before needing a tightening or adjustment. The working range or maximum flexibility of stainless steel and cobalt – chromium wires is low, that of b - titanium is medium and of nickel – titanium is high.

13 B Elastic recovery is a measure of an impression material's accuracy. This property is of utmost importance because the primary function of an impression material is to reproduce accurately and reliably the relationship between oral tissues. Therefore higher the value for elastic recovery, the more accurate is the material. Another term used to describe this property is permanent set, which describes the percentage of permanent change in shape that occurs during removal from undercuts. In this regard the materials with low values are most ideal. Elastic recovery of alginate is 97.3% and that of agar is 98.8%. Therefore agar is more accurate, and is the material of choice for crown and bridge work.

14 A Heat activation is not used to cause polymerization of dental polymers within oral cavity because the polymerization reaction is accompanied by evolution of a significant amount of heat, caused by the breaking of C = C bonds throughout the mass. Therefore the material heats up during hardening, and care should be taken not to burn one self or the patient. The material may reach a temperature of approximately 100°C. The evolution of heat has a significant effect on the dimensional stability of the material. Shrinkage normally accompanies the cooling process. This sets up additional internal stresses. The magnitude of the stress, and thus the overall distortion during stress relief depends upon maximum temperature and cooling rate.

15 C Steps involved in the preparation of alginate impression are proportioning, mixing, loading of tray and taking impression and cleanup and disinfection. After proportioning as per the manufacturer stir powder and water vigorously to wet powder completely. The powder and water are vigorously spatulated at a rate of 100-turns/minute for approximately one minute. During the process the mixture is stropped or wiped along the sides of the bowl, to push the air bubbles out and produce a homogenous mix. Care should be taken not to over mix, because this will limit the working time and breaks up the gel that is forming. Therefore mixing time should be kept up to 60 seconds. Metal or plastic trays with either holes or metal rim lock are used to carry the material to the mouth. Water-cooled trays are used for agar not alginate. It is important to seat the back portion of the tray first as the amount of material in the posterior region of the tray may be displaced down the patient's throat, stimulating a gag reflex. Therefore the tray is seated in the patient's mouth from the posterior region first to displace the material anteriorly in the patient's mouth. The tray should be held for additional 2-3 minutes until the material sets and complete gelation has occurred. The alginate will no longer be tacky and the impression will feel stiff and spring back rapidly on removal from undercuts.

16 C The rate of reaction of zinc phosphate cement depends upon powder to liquid ratio, temperature, water concentration in the mix and the mixing time.

17 B It would be inappropriate for a prophylaxis paste to contain diamond particles because diamond is the hardest substance with the hardness value of 10 on Moh's scale and enamel has the value of 5-6, and dentin has 3-4. Therefore the prophylaxis paste will remove the enamel or dentin.

18 D The word compomer is a contraction of composite and ionomer, suggesting a material with intermediate characteristics and properties. Compomers are packaged and handled much like composites. They have the same composition as composites with one exception. Compomers contain an additional molecule with carboxylic acid groups, similar to the molecules in conventional and resin modified GIC. This means that compomers can also undergo an acid-base setting reaction like GIC. Compomers however do not contain water (they are anhydrous). Compomers have properties that are intermediate to those of composites and resins modified GIC but are closest to composites.

19 B GIC are composed of an acidic polymer liquid (polyacrylic acid) that is mixed with a silicate glass powder containing calcium, aluminum and fluorine. When the powder and the liquid are mixed, the acidic liquid dissolves some of the powder, releasing metal ions with positive charges. These ions react with the negatively charged groups on the polymer molecules to form a hard matrix that holds the rest of the glass particles together. The hard matrix traps the fluoride ions released from the glass.

Various resin pit and fissure sealants, adhesive resins and dental composites have been formulated with fluoride containing compounds in the hope of producing cariostatic materials. In general these materials release fluoride in a manner similar to that of the glass ionomers except that fluoride is released from resin based materials less rapidly than from GIC, because the resin is less soluble in oral fluids.

20 A Direct gold restorations are done in a isolated tooth using incremental method. Cavity is filled using bulk forms of the material. It is common to use mat foil or chunks of mat or powdered gold. The key parameter is that gold be condensed with sufficient force to achieve excellent adaptation to the walls of the cavity and eliminate porosity, producing dense restoration. Direct gold can be placed with hand condensers by hammering pieces into the cavity with small mallet and condenser or with electrically operated mechanical condenser. The cavity must be built up in small increments to ensure that each increment is adapted and made dense. Since pure gold is very soft it is strain hardened with 10-15 pounds of condensation force. Another factor concerns the oral environment and the use of a material that must be welded during placement. Therefore it must be placed incrementally. The adhesion of one piece of gold to another will not take place in a cavity contaminated with moisture. Therefore the maintenance of dry field through rubber dam isolation is paramount. During manufacturing the foil is passed through a gas to adsorb a layer of ammonia onto their surface. The gas makes the surface non-adherent towards one another. The pieces will not weld together until this layer of contamination is removed, which usually is accompanied by passing the pieces of gold over the flame of an alcohol torch or by heating on an inert ceramic plate. Either treatment makes the gold cohesive.

21 B For the same reason that glass ionomers are attractive as restorative materials, they are attractive as liners. Their adhesive characteristics make them ideal for the sealing dentin under many types of restorations. They also release fluoride, which may give them anticarious properties. A very common technique is placement of GIC under composite, which is known as sandwich restoration seals all dentinal tubules thereby reduce the sensitivity.

22 B Investment materials expand on setting rather than contraction. Normal setting expansion is 0.7% and setting expansion under wet conditions (hygroscopic setting expansion) is double that of normal setting expansion (1.5%). All impression material undergoes contraction on setting. Elastomers undergo minimal shrinkage (0.05%) and have the ability to reproduce and resolve features at the level of 1 μm. During the burnout procedure the wax melts and flows out. During burnout there is no metal; hence there is no question of shrinkage of metal during burnout. Waxes do shrink on cooling due to high coefficient of thermal expansion, which may cause contraction on cooling.

23 B With the use of high viscosity, packable composite, it is felt that the heavy consistency aids to some extent in providing shape to the matrix for achieving the interproximal contact, although it is not nearly as proficient as amalgam in this regard. The heavy consistency also means that the packable composite will not flow and therefore filling gingival margins is more difficult. For this reason many clinicians place a low viscosity. Flowable composite as the first gingival increment to try to ensure good adaptation to the floor and the margins of the cavity.

24 A The distance between the tip of the curing light and the tooth is important, as the intensity of the light source is important. A minimum of 400-mW/cm^2 is required. It is recommended that the tip be placed as close to the surface to be cured as is physically possible (within 1 to 2 mm). The intensity of light is inversely proportional to the distance from the source. As a general rule each increment should be at most 1.5 to 2 mm thick. This will ensure complete penetration of the light and maximum curing of the composite at the bottom most portion of the cavity preparation.

25 B Nickel allergy is common. It is estimated that 9 to 10 % of women are allergic to nickel. The initial sensitization to the metal most likely originates from wearing costumes jewellery and piercing earrings. Only 1 to 2% of the male population appears to be allergic to nickel. Side effects caused by dental materials most often allergic reactions are most prevalent in orthodontics. This seems to be directly related to the wide use of nickel-containing stainless steel appliances in this speciality.

26 D Glazing produces the smoothest surface of ceramic. The benefit of glazing is that it produces a glassy surface on porcelain, which is the smoothest surface possible. Any instrumentation of a glazed surface removes the glaze and leaves the porcelain rougher and more abrasive.

Tin oxide is used as a polishing agent for polishing of teeth and metallic restorations in mouth. Aluminum oxide is used to make white stones that are commonly used for adjusting dental enamel and finishing metal alloys, resin based composites. Rouge is iron oxide it is blended with soft binders to form cake. It is used to polish high noble metal alloys.

27 B Several different color-measuring systems are available, with the most popular being the munsell and the CIE system. The CIE system uses somewhat expensive equipment to define how much red, blue and yellow a certain object appears to contain. Red, blue and yellow are referred to as the primary colors because adding the correct amount of each primary color can make any color. The Munsell system is based on a well-defined series of color tabs. This system is composed of three indices defined as hue, value and chroma. Hue refers to the dominant color of the object. Natural teeth do not vary much in terms of their hue, generally being in yellow to yellow-red range.

28 C The base under a metallic restoration serves a purpose of insulating the pulp from thermal insult. Thermal conductivity is the characteristic that determines the rate at which heat flows through a material. It is a function of the composition which determines the heat capacity (the amount of heat required to raise the temperature of an object by certain amount),

Of the magnitude of the temperature change, and

The thickness of the object.

Now amalgam has low heat capacity in other words it warms up and quickly transmits heat rapidly. Temperature variation in the mouth may be high up to 20°C. The thickness of the object can be increased by giving an insulating base of 0.75 to 1.0 mm to minimize the effects of a rapid and extreme change in temperature at the surface of amalgam during the ingestion of hot and cold food. A base of more than 1 mm is not advised because by increasing the thickness of the base would reduce the bulk of the amalgam that could be used to fill the cavity, resulting in shallow and weaker amalgam.

29 B The denture is placed into a water bath and cured by using either of the two methods. The first procedure involves heat processing at 75°C for 8 hours or more. The second method is quicker and includes a 1.5 to 2 hour soak in the 75°C bath followed by 30 minutes at 100°C. An important factor is that the heat should be generated slowly. Rapid heating raises the internal temperature of the denture above 100°C, especially in the thicker regions and causes uncured monomer to boil and produce porosity in the denture, because the boiling temperature of the monomer is 100.8°C.

30 A Important factors that affect cutting efficiency includes the hardness of the abrasive, the speed at which the abrasive moves, the object to be cut, size and shape of the abrasive, the pressure applied to the abrasive and the use of the lubricants. Amongst these factors the irregular particles will always abrade more than the regular or smooth spherical particles. And the more abrasive the particle on Moh's scales more abrasive it will be. Hence combining these two factors an irregular particle with hardness of 6 at Moh's scale will be more abrasive.

31 B The more common manifestation of a biologic response to dental restoration is the formation of secondary caries and pain associated with postoperative sensitivity. The importance of a seal between the restoration and the tooth tissue is important as its failure will lead to leakage of bacteria or their by-products, which cause secondary caries. The key factor in the reduction or elimination of secondary decay, other than the caries susceptibility and oral flora of the patient is probably the ability to seal completely the margins of the restoration.

32 B Agar is heated in one section of the heating unit to convert the gel to sol. The tubes of agar are placed into the conditioning chamber, which contains boiling water at 100°C. After the sol has been created it should be stored in storage bath that contains water at 65°C. At this temperature the sol will not transform to gel. When desired the agar can be removed from the storage bath and placed into the tempering bath which contains water at 45°C. The tempering bath reduces the temperature of agar to a level that will not burn the patient. Although agar will not immediately form a gel at this temperature, it will become rubbery in time, so care should be taken not to leave the agar in this bath for too long.

33 C Hardness is a measure of a materials ability to resist indentation. Several hardness scales exist to compare materials. One of them is Moh's scale – which ranks materials in terms of ability to resist being scratched. On Moh's scale relative value of the following materials is such:

Acrylic	-	2-3
Glass	-	5-6
Enamel	-	5-6
Metals	-	6-9
Gingival tissue	-	1-2

Therefore the only statement, which is true, is, the hardness of denture base acrylic is less than that of metals.

34 B High heat investment like phosphate-bonded investments are extremely resistant to high temperatures and greatly improves its strength. They are commonly used during the casting of high temperature alloys used in PFM.

Phosphate bonded investments contain the same silica refractory present in the gypsum bonded investment. The binder however is made of an acidic phosphate and magnesium oxide. High heat investments do not undergo lesser expansion than gypsum bonded investments.

35 A An example of base metal alloy (steel) is an alloy of iron with carbon. The carbon (1%) causes iron to become very hard, otherwise the iron is comparatively soft. The term cast iron is reserved for alloys of iron that contain more than 2.5 % carbon. These alloys are very hard but too brittle to be used in dentistry.

The typical steel used in dentistry is called as stainless steel. It is chromium in steel that makes it stainless, resistant to tarnish and corrosion. Chromium is very reactive towards oxygen. When an alloy containing sufficient chromium is exposed to air, it quickly forms an oxide film that serves as a passivating or protective coating. The coating is very thin and transparent, but it provides protection from corrosion for the metal.

36 C The polyvinyl siloxane is dispensed as two different colored pastes that must be mixed mechanically or by hand to produce a homogeneously colored and streak free material to ensure ideal accuracy and handling characteristics. First the catalyst paste is picked up on the spatula and added to the base paste, and the two are mixed together for 10 seconds with the circular motion. The material is then wiped across the entire surface of the pad with a pressing motion with the aim of producing a homogenous, creamy consistency. It is only after properly mixing the material it is loaded into the syringe. The material becomes rubbery after it sets completely; therefore the spatula should be cleaned only after the material has reached this stage so that it can be peeled off from the spatula.

37 C Inlay pattern waxes are hard at room temperature, so their surfaces are not easily damaged during preparation or smoothening of the wax pattern. Denture teeth are set into base plate waxes, which are supplied in sheets; they tend to be hard but brittle. Because this wax will be tried in the mouth once denture teeth have set in one of the first stages of denture making, it must remain relatively hard and not distort at oral temperature. The impression wax must be deformable at oral temperature to record the details of the oral tissue. Boxing wax or utility wax are soft and have low melting ranges.

38 B Pure gold has excellent resistance to tarnish and corrosion. It is also the most malleable metal. Therefore it was used first in dentistry. Pure gold however is not strong enough or hard enough to be used in stress bearing restorations. To enhance its properties gold was alloyed with copper and silver. Of course alloying reduced the costing rather than increasing.

39 C Polymers routinely absorb water and loose components demonstrate that they are not very stable. As they absorb water they expand (swell) which can lead to weight gain up to 2%. Most of this uptake of water usually occurs early but may continue for several weeks. This uptake may cause change in the fit. During soaking another process, which takes place, is the residual monomers that could be a source of irritation to the patient are dissolved out.

40 B Acrylics are the softest permanent restorative materials and must be treated with care. They have a Moh's hardness of 2-3 and can be abraded by even gypsum (Moh's value of 2). Amongst all the given materials quartz dust (7), ground glass (5-6), pumice stone (6) and talc powder (1), only talc powder has Moh's value less than acrylic therefore is least likely to scratch the surface of the acrylic.

41 B Intra oral repair of ceramic restoration is possible, though never as good as the original restoration. The key is to produce a rough surface for enhanced mechanical bonding. First step is to roughen the fractured surface with a diamond bur or to sandblast the surface using 50 um aluminum oxide particles. After roughening the surface is etched for 2-3 minutes with hydrofluoric acid, which etches or dissolves glass. Next a Silane solution is applied to the porcelain. The Silane serves the same purpose as the Silane coupling agent that bonds the resin matrix to the glass fillers in the dental composite restorative material. An adhesive primer is applied to the silated surface, as well to the exposed metal surface. Later the composite is applied and light cured.

42 C While replacing the enamel with composite high translucency is used. Today composite are made with varying degrees of translucency for use in specific portion of tooth. Opaquing agents, usually metal oxides particles are added to block the light penetration, often such material are used to cover up metal or discolored dentin to make it look white. Because enamel is more transparent than dentin. One's perception of the incisal edges of the anterior teeth is most influenced by the enamel. These edges are the most translucent portions of the teeth and actually appear bluish in color. Both the outer enamel shell and the inner dentin influence light passing through the middle portion of the tooth. Because the dentin is more opaque, less light passes through this portion of the tooth, and the tooth does not appear very translucent. If a tooth were replaced with a material of a uniform translucency it would not appear very natural.

43 C Electrochemical corrosion cell involves oxidation–reduction reaction takes place when two different materials are present in an electrolyte solution. Saliva acts as the electrolyte. As gold onlay is more corrosion resistant metal it serves as cathode and amalgam serves as anode. The surface of the metal referred to as anode is oxidized and metal ions are generated. The other metal serving as cathode or the site at which reduction occurs.

44 C After carving the amalgam is finished with stones, points and disks and use of the slow speed handpiece and water coolant. Care should be taken to rotate the bur from amalgam to the tooth to avoid chipping the brittle margins. These initial contouring steps actually may roughen the surface to values of 0.5 to 1.0 μm. Later the surface is smoothened by rubber points impregnated with abrasive particles. The lingual or buccal surfaces between teeth can be smoothened with abrasive disks. The interproximal strips are available to produce a final surface roughness of 0.1 to 0.3 μm in this region. Final, polishing can be achieved with a rubber cup or brush, first with slurry of pumice and then slurry of silex or tin oxide. These are used on the slow speed handpiece with light pressure. The tin oxide produces the smoothest surface with a roughness of 0.1 μm.

45 A The most biocompatible materials are the ceramics, the choice of ceramic for an implant would seem to be most ideal. Ceramic implant materials can be classified by the manner in which they interact with bone into two basic types, noncreative and bioactive. Typical noncreative ceramics such as aluminum oxide and sapphire are well tolerated by the bone tissue in much the same way as titanium. They have high strength, stiffness and hardness. Their fracture resistance is poor however especially when they are subjected to the bending forces. The problem with pure ceramic is that it does not entirely replace bone which also contains proteins; hydroxyapatite is brittle and cannot support the same types of forces as bone or a metallic implant. This has led to ceramic implants coated with calcium sulfate. Because bone is composed of a calcium phosphate ceramic, hydroxyapatite would seem most reasonable to replace it with a synthetic hydroxyapatite. Such implant undergo osseo-integration faster.

46 B When the mercury is mixed with the amalgam alloy, metal ions of silver, tin and copper dissolve from the outer surfaces of the particles into mercury. The ions then react with mercury to form new metal compounds. The most common reaction is between silver and mercury to form the crystalline matrix for the amalgam. This compound is called gamma –1. Gamma – 1 eventually occupies nearly 40% of the total volume of the amalgam and holds the original alloy particles together. Because only the surfaces of the original alloy particles dissolve, most of the rest of the volume of amalgam is occupied by these particles.

47 D Hardness refers to the ability of a material to resist forces of indentation. Hardness is often equated to the resistance to wear and abrasion.

Toughness is a measure of the amount of energy that a material can absorb without breaking.

Elastic modulus is a measure of the stiffness of the material. It is also referred to as the Young's modulus.

Percentage elongation or ductility is a measure of the amount of dimensional change that a wire can undergo before breaking.

48 D One of the die materials is epoxy polymer. Supplied as two components, an epoxy resin and a hardener. Die epoxies undergo little shrinkage in comparison to other polymers. These materials are stronger, less brittle and more abrasion resistant than is stone. They are not as accurate or as stable, because they shrink during hardening. Because water inhibits their curing, they cannot be used with hydrocolloid impression materials.

49 A There are two types of wear observed in composites. The first abrasive wear, takes place as a result of the movement of objects such as food and tooth paste, across the entire surface of the restoration. It is distinguished from the more aggressive degradation experienced in the area in which the opposing tooth makes direct contact with the restoration. This later wear is called as the contact or the attrition wear. If there is no contact on the restoration then wear is abrasive only and usually is of less concern. The abrasive wear characteristics for posterior composites have improved tremendously in the recent years. Initial formulations would undergo wear, usually measured at the margins, in increments of 50 to 100 μm/year or more recent composites undergo wear at the rate of 10 to 15 μm/year in contact free sites. This improvement is because of the inclusion of smaller particles in their formulations. Wear is most rapid for compositors having the largest filler particles.

Although the wear in contact free sites has been dramatically reduced by the development of composites with high levels of small fillers, concern remains over the relatively high rate of wear for the posterior composites in direct contact with opposing cusps.

50 C Composite is a mixture of two different classes of materials. Polymers and glass particles or fillers. They also contain chemicals to begin the hardening reaction and pigments to produce different shades. Composites originally were made with ground quartz because it produces good translucency and tooth like aesthetics when mixed with the resin. Chunks of quartz were grounded into irregularly shaped particles with an average size of 20 to 40 μm. The largest particles were 50 to 100 μm.

Composite class	*filler size (μm)*
Conventional	1-100
Microfilled	10-50
Small hybrid	0.1-3
Mid sized hybrid	0.1-10

51 C Provisional restorative materials are used to occupy a cavity preparation until such time when a more durable and permanent restoration can be placed. Typical provisional restorative materials in dentistry include ZOE cement, acrylic plastic, resin composite and aluminum crowns. Acid etched composite is not ideal as it would be difficult to remove it (it will take more time as well as it is not possible to remove it completely without cutting the healthy enamel or dentin). As a provisional restorative material all these materials should prevent further ingress of bacteria and their by products, should be strong enough to withstand occlusal forces, should be durable, should be easy to remove.

52 B The microfilled composites have unequalled esthetic results and their mechanical properties and abrasion resistance is adequate. The superb esthetic results of the microfilled composites are a function of the small particle size used in their fillers. When the particles are very small, polishing produces very smooth, mirror like surfaces that remain smooth over years. They mimic enamel well in this respect. Although hybrids approximate microfills in the size of their particles and their ability to take a smooth polish, they remain slightly rougher.

53 D Conventional heat cured poly methylmethacrylate contains a cross linking agent (usually 5-15% ethylene glycol dimethacrylate). The cross linking molecules are added to reduce the likelihood that small surface cracks will form in the denture when it is allowed to dry. These small cracks are called craze cracks and are produced by stresses created during the drying.

54 D The restoration of class IV cavities is more problematic, specially when incisal edges experience a significant amount of force during clenching or biting. This varies from patient to patient because of individual differences in the occlusion, but the longevity of class IV restoration in general would be expected to be less because of greater stresses and increased chances for fracture or chipping of the restoration. In this light it is seen that mid sized hybrids experience less failure than microfilled over 3 years period due to their greater strength and fracture resistance. A layered class IV restoration also is common. A stronger composite such as minifill or midfill is used as a dentin replacement to provide support whereas microfilled is overlaid on the hybrid to produce optimum surface smoothness and esthetic results.

55 D Advantages of polishing of amalgam restoration are:

It will feel more natural because of its smoothness,

Increased resistance to tarnish and corrosion, and

Less of plaque retention, therefore better oral hygiene.

But it does not affect the hardness of the amalgam and the wearing of the opposite tooth as that is directly proportional to the abrasiveness of the amalgam which remains unaffected by polishing.

56 D When mixing at a low powder to liquid ratio the pad is sufficient and a plastic spatula, similar to that used for self curing composites, can be used to mix the two components. Because of heavy consistency of the restorative materials however it is often helpful to mix it with a stiff spatula on a glass slab. One half of the powder is mixed into the liquid for approximately 10-15 seconds. The second half is then quickly added with the material folded in on itself until all of the powder is wetted by the liquid and it has a shiny, putty like consistency. The entire mixing time should not exceed 30 to 40 seconds to allow ample working time. These materials set rapidly, leaving a working time of approximately 2.5

minutes. When the mix no longer appears shiny it has reached the end of the working time. GIC can be mixed on a chilled glass slab to prolong the working time when desired. Working time is enhanced when the mixing time is less. Greater energy supplied during mixing causes the setting to be somewhat accelerated.

57 A Most recent dentin bonding materials are designed to be hydrophilic. These adhesives are supplied as either one component or multicomponent systems. Multicomponent systems usually contain three separate components etchant, primer and adhesive resin. The etchant is usually phosphoric acid gel. The primer is usually a hydrophilic monomer that serves as an agent to wet and penetrate the etched dentin, preparing it to receive the adhesive. One component system have a combined etchant and primer (so called self etching primer) or a combined primer and adhesive in the latter an acid etch is usually used in the first step and the primer/adhesive is applied after the In Etch has been washed off. Therefore some one component systems actually require two steps. Antimicrobial agent is not a part of a dentin bonding agent.

58 C One component systems have a combined etchant and primer (so called self etchant primer) or a combined primer and adhesive. In the latter an acid etch is usually used as the first step and the primer/adhesive is applied after the etch has been washed off. Therefore some one component systems actually require two steps. It seems that one component and multicomponent systems produce similar adhesion to dentin and enamel and have similar costs. Typical three component system involves three steps as follows:

Step one – application of etchant.

Step two – application of separate primer to the dentin.

Step three – application of adhesive.

59 A Bases are placed in relatively thick layers atleast 0.75–1 mm to provide thermal insulation under deep (less than 1 mm of dentin remaining) metallic restorations. Bases can also seal the dentin at the same time, especially if they are made from GIC or resin modified GIC.

60 B The rate of reaction depends upon several variables including the powder to liquid ratio, temperature, water concentration in the mix and the mixing time. The reaction is exothermic meaning it gives off heat. When enough powder becomes dissolved in the acidic liquid the acid becomes neutralized and gives off heat. Because the heat accelerates the setting reaction it is important to slow the interaction between the powder and the liquid. Therefore the mixing should be done on a chilled glass slab. The chilled glass slab slow the setting reaction by reducing the mixing temperature. The glass slab can be chilled by placing it in a refrigerator or under cold water for 5 minutes. In any case the slab has to be absolutely dry before mixing because moisture on the slab wili cause the cement to set faster.

61 B The solubility of the cements is a major concern. A primary cause of failure of dental castings is related to the washout or dissolution of the cement at the margins of a restoration. This cement loss contributes to leakage, secondary decay and loosening of restoration. The solubility of the cement in water does not reflect their solubility in the oral cavity, however, with one exception of resin containing cements, which are most insoluble of all the cements. In the salty and acidic environment of oral cavity glass ionomers are the least soluble of the non-resin cements followed by zinc phosphate and zinc polycarboxylate. ZOE is the most soluble cement in the oral cavity, which limits their use to temporary cement.

62 C ZOE, GIC and calcium hydroxide all three materials are used as cavity liners. Calcium hydroxide is a basic compound with a pH of 11. It is mildly irritating to vital pulp tissue. It also has bacteriostatic properties. All these properties make it a good lining material for restorations in close proximity to the pulp. It is also believed that it promotes the formation of secondary dentin that served to wall off and protect the pulp from external insults. The high pH provides a stimulus for the tooth to repair itself in the absence of bacterial infection.

63 D GIC is often used as a base under the amalgam restoration because they adhere both to enamel and dentin, it is a good insulator, it can tolerate condensation force of 5 to 6 pounds during condensation, it has a rapid setting time. The compressive strength of GIC is around 85 MPa (zinc phosphate 70–100 MPa) so therefore it can not be said to be twice as strong as other bases. GIC is soluble in oral fluids. But it has a unique property of fluoride release.

64 C There are two types of reinforced ZOE, one containing a polymer and the other aluminum oxide particles with the chemical ethoxybenzoic acid (EBA) both are powder liquid system. The powder is a zinc oxide formulation with aluminum oxide reinforced particles a 2:1 ratio. The EBA helps to produce a stronger matrix to hold the particles together, thus creating a stronger base. These reinforced ZOE bases often have been used for patients with sensitive teeth. The rationale has been that the pulp would be less affected by the neutral ZOE than it might be by the acidity of other common base materials, such as GIC or zinc phosphate.

65 B The specific objectives for condensation are to adapt the amalgam intimately to the walls of the cavity to minimize the porosity within the amalgam and to express excess mercury not needed for the chemical reaction. Many factors that determine the handling characteristics of amalgam are shape of the alloy particles, ratio of mercury to alloy powder, time and speed used to mix the two components. Usually greater condensation forces (4 to 6 pounds) are required to be applied for the condensation of the lathe cut amalgam alloy particles. Little resistance is offered by the spherical particles therefore lighter forces (2 to 3 pounds) are necessary for compacting amalgam because the spheres roll away from the condenser efficient packing can be accomplished only by the use of condenser with large heads.

66 A Powder consists of acid soluble calcium fluoroaluminosilicate glass. It also contains strontium, barium or zinc oxide to provide radiopacity. The liquid contains polyacrylic acid in a concentration of 40-50%. Also copolymers of itaconic, maleic or tricarboxylic acid are added. These copolymers are added to increase the reactivity and reduce the viscosity of the liquid. Tartaric acid is also added to the liquid to increase the handling characteristics and increase the working time.

Eugenol is the only component that is not a part of GIC.

67 D Several materials have been used as sealants for pit and fissures. The most common is the resin component of dental composites. This resin is composed of a specific organic monomer often abbreviated as bis-GMA in addition to other monomers such as triethylene glycol dimethacrylate. The other monomers are added to dilute the viscous bis-GMA and enhance its flow and mixing characteristics. Fillers are added to these resins to improve the physical properties. To enhance the bonding between the fillers and the monomers the silane coupling agents are used. Phosphoric acid is commonly used as etchant prior to use of the bonding agent.

68 D For the indirect technique, a separating medium such as petroleum jelly or liquid tinfoil substitute is coated onto the plaster cast. (Plaster cast of the prepared teeth and for this an impression of the prepared teeth is a must). The template is then filled approximately three quarters full with the proper shade of an acrylic provisional material that has been mixed to a creamy consistency. The filled crown is placed on the prepared tooth and held in place until the polymer begins to increase in viscosity and becomes doughy. The crown is then removed from the tooth and held for a few seconds before reseating. This technique is called as the on and off technique. A plaster model of unprepared teeth is always required for the initial diagnosis and treatment planning.

69 D Polyvinyl siloxane is the material of choice because of their excellent physical properties and accuracy. It is known that the setting of these materials is inhibited when they contact rubber dam or latex gloves. The sulfur compounds are supposed to be responsible for the inhibition of setting of polyvinylsiloxane. Therefore it is prudent to avoid touching the impression material with a glove as well as to avoid touching any surface to be impressed with the gloves. Some organic chemicals such as methacrylates from temporary restorative materials also have the same effect. Therefore it is recommended that the impression be made of a prepared tooth before making a temporary. Otherwise the surface of the impression material in contact with the prepared tooth may not completely set and may have a wrinkled surface.

70 B Condensation polymerization is a type of polymerization, in this process a small molecule such as water or alcohol is released as a by product of the reaction between the two monomer units. One of the examples is polysulfide rubber impression material.

Some materials made of monomers polymerize by a mechanism called ring opening. Simply stated, a molecular ring of atoms at the reactive end of the molecule is forced to open up during the polymerization reaction. Because of the ring opening, two reacting molecules actually elongate and increase their volume at the same time that the total volume is decreased by their formation of covalent bond.

Addition polymerization usually involves monomers containing carbon-carbon double bonds. The reaction as the name implies, monomers are added one after the other to make the long polymer chains. There are no by-products.

71 D The introduction of the high-speed amalgamator or triturator eliminated the need of hand mixing. Mixing is accomplished by briefly shaking the alloy powder together with the liquid mercury in a closed plastic capsule at high speed. Complete mixing usually is accomplished by triturating for 5 to 20 seconds at speeds of 2000 to 4500 cycles/minute. The exact conditions depend upon the type of triturator and amalgam, and specific directions are supplied with each alloy. Faster speed or longer trituration times generally hasten the setting of the amalgam and produce hotter mixes that tend to be shiny and sticky. The extra energy of mixing under these conditions is transferred to the amalgam causing the reaction to take place faster.

72 B A preventive resin restoration (PRR) involves placement of a dental composite within an incipient lesion of the pits and fissures, with minimal excavation of the tooth. Application of composite is followed by sealing the entire occlusal surface of the tooth with a pit and fissure sealant. The PRR is typically done on premolars and molars. The restoration is more conservative than amalgam restoration. As only 5% of the occlusal surface is involved in preparation for a PRR compared with 25% for typical amalgam restoration.

In a recurrent decay around an existing amalgam restoration there is no question of a preventive restoration.

73 A The invested mold is heated to eliminate the wax and make room for the liquid metal. The ring is placed with the sprue hole down so that no contaminants can fall into the hole. The slow heating is carried on to ensure that the investment material will not crack. Heating of investment removes all the wax, it also performs another function that as the investment is heated to (650°C) it undergoes thermal expansion of 1.25% thus the total expansion of the investment material is approximately 1.95% (setting expansion = 0.7% + thermal = 1.25%) this creates a larger cavity for the metal to fill in the next step. Another aspect of heating of investment is that it raises the temperature of the investment to a level closer to the temperature of the molten metal that will be cast into it. If the thermal shock produced by a very hot liquid metal hitting a very cold ceramic mold is too great the mold will crack and cause a defective casting.

74 B Mouth guards generally are made from semi-rigid but soft plastics; a common material is a polymer of polyvinyl acetate and polyethylene. The material generally comes in thin sheets less than 1/8 inch thick that can be custom fitted to the dentition by heating and forming within the mouth. These materials possess the characteristics of being thermoplastic, means that they become softened and moldable on heating but become rigid enough to hold their shape when cooled. The material has only minimal strength and resistance to tearing.

75 B In metallic bond many atoms share all of their outer or valency electrons with their neighbors. This kind of arrangement is very strong and stable, with the shared electrons free to move between and among the billions of atoms that make up a solid, never being tightly held to a specific atom. This accounts for the ability of a metal to conduct electricity and heat readily.

76 D Remove bulk excess with spatula and discard in trash, if the material has hardened by this point, flex the bowl to break up gypsum, and discard pieces in trash. Gypsum fractures as it is a brittle material with poor strength in thin sections.

Wipe insides of bowl with paper towel to remove residual mix. Wipe spatula clean with paper towel.

77 B The deterioration of a metal by a chemical or an electrochemical reaction is called corrosion. A type of deterioration that involves only the surface of the metal and whose end result is usually discoloration is called as tarnish. The difference between corrosion and tarnish is basically of the extent, with corrosion being irreversible and of much greater concern. In corrosion there is active deterioration that produces ions at a faster rate, where as tarnish involves passive loss of ions.

78 C Factors affecting the rate of abrasion are:
Difference between the hardness of abrasive and the hardness of the substrate, greater the difference more the rate of abrasion.
Shape—more irregular and with sharp edges is the shape of the abrasive more the rate of abrasion.
Size—larger particles abrade the surface more rapidly than smaller ones because the larger particles plough deeper groves or cuts into the surface.

Pressure—use of a greater force during finishing causes a more rapid removal of material by forcing the abrasive to cut deeper to the surface.

Speed–greater the speed of abrasion more is the rate of abrasion.

79 A As the names imply, inelastic materials are not elastic and exhibit little to no spring like quality when deformed. In other words they are rigid materials with a low maximum flexibility; any significant deformation produced permanent change in their shape. In contrast elastic material behaves like rubber band. They can be bent and stretched appreciably without suffering a permanent change in dimension.

80 D Fluoride gels usually contain 1.25 % fluoride. The gels are called APF which stands for acidulated phosphate fluoride. The gels also contain small amount of phosphoric acid. Gels have a pH values near 3 to 5. The gels are applied in soft trays like mouth guards and are held in mouth for several minutes. The existing composite restorations can become slightly etched and roughened during the application of APF gel. Fluoride gel is applied in office adjunct to normal home cleaning with fluoride tooth paste and dietary fluoride supplementation.

81 B Light cured composites are activated by light with a peak wavelength of 470 nm. The photo activator used is such as camphorquinones added in amounts varying from 0.2%-1% the reaction is accelerated by the presence of an organic amine containing a carbon double bond.

Chemical cured composites are activated by organic amine reacting with peroxide.

82 B Maximum amount of mercury vapor allowed in the workplace as per the OSHA (occupational and safety health administration) is 0.05 mg/m^3. Fetuses exposed to mercury concentration of 5 mg/m^3 were stillborn. The lowest dose of mercury that elicits a toxic reaction is 3 to 7 µg/kg body weight. Paresthesia occurs at about 500-µg/kg body weight of body weight. Ataxia at 1000-µg/kg body weight, joint pains at 2000 µg/kg body weight and hearing loss and death at 4000-µg/kg body weight.

83 D The final polishing of amalgam is commonly done in second appointment after careful carving in the first appointment. This final polish by use of fine stones and abrasive disks or strips. To develop the final polish, a rotating soft brush is used to apply a suitable polishing agent such as extra fine silex, followed by a thin slurry of tin oxide. Because the amalgam is weak in tensile and shear resistance it should not be drawn over the margin by burnishing.

84 D For final finishing of microfilled composites abrasive impregnated rubber rotary instruments or rubber cups are used with polishing pastes. Finishing is ideally done in wet field. Polishing can be performed with aluminum oxide abrasives. But the smoothest surface is achieved by use of Mylar matrix.

85 C Calcium hydroxide has many favorable properties; the pH of calcium hydroxide is between 9-11. Free calcium hydroxide in excess of that necessary to form the calcium disalicylate stimulates secondary dentin formation in proximity to the pulp and shows antibacterial activity. Calcium hydroxide is strong enough to support the forces of condensation of amalgam. Their compressive strength ranges from 6.5 to 14.3 MPa. They provide thermal insulation to the pulp if used in sufficient layer of 0.5 mm. The solubility varies from 0.4% to 7% in distilled water at 37°C.

86 C The values of modulus of elasticity of commonly used cements are

GIC	– 3.5-6.5 GPa
Zinc polycarboxylate	– 4.0-4.7 GPa
Zinc phosphate	– 9.3-13.4 Gpa
Hybrid ionomer	– 2.5-7.5 GPa
Composite	– 4.5-6.5 GPa
Zinc oxide eugenol	– 5 GPa

87 C The quality of ceramic depends on the choice of ingredients. Only the purest ingredients are used in the manufacture of dental porcelain because of stringent requirements of color, toughness without brittleness, insolubility and translucency. In the mineral state, feldspar is the main raw ingredient; it is crystalline and opaque with an indefinite color between gray and pink. Chemically $K_2O.Al_2O_3.6SiO_2$. Iron and mica are commonly found as impurities in feldspar. Pure quartz SiO_2 crystals are used in dental porcelain and ground to the finest grain size. Silica is added and contributes stability to the mass during heating by providing a glassy framework for the other ingredients. Alkali metal carbonates are added as fluxes.

88 C Heat pressing relies on the application of external pressure to sinter and shape the ceramic at high temperature. Heat pressing is also called as high temperature injection moulding. Heat pressing helps in avoiding large pores and promotes a good dispersion of crystalline phase within the glass matrix. The mechanical properties of many ceramic systems are maximized with high density and small crystal size. Heat pressed system may be either Leucite based ($KAlSi_2O_6$) or lithium dislocate based ($Li_2Si_2O_5$). The usual advantages of heat pressed ceramics include good aesthetics, high strength, and ability to use the well known lost wax technique. The processing times are short and the marginal accuracy is within the acceptable range.

89 C To mimic natural teeth the metallic pigments are added. Titanium oxide–yellow brown, magnesium oxide–lavender, iron oxide–brown, cobalt oxide-blue, copper or chromium oxide-green and nickel oxide–brown.

90 C Varnish is used to provide a barrier against the passage of irritants from cements or other restorative materials and to reduce the penetration of oral fluids at the tooth-restoration interface into underlying dentin. Varnishes are not used under composite restorations, because bonding agents effectively seal the dentin tubules.

91 C ADA specification 1 is for alloys of dental amalgam.
ADA specification 3 is for dental mercury.
ADA specification 57 is for endodontic sealing materials.
ADA specification 3 is for impression compound, which is now obsolete.

92 B The density of fully sintered feldspathic porcelain is around 2.45 g/cm^3 and varies with the porosity of the material. The density of ceramic also depends upon the amount of crystalline phase present. Usually the density of all ceramic materials is around 2.4-2.5 g/cm^3.

93 D Corrosion resistant steel is because of chromium. Iron cannot be used without chromium because rust or iron oxide is not adherent to the bulk of the metal. Approximately 11% chromium is needed to produce corrosion resistance in pure iron. Chromium resists corrosion by forming strongly adherent coating of oxide on the surface that prevents further reaction with the metal below the surface. The formation of such an oxide layer is called passivation. In 18-8 steel the chromium composition must be between 13-28%. If the chromium concentration is less than 13 % the adherent chromium oxide layer does not form and if the concentration of chromium is more than 28% chromium carbide is formed at the grain boundaries and embrittling the steel.

94 D Osmium has the highest melting temperature amongst these elements.
Osmium – 3045°C
Iridium – 2410°C
Gold – 1064°C
Platinum – 1772°C

95 B COTE of ceresin between 27°C and 34°C is 849 × 10^{-6}/°C.
COTE of paraffin between 27°C and 34°C is 1631 × 10^{-6}/°C.
COTE of beeswax between 27°C and 34°C is 1048 × 10^{-6}/°C.
COTE of inlay wax between 27°C and 34°C is 323 × 10^{-6}/°C.

96 D Waxes obtained from plant kingdom are carnauba, candelilla, Japan wax, cocoa butter and ouricury. Beeswax is obtained from insect source.

97 B The maximum allowable level of mercury in the blood is 3 µg/l. amalgam restorations elevate blood mercury levels to 1 to 2 µg/l. the urine mercury is below 1 µg/l. maximum amount of mercury vapor allowed in the workplace as per the OSHA (occupational and safety health administration) is 0.05 mg/m^3. Fetuses exposed to mercury concentration of 5 mg/m^3 were stillborn. The lowest dose of mercury that elicits a toxic reaction is 3 to 7 µg/kg body weight.

Notes

Syllabus

I. Pathology

1. Introduction to pathology as a scientific study of disease, and some techniques used in the same.
2. Causes of disease with special reference to our prevailing conditions.
3. Cellular structure and Metabolism.
4. Disturbances in Metabolism of cells.
5. Retrogressive changes–Degeneration, Necrosis and Gangrene, Amylodosis, Lipidosis and disorders of Pigmentation, calcification.
6. Inflammation–Acute and chronic inflammation, Repair with special emphasis on repair of bones, wounds and the effects of modern treatment on repair.
7. Hypersensitivity and Allergic reactions.
8. Haemorrhage, shock, reaction of body to injury.
9. Circulatory disturbance and Hypertension.
10. Pathology of Bacterial Infections with reference to the common diseases prevalent in our country, e.g. Pyogenic infection, Enteric fever, Toxemias Tuberculosis Leprosy, Syphilis and some examples of epidemic infections of public health interest and hospital infections. Common diseases of the bone. Injuries due to chemical and physical agents including ionising radiations. Disturbances of nutrition with special reference to Indian conditions. Metabolic disorders, e.g. Rickets, Scurvey, Diabetes, Mellitus, etc.
11. Clinical pathology comprising Anemias and their laboratory investigations, blood disorders including Leukemias, bleeding disorders and their Investigations. Laboratory Investigations commonly required by Dental Surgeons.

II. Microbiology

1. General Bacteriology and elementary virology, mycology and parasitology.
2. Introduction to Bacteriology with special reference to Medical and Dental Bacteriology including public health and preventive aspect of infection and infectious diseases.
3. Pyaemia, septicemia and toxaemia.
4. Immunity and immunising agents–vaccines, sera.
5. Auto–immunity with special emphasis on practical application.
6. Morphology, Physiology and classification of micro–organisms in general and of the following in particular pus forming organisms–cocci and bacilli.
7. Normal flora of the mouth and upper and lower respiratory tracts.
8. Organisms causing meningitis diptheria, tetanus, gas gangrene, tuberculosis, syphilis.
9. Organisms related to dental caries.

Chapter 4

General Pathology and Microbiology

1. The migration of leukocytes towards a foreign antigen is labelled as
A. Diapedisis B. Chemotaxis
C. Opsonisation D. Margination

2. In response to an injury the hypertrophic, collagenous tissue reaction is
A. Callus B. Cicatrix
C. Keloid D. Contracture

3. Characteristic feature of a malignant lesion include
A. Necrosis
B. Apoptosis
C. Decrease in size of tumor
D. Lowered vascularity

4. *Olliers syndrome* is related to
A. Choristoma B. Teratoma
C. Hematoma D. Hamartoma

5. Benign neoplasms are likely to
A. Interfere with organ function
B. Metastasize
C. Cause necrosis
D. Cause extensive bleeding

6. Lack of differentiation is known as
A. Aplasia B. Anaplasia
C. Hypoplasia D. Neoplasia

7. One of the complications of inflammatory process is
A. Isolation of infected mass
B. Neutralization of toxins
C. Fistula formation
D. Removal of necrotic tissue

8. A strict vegetarian will have deficiency of
A. Vitamin B_{12} B. Vitamin C
C. Vitamin D D. Vitamin E

9. *Blebs* form at the cell surface during
A. Inflammation B. Repair
C. Cell injury D. Mitosis

10. Central factor in pathogenesis of irreversible cell injury is
A. Cell membrane damage
B. Nuclear damage
C. Damage to ribosomes
D. Damage to mitochondria

11. Conversion of one adult cell type into other adult cell type is
A. Metaplasia
B. Dysplasia
C. Dyskeratosis
D. Neoplasia

12. *Opaque Tombstone* appearance of cells is seen in
A. Coagulation necrosis
B. Fat Necrosis
C. Caseous necrosis
D. Gangrenous necrosis

13. Fat necrosis is most commonly seen in necrosis of
A. Liver B. Pancreas
C. Tooth pulp D. Brain

14. Caseous necrosis is a combination of
A. Fat and Gangrenous necrosis
B. Coagulative and Liquefactive necrosis
C. Fat and Caseous necrosis
D. Fat and Coagulative necrosis

15. Fatty changes in cells of liver begin as collection of
A. Liposomes B. Ribosomes
C. Mitochondria D. Centromeres

16. Excess collection of iron in parenchymal cells of liver can result in its
A. Fibrosis B. Hemorrhage
C. Hyperplasia D. Neoplasm

17. *Psammamo bodies* refer to
A. Metastatic calcification
B. Dystrophic calcification
C. Multinucleated giant cells
D. Russel bodies

18. Nephrocalcinosis results due to
A. Dystrophic calcification
B. Metastatic calcification
C. Hypocalcemia
D. None of the above

19. Red infarcts are seen usually with
A. Arterial occlusion
B. Solid tissues
C. Loose or solid tissues
D. Venous occlusion

20. *Blooms syndrome* is associated with
A. Chromosomal mosaicism
B. Chromosomal breakage, loss and rearrangement
C. Chromosomal translocation
D. None of the above

21. Glucocerebroside deficiency is seen in
A. Gauchers disease
B. Niemann–Pick disease
C. Tay-sachs disease
D. Mucopolysaccharidoses

22. Anaplastic cell may show the following nuclear–cytoplasmic ratio
A. 1: 1 B. 1: 4
C. 1: 16 D. 1: 10

23. Resistance to invasion by a malignant neoplasm is offered by
A. Collagen fibres
B. Blood vessels
C. Reticulin fibres
D. Basement membrane

24. Grading of cancers is based on
A. Clinical features
B. Histological features
C. Only metastasis
D. Nodal involvement

25. *Anchorage–independence* is not a feature of the following, *except*
A. Neoplastic cell
B. Inflammatory cell
C. Dyskeratotic cell
D. None of the above

26. Reduced cohesiveness of a neoplastic cell is brought about by
A. Alterations in cell surface proteins
B. "A" and certain glycoproteins
C. Proteoglycans
D. None of the above

27. *Wilms tumor* occurs more in
A. Childhood B. Middle age
C. Elderly age D. None of the above

28. Squamous cell carcinoma of uterine cervix contains
A. HPV B. EBV
C. CMV D. Hepatitis virus

29. DNA content of tumor cells can be measured by
A. Exfoliative cytology
B. DNA flow cytometry
C. Immunohistochemistry
D. None of the above

30. *Ghons complex* represents
 A. Secondary tuberculosis
 B. Primary lung lesion
 C. Primary lung lesion and lymph node involvement
 D. Only lymph node involvement

31. *Lepra cells* are
 A. Macrophages laden with bacteria
 B. Macrophages laden with lipid and bacteria
 C. Macrophages laden with necrotic debris only
 D. None of the above

32. **Tuberculosis is immunologically mediated disorder of**
 A. Autotoxic type
 B. Immune complex disease
 C. Delayed hypersensitivity
 D. Anaphylactic type

33. **Helminthic infections invoke inflammation characterized by**
 A. IgE antibodies
 B. IgA antibodies
 C. IgM antibodies
 D. None of the above

34. **Macrophages with engulfed fibers are seen in**
 A. Asbestosis
 B. Pneumoconioses
 C. Berylliosis
 D. None of the above

35. *Reedsternberg cell* **is a feature of**
 A. Hodgkins lymphoma
 B. Non-Hodgkins lymphoma
 C. Leukemia
 D. All of the above

36. **Lungs are more affected by**
 A. Primary carcinomas
 B. Primary sarcomas
 C. Metastatic neoplasms
 D. All of the above

37. **Mesiothelioma is a neoplasm of**
 A. Pleura
 B. Embryonic germ layer
 C. Skin
 D. Only pericardium

38. **Malignant gastric ulcers are common in**
 A. Young adults
 B. Neonates
 C. Elderly
 D. All age groups

39. **Progressive Alcoholic cirrhosis is characterized by**
 A. More of fat
 B. More of fibrous tissue
 C. More of mucous tissue
 D. Mixture of fibrous and fatty tissue

40. **Thyroglossal tract cyst forms from**
 A. Thryoglossal duct
 B. Foramen Cecum
 C. Hyoid bone
 D. Lymph nodes

41. **HIV usually infects**
 A. CD8 cells B. CD4 cells
 C. NK cells D. Red cells

42. **The following disorder manifests antibodies to centromeres in**
 A. CREST syndrome
 B. SLE
 C. Sjögren syndrome
 D. Pemphigus

43. **The simulating features of Thalassemia major and Thalassemia minor are**
 A. Familial occurrence
 B. Anemia
 C. Homozygous form
 D. Life span

44. **The typical lesion of rheumatic fever is**
 A. Negri bodies
 B. Anitschkow cell
 C. Aschoffs body
 D. Tzanck cells

45. **The common type of Esophagitis is**
 A. Reflux B. Viral
 C. Fungal D. Corrosive

46. Giant cell tumor is common in
A. Jaws B. Long bones
C. Skull D. Pelvic bones

47. The virus that has direct cytopathic effects on hepatocytes is
A. HBV
B. HDV
C. Hepatitis C virus
D. Hepatitis E virus

48. The most common type of testicular germ cell tumor is
A. Seminoma B. Choristoma
C. Teratoma D. Yolk cell tumor

49. Liposarcomas frequently arise from
A. Superficial tissues
B. Deeper tissues
C. Oral mucosa
D. Pre-existing lipomas

50. Rhabdomyosarcomas occur
A. More commonly than rhabdomyomas
B. Less commonly than rhabdomyomas
C. Equal to rhabdomyomas
D. Never in young children

51. Spirochaetes are demonstrated by
A. Simple stain
B. Negative staining
C. Simple or negative staining
D. None of the above

52. Mycoplasmas are the bacteria that have
A. Stable morphology
B. Deficient cell wall
C. Prominent cell wall
D. None of the above

53. Spores of all the bacteria (medically important) are destroyed by
A. 100°C for 10 mts
B. 120°C for 15 mts
C. 160°C for 20 mts
D. 100°C for 5 mts

54. Bacterial growth curve follows following phases in sequence
A. Lag phase, stationary phase, phase of decline
B. Phase of decline, lag phase, log phase
C. Lag phase, log phase, stationary phase, phase of decline
D. None of the above

55. Sudden exposure of bacteria to hypertonic solutions causes
A. Osmosis B. Reverse osmosis
C. Plasmolysis D. None of the above

56. In hot air oven method of sterilization, the temperature used is
A. 160°C for 3 hours
B. 160°C for 2 hours
C. 160°C for 1 hour
D. None of the above

57. The effective concentrations of alcohols as antiseptic is
A. 20-80% in water
B. 60-70% in water
C. 10-20% in water
D. None of the above

58. The appropriate example of Anaerobic media is
A. Robertson's cooked meat medium
B. Staurt's medium
C. Mac Conkeys media
D. Blood agar

59. A convalescent carrier is one
A. Who has recovered from the disease but continues to harbour microorganism
B. Who is having the disease but harbours no microorganism
C. Who acquires pathogen from other carrier
D. None of the above

60. Exotoxins are
A. Heat Labile and weakly antigenic
B. Weakly antigenic
C. Heat Labile and highly antigenic
D. None of the above

61. Which of the following organism might not be found in a patient with acute suppurative arthritis?
- **A.** Mycobacterum tuberculosis
- **B.** Neisseria
- **C.** Typhoid
- **D.** Pneunio cocci

62. Gonorrhoea
- **A.** Is due to Neisseria gonorrhoea which is a gram positive coccus
- **B.** Can cause acute suppurative arthritis
- **C.** Begins by peretration by the gonococcus of the epithelium of the glans penis
- **D.** Often presents as acute retention of urine

63. Antisepsis depends entirely upon
- **A.** Carbolic acid
- **B.** Iodine
- **C.** A commitment against all infection caused by trauma or operation
- **D.** Theatre ventilation

64. Which is the most common cause of sub-acute bacterial endocarditis?
- **A.** Chlamydia **B.** Staphylococcus
- **C.** Gonococcus **D.** Pseudomonas

65. Syphilis (Which is incorrect)
- **A.** Is caused by the trepanosome
- **B.** Appears as a primary sore 3-4 months after infection
- **C.** Is diagnosed in the primary chancre by finding the organisms by dark field microscopy
- **D.** If in the secondary stage is non-infective as it is an immune response and does not feature the spirochetes

66. Regarding tetanus infection (Which is incorrect)
- **A.** The disease is produced by the endotoxin of bacillus tetani
- **B.** The toxin travels along nerves to the central nervous system
- **C.** A child under the age of one year has an inborn immunity to the disease
- **D.** Acute immunity is conferred by giving ATG (Human antitetanus globulin)

67. Concerning the principle organism of sepsis
- **A.** The pathogenic stephylococcus aurens is coagulase negative
- **B.** Group A haemolytic streptococci occur in clusters
- **C.** Escherichin coli are resistant to penicillin
- **D.** Proteus in a urinary infection makes the urine acid

68. Which of the following is not a worm?
- **A.** Taenia solium
- **B.** Taenia coli
- **C.** Taenia saginata
- **D.** Taenia echinococcus

69. In some 80% of cases of infection of the hand the organism is
- **A.** Gram negative bacillus
- **B.** Streptococcus pyogenes
- **C.** Staphylococcus aureus
- **D.** A clostridium

70. One of the following is an acute specific infection
- **A.** Diphtheria
- **B.** Actinomycosis
- **C.** Tuberculosis
- **D.** Leprosy

71. The main causative organism Ludwig's angina is
- **A.** Streptococcus viridans
- **B.** Staphylococcus albus
- **C.** Staphylococcus aurens
- **D.** Streptocococcus haemolyticus

72. Virus responsible for infectious mono-nucleosis is
- **A.** RNA paramyxo virus
- **B.** Varicella zoster virus
- **C.** Epstein Barr virus
- **D.** Coxsackie virus A 16

73. Slide flocculation test represents
- **A.** VDRL test **B.** Tube test
- **C.** Ring test **D.** Immuno diffusion

74. Complement constitutes or is comprised
A. 10-20% of human serum globulins
B. 10-15% of human serum globulins
C. 50-60% of human serum globulins
D. 0-10% of human serum globulins

75. The example of immediate hypersensitivity is
A. Atopy
B. Infection (tuberculin) type
C. Contact dermatitis
D. B and C both

76. The example of type III hypersensitivity reaction is
A. Immune complex or toxic complex diseases
B. Reaginic
C. Delayed hypersensitivity
D. Cytotoxic

77. Lancefield serological group is done for
A. Streptococci B. Salmonella
C. Staphylococci D. Vibrio

78. Crystal violet is used as a preparation of selective media for
A. Staph. aureus
B. Str. pyogenes
C. A and B both
D. None of the above

79. Aryl sulphatase test is the biochemical test used to identify
A. Streptococci
B. Staphylococci
C. Myobacterium
D. Pneumococci

80. In Mantaux test the positive reaction is indicated by
A. Edema at the infected site
B. Induration within 24 hours
C. Edema and induration at the injected site after 48-72 hours
D. None of the above

81. Treponema Pallidum is a delicate spirochete measuring
A. 0.1-0.4 μ wide
B. 0.1-0.5 μ wide
C. 0.1-0.2 μ wide
D. 4-14 μ wide

82. The 'Pallidum' in Treponema Pallidum referes to
A. Metalic staining
B. Pale staining
C. Pink staining
D. A and B

83. Viruses contain
A. Only DNA
B. Only RNA
C. Either single or double stranded DNA or RNA
D. None of the above

84. Polio virus can attach itself to
A. Primate cells or rodent cells
B. Primate cells
C. Rodent cells
D. None of the above

85. The time taken for a single cycle of replication by a bacteriophage is
A. 0-10 mts
B. 15-30 mts
C. 15-30 hours
D. 72 hours

86. Virods are referred to
A. Virus within a bacteria
B. A bacteria
C. Sub viral agents having genome smaller than known viruses
D. Viral types having genomes larger than known viruses

87. Prions are
A. Unconventional bacterias
B. Proteinaceous infected particle virus like
C. Not sensitive to proteases
D. A and C both

88. Herpes viruses are seen as inclusion bodies in
A. Cytoplasm of the cell
B. Nucleus of the cell
C. Mitochondria of the cell
D. A and C both

89. Rhinoviruses are the viruses that
A. Are inactivated in GIT
B. Cause infections of GIT
C. Are not enveloped
D. None of the above

90. The viruses that enter through the skin abrasions are
A. Arbovirus
B. Papilloma virus
C. Type B hepatitis
D. Rabies virus

91. Papillomas and molluscum contagiosum may have
A. Short incubation period
B. Long incubation period
C. Long or short incubation period
D. None of the above is correct

92. Herpes viruses particle consists of
A. Capside with 162 capsomers
B. Capside with 100 capsomers
C. Capside with 200 capsomers
D. Capside with 10 capsomers

93. Passenger viruses isolated from lymphoma a cells are known as
A. Herpes simplex
B. Epstein Barr virus
C. Cytomegalo virus
D. A or B

94. A 22 mm in size nonenveloped RNA virus is labelled as
A. HAV B. HIV
C. HBV D. B and C

95. Retroviruses HTLV-cause
A. Hepato cellular carcinomas
B. Adult T-cell leukaemia
C. Urogenital tumors
D. Burkitts lymphoma

96. The viral oncogene V-src is located on
A. Chromosome 20
B. Chromosome 11
C. Chromosome 8
D. Chromosome 22

97. The commensals from the normal flora of mouth
A. Never enter the blood and tissues
B. May enter the blood and tissues
C. Always enter blood and tissues
D. None of the above

98. In toxin type of food poisoning the incubation period is
A. 10-20 hours B. 1-6 hours
C. 6-12 hours D. 0-72 hours

99. The interval between the Ist and IInd subcutaneous injection of DPT vaccine is
A. 8-12 weeks B. 4-8 weeks
C. 6-7 days D. 10-12 months

100. The biological vectors are the pathogens that
A. Only multiply in the body of vectors
B. Multiply and undergo a developmental cycle and transmit infection
C. Never multiply in the body of vector but transmit injection
D. None of the above

Answers

1 B Diapedisis refers to the emigration through the gaps of endothelial cells. These cells fall from the central column of blood to come in contact with endothelial cells before diapedisis. Chemotaxis is the migration of cells towards an attractant in one direction.

2 C Keloid is abundant collagen formed during healing process leading to scar. Contractures and adhesions lead to abnormal adherence to the structures, while callus is formed as a result of hyperplasia of stratum corneum of superficial skin. These are formed in areas of repeated friction of skin.

3 A Necrosis, recurrence, multinodularity, increase in size of tumors are some features of malignancy. The neoplastic cells need nutrition to survive as such the vascularity may be increased.

4 A Teratoma is a benign tumor derived from all the germ layers, while hamartoma is a disorganized growth of tissues in an uncoordinated fashion native to the site. Hematoma is the collection of blood in extravascular spaces. Multiple chondromas, that are the growth of disorganized tissue in a haphazard pattern alien to site, are associated with Olliers syndrome.

5 A Benign neoplasms likely interferes with the organ functioning. The malignant tumors metastatize. The benign lesions do not expand to rupture the blood vessels and do not cause ulceration and necrosis. Also no recurrence and multinodularity is seen with benign lesions.

6 B The aplasia means lack of development of an organ or a tissue, the hypoplasia refers to partially formed tissue. The anaplasia is labelled as lack of differentiation i.e. nonresemblance of cells to the parental origin. Neoplasia refers to the new growth of tissues.

7 C The choices A, B, D are the useful facets of inflammation while fistula formation is a complication.

8 A

9 C Blebs are formed during the reversible injury of cell at its surface. Cell injury begins with the herald of hypoxia, which lead to failure of the cells aerobic respiration.

10 A Studies have shown that the central factor in pathogenesis of irreversible injury is damage to cell membrane.

11 A Dysplasia means disordered growth, size, shape of cells. Dyskeratosis refers to abnormal keratinisation while neoplasia is a new growth.

12 A In coagulation necrosis, the changes that take place in a cell are typically acidophillic conversion and opaque tombstone like appearance.

13 B Fat necrosis is a morphological pattern of cell death in adipose tissue due to the action of lipases especially seen in pancreas.

14 B Caseous necrosis is seen in the tuberculous lesion and results due to the coagulative and liquefactive necrosis.

15 A Liposomes are small membrane bound inclusions that are closely in contact with endoplasmic reticulum. With time more of these vacuoles are formed, which coalesce together and displace the nucleus away.

16 A Excessive collection of the iron in a disease called hemochromatosis results in fibrosis of liver and diabetes.

17 B Psammoma bodies are the form of dystrophic calcification that accumulate in layers around the necrotic body in a lamellated pattern and resemble grains of sand.

18 B Mineral salt when collected in excess in lungs can result in respiratory deficiency and the collections in kidneys can cause the renal damage.

19 D An organ that shows ischemia, may lead to eventually to necrosis. This localized area of tissue damage is referred to an infarct.

20 B Mosaicism refers to aberrations at the molecular level of cell in its early development resulting in two or more populations of cells in the same person. The translocation is the cytogenic disorder which manifests as transfer of one part of chromosome to the other. The choice B involves the structure of the chromosome. Usually this is manifested as breakage of chromosome and rearrangement and is seen in Blooms syndrome, Fanconis anemia.

21 A This disorder results due to deficiency of an enzyme glucocerebrosidases which normally cleaves glucose from ceramide. The plenty of glucocerebroside accumulates within phagocytes and in CNS.

22 A

23 C

24 B Staging is based on clinical features, while the grading of tumors is based on histopathological features. The metastasis is the spread of tumor to other part of body. The nodal involvement is one of the criteria of clinical staging.

25 A Mostly the normal cells will only grow on solid surface. One of the properties of a neoplastic cell is the anchorage independence.

26 A

27 A The occurrence of cancers varies with the age. Certain cancers have propensity to occur in childhood only.

28 A Viruses have been long implicated in the causation of cancers e.g. papilloma was the first benign lesions to be reported to occur in association with viruses. In most of the cases the squamous cell carcinoma shows the evidence of HPV virus.

29 A Exfoliative cytology involves scraping of the tissue to screen the cellular changes while immunohistochemistry involves the study of antigens by various antibodies. Flow cytometry measures the DNA content of a cell in usually various tumors where it may be altered.

30 C The infection of tubercular bacilli results in the lesion primarily in lower part of upper lobes or upper part of lower lobes of lungs. The nodal involvement together with lung involvement is referred to as Ghons complex.

31 B Lepra cells are seen in response to the mycobacterium leprae. These are mainly the macrophages laden with lipid and microbes and are seen localized in the cooler tissue. Such reaction also evokes the development of macules, papules and nodules in the skin.

32 C

33 A Parasitic infections often evoke the immune response that is humoral and is usually comprise IgE.

34 A Asbestos comprises fibres that may be serpentine, curled, flexible or brittle and straight. The small long, flexible fibres do not fracture and resist air flow and tend to deposit in the lungs, when inhaled. In lungs these fibres are engulfed by macrophages. Pneumoconioses results due to inhalation of any aerosol e.g. inhalation of dust.

35 A

36 C The sarcomas as well as carcinomas spread to lungs by direct infiltration, lymphatics or by blood.

37 A Teratomas arise from germ layers. The mesitheliomas arise from visceral and parietal pleura.

38 C

39 B The initial stage of alcoholic cirrhosis is characterized by accumulation of fat. At this stage the liver is macronodular, but over a period of years with continuation of alcohol intake the liver shrinks to form micronodular. This is characrerized by excessive fibrous deposition.

40 A Thyroglossal duct is a developmental anomaly resulting due to the cystic degeneration of the thyroglossal duct remnant during embryogenesis. The cyst can form anywhere along the foramen caecum and the hyoid bone.

41 B The HIV binds specifically to the receptors on T helper cells via a glyco protein that is present on the viral enevelope.

42 A

43 A The thalassemia syndromes are characterized by the defecient synthesis of either alpha or beta chain of hemoglobin. Both the T. major and T. minor are genetically determined.

44 C Aschoff bodies are localized areas of necrosed tissue infiltrated with inflammatory cells e.g. lymphocytes, macrophages and plasma cells. These are found predominantly affecting heart. Negri bodies are bullet shaped aggregates of rabies viruses found usually in neurons.

45 A Viral and bacterial infection is seen more common in immunocompromised individuals.

46 B Giant cell granulomas are common in jaws while the giant cell tumors affect the long bones.

47 B HDV is a Delta virus. It is small defective RNA virus.

48 A Seminomas are the most common type of germinal tumors present in fourth decade of life.

49 B

50 A These are one of the most common sarcomas seen in children.

51 B

52 B Mycoplasma refers to fungus like form of branching filaments. Their characteristic feature is absence of cell wall.

53 B

54 C

55 C

56 C It is widely used method of sterilisation by heat and is used to sterilise glasswares, forceps, scalpel.

57 B

58 A This media is used to test special properties e.g., urease production.

59 A

60 C

61 A

62 B Gonococcus was first described in Gonococcus pus by Neisser in (1879).

63 C

64 C

65 A

66 B Toxin produced is absorbed by motor nerve endings and transported to the Central Nervous System along the axis cylinders of peripheral nerve.

67 A

68 A

69 A

70 A

71 A

72 C

73 A

74 B Complement is a system of factors comprising nine different fractions.

75 A Types of hypersensitivity are immediate and delayed.

76 A

77 A

78 B

79 C

80 C

81 C

82 B

83 C Viruses do not have a cellular organization, they contain only one type of Nucleic acid either RNA or DNA but never both.

84 B

85 B

86 C Viroids are subviral agents showing apparent absence of extracellular dormant phase (vision) and by a genome much smaller than those of known viruses.

87 B Prions are referred as virus-like agents proteinaceous infectious particles.

88 B Herpes virus is about 100-200 nm in diameter consisting of icosohedral capsid with 162 capsomers surrounded by lipid envelope.

89 A

90 B

91 B

92 A

93 B

94 A

95 B

96 A

97 B

98 B

99 B

100 B

Syllabus

Development and growth of jaws. Development of the teeth and surrounding structures and calcifications (including theories) of hard tissues. Microscopic anatomy of hard and soft tissue of the tooth and surrounding structures oral mucous membrane, the lips, tongue, floor of the mouth; palate and the salivary glands.

- Eruption and shedding of teeth.
- Morphology of teeth Occlusion.
- Saliva, Calcium metabolism. Mastication and deglutition.
- Age changes in teeth and surrounding structures.

I. General Medicine

1. Introduction:
   a. Aims of Medicine.
   b. Definition of diagnosis, prognosis and treatment.
   c. History taking and physical examination of a medical case.
   d. Medical emergencies in dental practice.
2. G.I. Disorders:
   - Stomatitis, glossitis, gastritis, Diarrhoea, Amoebiasis, Ascites, malabsorption syndrome.
3. Liver:
   - Jaundice, Viral hepatitis, cirrhosis liver, Tender hepatomegaly.
4. Cardiovascular System:
   a. Congenital heart disease, classification Rheumatic heart disease subacute bacterial endocarditis.
   b. Congestive heart failure left ventricular failure.
   c. Hypertension.
   d. Coronary artery disease.
5. Respiratory System:
   - Pneumonia, Bronchitis, Emphysaema, Lung, Abscess, Eosinopbilia, Plumonary Embolism, Pulmonary Tuberculosis, Respiratory failure.
6. Renal Disease:
   - Nepuritis, Nephrotic Syndrome.
7. Hematology:
   a. Anaemia, Coagulation defects, Bleeding disorders.
   b. Agranulocytosis, Leukaemia, Oral manifestations of hematological disorders, Lymphadenopathy and splenonegaly.
8. Central Nervous System:
   - Meningitis, Facial Palsy, Facial pain Epilepsy, Headache, Syncope.
9. Nutritional and Metabolic:
   a. Balanced diet Normal daily.
   b. Protein caloric malnutrition requirements.
   c. Avitaminosis.
   d. Diabetes melitus.
   e. Calcium homestasis.
10. Endocrine Disorders:
    a. Thyroid-Hypo and hyper pituitary.
    b. Hypo and hyper parathyroid.
11. Infections:
    a. Enteric fever.
    b. Mumps.
    c. Viral exanthemata.
    d. Diphtheria.
    e. Syphilis.
    f. Gonorrhaeo.

II. Miscellaneous

1. Infections:
   a. Allergy.
   b. Drug reactions.
   c. Drug interactions.
   d. Evaluation of a case for general anaesthesia.

Chapter 5

Human Oral Anatomy including Embryology and Histology

1. The rate of epithelial cell proliferation in gingival epithelium (turnover time) is
- A. 52-75 days
- B. 4-14 days
- C. 41-57 days
- D. 1-10 days

2. The following cellular structure depict the cell of epithelial origin
- A. Nucleus
- B. Vimentin
- C. Tonofilaments and desmosomes
- D. Ribosomes

3. Lectins are used as markers of
- A. Mesenchymal cells
- B. Epithelial cells
- C. Cell surface carbohydrate antigen of epithelial cells
- D. None of the above

4. Desmoplakin is present in
- A. Desmosomes
- B. Hemidesmosomes
- C. Anchoring fibrils
- D. Anchoring filaments

5. Tono filaments in non keratinized epithelium are
- A. More dense
- B. Arranged in bundles
- C. Are less conspicuous
- D. Arranged in pile

6. Filaggrin is associated with
- A. Keratohyalin granules of epithelial cells
- B. Mesenchymal cells
- C. Nerve cell
- D. Hemidesmosome

7. Birbecks granules are seen in
- A. Any dendritic cells
- B. Merkels cells
- C. Langerhan cells
- D. Langhan cells

8. A siderophage is the macrophage cell that can ingest
- A. Melanin
- B. Hemosiderin derived from RBC's
- C. Melanin and bilirubin
- D. None of the above

9. The submucosa of floor of the mouth consists of
- A. Loose fibrous connective tissue containing fat and minor salivary gland
- B. Fibrous connective tissue with less fat
- C. Elastic fibres and sebaceous glands
- D. Sebaceous glands and salivary glands

10. Gustin, a protein in saliva helps in
- A. Only in digestion of carbohydrates
- B. Growth and maturation of taste buds
- C. Tonicity of saliva
- D. Maintaining pH

11. Statherins inhibits
- A. Calcium phosphate deposition in saliva
- B. Increase pH levels of saliva
- C. Inhibits decrease levels of pH in saliva
- D. Calcium phosphate and acidic proline-rich proteins

12. **The Golgi bodies are more prominent in mucous cell because of**
A. Increase in protein synthesis
B. Increase in carbohydrate metabolism
C. Increase in glyco protein complex
D. A and B

13. **Demilunes are the**
A. Mucous cells seen in salivary gland acini
B. Mucous cells seen with serous cells
C. Mucous cells often capped by a crescentic serous cell
D. Striated duct cells

14. **Oncocyte, are the cells that are seen in the salivary gland ducts, often represent**
A. An overload of mitochondria
B. An overload of lysosomes
C. An overload of immuno globulins
D. Lectins

15. **The total volume of salivary secretion daily is**
A. 10-20 ml B. 600-1200 ml
C. 20,000 ml D. None of the above

16. **Sublingual gland is**
A. A mucous secreting gland
B. Sero mucous secreting gland
C. Serous salivary gland
D. All of the above

17. **During dentinogenesis the following is obligatory**
A. A good blood supply
B. A good blood and nerve supply
C. A good blood supply and alkaline phosphatase
D. Alkaline phosphatase or blood supply

18. **When the tooth erupts to its functional position?**
A. 1/3rd of root dentin is formed
B. 1/2 of root dentin is formed
C. 2/3rd of root dentin is formed
D. Root dentin is not formed

19. **The open apex in a deciduous erupted teeth is seen**
A. Till 12 months after eruption
B. Till 18 months after eruption
C. Till 6 months after eruption
D. Till 2-3 years after tooth eruption

20. **The cell rests of serre's are**
A. The cell remnants or residues when enamel organ detaches from overlying epithelium
B. Seen in Hertwigs epithelial root sheath
C. Seen in periodontal ligament
D. None of the above

21. **The only dendritic cells that are attached to each other by desmosomes are**
A. Merkel cells
B. Melanocytes
C. Langerhans cells
D. None of the above

22. **Oral mucosa does not play important role in**
A. Sensation B. Secretion
C. Protection D. Thermal regulation

23. **Laminin and bullous pemphigoid antigen is present in respectively**
A. Lamina densa and lamina lucida
B. Lamina lucida and anchoring fibrils
C. Reticular layer and collagen
D. Lamina propria and submucosa

24. **Secretory odontoblast cells have**
A. Open faced nuclei
B. Closed faced nuclei
C. Pyknotic nuclei
D. None of the above

25. **Incremental lines of Dentin are formed at a rate of**
A. 8.5 μm daily B. 3 μm weekly
C. 14.5 μm daily D. 4 μm daily

26. **The mineralisation of dentin occurs in a**
A. 4 hourly cycle
B. 12 hourly cycle
C. 24 hourly cycle
D. Once a weekly cycle

27. Vorn korff fibres are seen as
A. Process of odontoblasts in enamel
B. Collagen fibres in dentin
C. Extra cellular matrix
D. None of the above

28. In DEJ, the convexities face towards
A. Enamel
B. Dentin
C. Cementum
D. None of the above

29. The Dentinal tubules are
A. Straight in coronal dentin
B. S-Shaped in root dentin
C. Straight in root dentin
D. None of the above

30. The S-shaped curve of dentin is least pronounced in
A. Cervical 1/3rd of the root
B. Cervical 2/3rd of the root
C. Middle 1/3rd of the root
D. Coronal dentin

31. The range of odontoblasts has been found in root dentin is
A. 59,000 to 76,000 per square mm
B. 20,000 to 28,000 per square mm
C. 10,000 to 25,000 per square mm
D. 80,000 to 1 lakh per sq mm

32. Weibel palade granules are seen in
A. Cytoplasm of epithelial cells
B. Cytoplasm of endothelial cells
C. Cytoplasm of merkel cells
D. Cytoplasm of fibroblast cells

33. The majority of enamel proteins that constitute 90% is
A. Enamelin B. tuftelin
C. Amelins D. Amelogenins

34. The primary stage of enamel mineralisation forms
A. 90% of enamel
B. 20% of enamel
C. 30% of enamel
D. 40% of enamel

35. Rod sheaths are formed as
A. Covering of enamel rods
B. The boundary where the crystals of rod and inter rod meet
C. A result of protein sheath covering the crystals
D. None of the above

36. Collagen of PDL constitutes mostly
A. Collagen type I
B. Type II
C. Type I and III
D. Type IV

37. The surface area covered by maxillary teeth in an alveolus is
A. Less than the area covered by mandibular
B. Equal to that of the mandibular teeth
C. More than the area covered by mandibular teeth
D. None of the above

38. Ectomesenchyme has an origin from
A. Mesenchyme
B. Epithelium
C. Endoderm
D. Neuroectoderm

39. The tongue development begins
A. During 1st week of intra-uterine life
B. During 7th week of intra-uterine life
C. During 4th week of intra-uterine life
D. During 1st to 4 weeks of life

40. The transmembrane linkers present between the adjacent gaps are called
A. Cadherins
B. Cytokeratin
C. Vimentin
D. None of the above

41. The only fibroblast cell to cell contact is seen in
A. Fibrosis
B. Embryonic tissue and PDL
C. Matured tissue and PDL
D. None of the above

42. The movement of the cell is brought about by
A. Expression of cytokeratin along the migratory pathway
B. Expression of *tenascin* along the pathway
C. Expression of perlecan along the pathway
D. Expression of versican

43. The α-polypeptide unit of an integrin
A. Confers ligand specificity
B. Interacts with actin filaments of cyto skeleton
C. Both A and B
D. Attaches to vineculin and talin

44. During mineralisation process of bone further growth of hydroxyapatite crystals is stopped by
A. Phosphate accumulation
B. Pyrophosphate accumulation on crystal
C. Phospholipid accumulation on crystal
D. None of the above

45. Osteoclasts are generally seen
A. In clusters
B. Singly
C. As multinucleated cell in clusters
D. None of the above

46. The leading edge of a resorbable bone is called
A. Cutting edge
B. Several lines
C. Filling cones
D. None of the above

47. The osteogenic layer of suture is referred to as
A. Capsule
B. Cambium
C. Both A and B
D. Periosteum

48. Areas of deficient calcified dentin is called
A. Interglobular dentin
B. Intraglobular dentin
C. Incremental lines of dentin
D. A and B

49. The only dendritic cell that are joined by desmosomal attachment is
A. Melanocyte
B. Merkel cell
C. Langerhan cell
D. B and C

50. Wheat shafing or clumping of odontoblasts cells occurs due to
A. Apoptosis of cells
B. Vacuolisation of cells
C. Inadequate fixation
D. Degeneration

51. The maxillary permanent central incisor shows
A. More convex distal outline of the crown than mesial outline
B. More concave mesial outline than distal outline
C. Mesial outline more convex than distal outline
D. Mesial outline straighter than the distal outline

52. The two forms of permanent maxillary central incisors can be differentiated on the basis of
A. Labio-lingual dimension at cervix
B. Labio-lingual dimension at contact area of crown
C. Mesiodistal dimension at cervical line and mesiodistal dimension at the contact area
D. None of the above

53. The lingual incisal ridge of crown of maxillary central permanent incisior is
A. At level with the marginal ridges mesially and distally
B. Is not at level with the marginal ridges mesially and distally
C. At lower level with the marginal ridges mesially and distally
D. A and C

54. Labiolingual dimension of the crown of permanent maxillary central incisors
- **A.** Is equal to the mesiodistal dimension of crown
- **B.** Is lesser than the mesiodistal dimension of crown
- **C.** Is more than the M-D dimension of crown
- **D.** May or may not be greater than M-D of dimension of crown

55. The crest of contour of permanent maxillary lateral incisor mesially is
- **A.** At the junction of middle and incisor thirds
- **B.** At the cervical 1/3rd
- **C.** At the middle third
- **D.** At the middle and cervical 1/3rd

56. The permanent mandibular central incisors are
- **A.** Smaller than mandibular lateral incisors
- **B.** Greater than mandibular lateral incisors
- **C.** Same dimensions when compared to mandibular lateral incisors
- **D.** None of the above

57. The occlusal contact of anterior teeth features
- **A.** Anterior teeth in contact with mandibular arch in protrusive occlusal relation
- **B.** Anterior teeth in contact with a mandibular arch in retrusive occlusal relation
- **C.** Anterior teeth in contact with a mandibular arch in lateral occlusal relation
- **D.** None of the above

58. The mesial slope of maxillary canine is
- **A.** Longer than distal slope
- **B.** Shorter than distal slope
- **C.** Equal to distal slope
- **D.** None of the above

59. The line bisecting the cusp of permanent maxillary canine is
- **A.** Lingual to the line bisecting root
- **B.** Labial to the line bisecting the root
- **C.** In line with the axis of the crown
- **D.** In line with the axis of the root

60. The developmental depressions on the distal side of the root of permanent maxillary canine
- **A.** Is very shallow
- **B.** Is more pronounced
- **C.** May or may not be present
- **D.** None of the above is correct

61. Incisal aspects of maxillary canines or mandibular canines can be outlined by series of arcs with help of
- **A.** French curve
- **B.** Curve of Spee
- **C.** Curve of Monson
- **D.** Curve of Wilson

62. The lingual surface of the root of mandibular canine is
- **A.** Narrower than root of maxillary canine (lingual surface)
- **B.** Broader than lingual portion of root of maxillary canine
- **C.** Equal to the lingual portion of the root of maxillary canine
- **D.** None of the above

63. The cusp tip and mesial cusp ridge of mandibular canine are
- **A.** Inclined in a buccal direction
- **B.** Inclined in a lingual direction
- **C.** Inclined in a mesial direction
- **D.** Inclined in a distal direction

64. The maxillary permanent premolars are developed from
- **A.** 2 lobes
- **B.** 3 lobes
- **C.** 4 lobes
- **D.** 5 lobes

65. The maxillary premolar crown are
- **A.** Shorter than those of maxillary canines
- **B.** Longer than those of mandibular canines
- **C.** Equal to those of maxillary canine
- **D.** None of the above

66. The contact point of maxillary first premolars are at
A. Same level
B. Unequal level
C. Contact is towards the cervical line
D. None of the above

67. Posterior teeth generally have
A. Narrow contact areas
B. Broader contact areas
C. Minimal contact areas
D. None of the above

68. Buccal aspect the crown of permanent first premolar roughly look like a
A. Trapezoid B. Rectangular
C. Rhomboid D. Ovoid

69. Mesial slope of permanent maxillary premolar cusp is
A. Equal to distal slope
B. Is longer than distal slope
C. Is shorter than distal slope
D. May be shorter or longer than distal slope

70. Distal slope of permanent premolar cusp is
A. Shorter and curved
B. Longer and curved
C. Curved
D. None of the above

71. Permanent posterior teeth have
A. Mesiodistal dimension (MD) greater than buccolingual (BL)
B. MD dimension equal to BL dimension
C. BL dimension greater than MD dimension
D. None of the above statement is true

72. The lingual cusp of maxillary first premolar is
A. Equal to its buccal cusp
B. Shorter than buccal cusp
C. Longer than buccal cusp
D. May or may not be shorter than buccal cusp

73. The tip of cusp tips in a posterior teeth are
A. Within the confines of a root trunk
B. Labial to root trunk
C. Lingual to root trunk
D. None of the statement is true

74. The occlusal surface of first maxillary premolar resembles
A. A hexagon B. A pentagon
C. A heptagon D. A triangle

75. The occlusal aspect of a first maxillary premolar shows a hexagonal figure of which
A. Two buccal sides unequal and Mesiolingual < Distolingual side
B. Two buccal sides nearly unequal
C. Two buccal sides are nearly equal and mesial side is shorter than distal side
D. Distal side is shorter than mesial side

76. The maxillary 2nd premolar is
A. More angular than maxillary 1st premolar
B. More rounded than maxillary 1st premolar
C. May or may not be angular than maxillary first premolar
D. A and B

77. The mandibular first premolar shows
A. Mesial contact area broader than distal contact area
B. Distal contact area broader than mesial contact area
C. Mesial contact area of same dimension to that of distal contact area
D. None of the above

78. Occlusal surface of mandibular first premolar is
A. Diamond shaped
B. Trapezoid shaped
C. Hexagonal shaped
D. Spheroid shaped

79. Occlusal surface of first mandibular premolar shows
- A. Mesial and lingual fossa
- B. Mesial and distal fossa
- C. Distal fossa and lingual fossa
- D. Lingual fossa and buccal fossa

80. The occlusal aspect of 2nd mandibular premolar shows
- A. The mesiolingual line angle sharper than distolingual line angle
- B. The Mesiolingual line angle and Distolingual line angle rounded
- C. The Mesiolingual line angle and Distolingual line angles are angular
- D. None of the above

81. The mesiobuccal (MB) root of maxillary 1st molar is
- A. Broader buccolingually as compared to other roots
- B. Narrower buccolinguallly as compared to other roots
- C. Broader in dimension as compared to other roots
- D. None of the above

82. The maxillary 1st molar exhibits
- A. Mesiobuccal (MB) cusp broader than Distobuccal (DB) cusp
- B. MB cusp narrow than DB cusp
- C. MB cusp equal to DB cusp
- D. None of the above

83. The maxillary 1st molar exhibits
- A. Distobuccal (DB) cusp sharper than Mesiobuccal (MB) cusp
- B. MB cusp sharper than DB cusp
- C. DB cusp of same shape as DB cusp
- D. None of the above

84. The distal contact area of 1st maxillary first molar shows from buccal aspect
- A. Distal contact area is in the middle of middle third
- B. Distal contact area in the occlusal third
- C. Distal contact area in the cervical third
- D. None of the above

85. The maxillary first molars show
- A. Axes of roots are inclined distally
- B. Axes of roots are inclined mesially
- C. Axes of roots are inclined buccally
- D. Axes of roots are inclined lingually

86. Protusion of the mandible without occlusal contact results from
- A. Contraction of lateral and medial pterygoid muscles and masseter muscle
- B. Contraction of temporalis muscle
- C. Contraction of suprahyoid
- D. Contraction of infra hyoid

87. The Mesiolingual (ML) cusp is
- A. About 3/5th of Mesiodistal (MD) crown diameter
- B. About 1/3rd of MD of crown diameter
- C. About 2/3rd of MD of crown diameter
- D. None of the above

88. Distolingual cusp occupies
- A. About 2/3rd of Mesiodistal (MD) of crown diameter
- B. About 2/5th of MD of crown diameter
- C. About 1/5th of MD of crown diameter
- D. About 1/2 of MD of crown diameter

89. The occlusal surface of 1st maxillary molar exhibits
- A. Rounded distolingual cusp
- B. Rounded mesiobuccal cusp
- C. Rounded distobuccal cusp
- D. Rounded mesiolingual cusp

90. Maxillary first molar shows
- A. Mesiolingual (ML) cusp as the largest cusp
- B. Mesiobuccal (MB) cusp as the largest cusp
- C. Mesiolingual (ML) cusp as the smallest cusp
- D. Distobuccal (DB) cusp as the largest cusp

91. Occlusal aspect of 1st maxillary molar resembles a figure of

A. Rhomboid B. Trapezoid
C. Spheroid D. Square

92. Occlusal aspect of 1st maxillary molar shows major fossa that is

A. Distal to oblique ridge
B. Mesial to oblique ridge
C. Buccal to oblique ridge
D. None of the above

93. Oblique ridge of 1st maxillary molar occlusally is formed by

A. Union of ridge of Distobuccal (DB) cusp and ridge of Mesiopalatal (MD) cusp
B. Union of ridge of Mesiodistal (MD) and Distolingual (DL) cusps
C. Union of Distolingual (DL) cusp and mesiobuccal cusps
D. None of the above

94. The crown of 2nd maxillary molar is

A. Shorter cervico inciso-cervically and same bucco-lingually when compared to 1st maxillary molar
B. Longer inciso-cervically as compared to 1st maxillary molar
C. Broader bucco-lingually when compared to maxillary 1st molar
D. Shorter bucco-lingually when compared to 1st maxillary molar

95. Occlusally the 3rd maxillary molar is

A. Heart shaped
B. Rhomboid shaped
C. Trapezoid
D. Spheroid

96. DL cusp of maxillary 3rd molar is

A. Well developed
B. Poorly developed
C. Mostly absent
D. Poorly developed and may be absent

97. Mandibular molars have crown exhibiting

A. Mesiodistal dimension > Buccolingual
B. Buccolingual dimension > Mesiodistal
C. Mesiodistal dimension equal to Buccolingual
D. May be A or C

98. Mesiolingual cusp of maxillary first molar contact with

A. Central fossa of mandibular first molar
B. Central groove of mandibular first molar
C. Distolingual cusp of mandibular molar
D. Buccal cusp of mandibular molar

99. Distolingual cusps of maxillary molars are in apposition to

A. Distal triangular fossa of mandibular molar
B. Mesial triangular of mandibular fossa molar
C. Distal triangular fossa, marginal ridge
D. Mesial triangular fossa of mandibular molar

100. The outline of the arch of the teeth

A. May correspond to the outline of the arch of bone
B. Does not correspond to the outline of the arch of the bone
C. May or may not correspond to the outline of the arch of bone
D. None of the above

Answers

1 C The turnover time refers to the time taken by epithelial cell to divide and pass through the entire epithelium. In skin the turnover time is 52-75 days while in the gingival mucosa it is 41-75 days and it is 25 days in cheek mucosa.
2 C Vimentin is protein in mesenchymal cells.
3 C
4 A The protein desmoplakin forms the attachment plaque and is found only in desmosomes. Some vesiculo-bullous disorders manifest breakdown of desmosomal components.
5 C This cell is found in the deeper epithelium as well as in upper part. The cell shows small rod shaped or flask shaped granule.
6 A
7 C
8 B
9 A The inclusion of sebaceous glands is rarely seen usually in cheek mucosa and is referred to as Fordyces granules.
10 B
11 D Statherins maintain the integrity of tooth structure by their function.
12 B Increase in the content of golgi bodies reflects the secretory activity of carbohydrate in mucous cells.
13 C
14 A
15 B
16 A
17 C
18 C
19 B
20 A
21 A
22 D Thermal regulation is the function of oral mucosa seen in the animals usually.
23 B The basal lamina is the highly organized complex which shows ultrastructurally lamina lucida and lamina densa. The lamina lucida is electron lucent situated towards epithelium while lamina densa is electron dense and is electron dense. Laminin is present in lamina densa along with type IV collagen. The lamina lucida shows glycoproteins including bullous pemphigoid antigen.
24 A
25 D
26 B
27 D Vorn korffs fibres are not the actual fibrous structures. The extra cellular compartment between the newly differentiated odontoblasts take up the silver stain which under the light microscope appears as negative outline of the odontoblasts and simulate the fibre like structure.
28 D
29 C
30 A
31 A
32 B
33 D
34 C
35 B
36 C
37 C
38 D Embryonic connective tissue is derived from mesenchyme but the primitive mesenchyme of head and neck is derived from neuroectoderm.
39 D
40 A
41 B
42 B
43 A
44 B
45 C
46 A
47 B
48 A
49 B
50 C
51 A
52 C
53 A
54 B
55 A
56 A
57 B
58 A
59 B
60 A
61 A
62 B
63 C
64 C
65 A
66 B
67 A
68 B
69 A
70 C
71 B
72 A
73 A
74 C

75 B
76 B
77 B
78 B
79 B
80 A
81 A
82 A
83 A
84 A
85 A
86 A
87 B
88 A
89 A
90 A
91 B
92 A
93 A
94 A
95 D
96 A
97 A
98 C
99 B
100 C

Syllabus

I. General Pharmacology:

1. General principles of pharmacology; dosage forms; prescription writings; pharmacokinetics (absorption, distribution, metabolism and excretion of drugs), mode of action of drugs, factors, modifying drug response, adverse drug reactions; drug interactions.
2. CNS drugs; General anaesthetics, hypnotics, analgesics, psychotropic drugs, antiepileptics muscle relaxants, analeptics, local anaesthetics.
3. Autonomic drugs: Sympathomimetics, antiadrenergic drugs, parasympethomimetics, parasympatholoytics, histamine and antihistaminics.
4. Cardiovascular drugs: Cardiac stimulants and antiarrhythmic drugs; antihypertensive drugs; vasopressor agents and treatment of shock.
5. Drugs acting on blood: Coagulants and anti-coagulants, hematinics.
6. GIT Drugs: Purgatives, anti-diarrhoeal, anticids, anti-emetics.
7. Endocrines: Emphasis on treatment of diabetes and adrenal cortical steroids.
8. Chemotherapy: Sulfonamides and antibiotics, chemotherapy of tuberculosis, leprosy and malignancy.
9. Vitamins.
10. Miscellaneous drugs: Such as diuretics, heavy metal antagonists (BAL and EDTA) etc.

II. Dental Pharmacology and Therapeutics:

1. Anti-septics, astringents, obtundents, mummifying agents, bleaching agents, styptics, disclosing agents, dentifrices and mouth washes.
2. Treatment of common oral condition.

Chapter 6

General and Dental Pharmacology and Therapeutics

1. **Which of the following is not a nucleoside reverse transcriptase inhibitor?**
   A. Zidovudine
   B. Lamivudine
   C. Nevirapine
   D. Didanosine

2. **Which of the following antimicrobials has antipseudomonal action**
   A. Cefpodoxime proxefil
   B. Ceforamicle
   C. Cetazidine
   D. Cefo perazone

3. **Which of the following fluoroquinolones does not require dose adjustment in a patient with creatinine clearance of < 50 mg/min?**
   A. Ciprofloxacin
   B. Norfloxacin
   C. Lomefloxacin
   D. Sparfloxacin

4. **Which of the following statements is not true regarding sulfonamides?**
   A. Sulfasolazine is absorbed well from gastrointestinal tract
   B. Crystalluria can occur with sulfonamide administration
   C. Sulfonamide administration to newborn may cause kernicterus
   D. Sulfonamides are of value in treatment of infections due to nocardia species

5. **Which of the following actions is ascribed to delta type of opioid receptors, *except***
   A. Supraspinal analgesic
   B. Respiratory depression
   C. Euphoria
   D. Reduced intestinal motility

6. **The main excitatory neuro transmitter in CNS is**
   A. Glycine
   B. Acetyl choline
   C. Aspartate
   D. Glutamate

7. **A 37-year-old multipara construction labourer has a blood picture showing hypochronic *anisocytosis.* This is most likely indicative of**
   A. Iron deficiency
   B. Folic deficiency
   C. Malnutrition
   D. Combined iron and folic acid deficiency

8. **Which of the following does not bind to GABA receptor chloride channels?**
   A. Ethanol B. Alphaxdone
   C. Zolpidem D. Buspirone

9. **Which of the following is not an important cause of hyponatremia?**
   A. Gastric fistula
   B. Excessive vomiting
   C. Diarrhoea
   D. Prolonged Ryle's tube aspiration

10. Which of the following is the earliest manifestation in Cushing's syndrome?
- A. Loss of diurnal variation
- B. Increased ACTH
- C. Increased plasma cortisol
- D. Increased urinary metabolites of cortisol

11. The presence of higher amounts of proline-rich proteins (PRP) can have what kind of effect on caries causation?
- A. Caries promoting since they help in bacterial adherence
- B. Make tooth surface resistance to caries since it enhanced fluoride action
- C. It has role during tooth mineralization only therefore no effect on caries
- D. Aid in super saturation of saliva therefore make tooth resistant to caries

12. Which of the following is the first drug of choice in anaphylactic reaction?
- A. Epinephrine 1: 1000
- B. Dexamethasone 8 mg
- C. Hydrocortisone 8 mg
- D. Epinephrine 1:1,00,000

13. The role of sodium metabisulfite in local anaesthetic agent is
- A. Preservative
- B. Fungicide
- C. Reducing agent
- D. Vasoconstrictor

14. Which of the following antibiotic prescribed in case of juvenile periodontitis?
- A. Tetracycline B. Erythromycin
- C. Sulfadiazine D. Cephalexin

15. Microabrasion involves the use of
- A. Sulphuric acid
- B. Acetic acid
- C. Phosphoric acid
- D. Hydrochloric acid

16. Which of the following elements is known to influence the body's ability to handle oxidative stress?
- A. Calcium
- B. Iron
- C. Potassium
- D. Selenium

17. All of the following are used as proxy measures for incubation period except
- A. Latent period
- B. Period of communicability
- C. Serial interval
- D. Generation time

18. Which of the following volatile anaesthetic agents should be preferred for induction of anaesthesia in children?
- A. Enflurane B. Isoflurane
- C. Sevoflurane D. Desflurane

19. Which of the following is the test indication for propofol as an intravenous induction agent?
- A. Neurosurgery
- B. Day care surgery
- C. Patients with coronary artery disease
- D. In neonates

20. The drug that causes intrinsic staining of teeth due to calcium chelation is
- A. Alizarin B. Ampicillin
- C. Tetracycline D. Erythromycin

21. Which of the following medications shortens the recovery period of primary herpetic gingivostomatitis?
- A. Acyclovir
- B. Ziduvidine
- C. Kenalog in orabase
- D. All of the above

22. Radioisotopes are used in the following techniques except
- A. Mass spectroscopy
- B. RIA
- C. ELISA
- D. Sequencing of nucleic acid

23. A highly ionized drug
- A. Is excreted mainly by the kidneys
- B. Crosses the placental barrier easily
- C. Is well absorbed from the intestine
- D. Is highly protein bound

24. Hair and nails are usually preserved in poisoning from
A. Arsenic
B. Phosphorous
C. Barbiturates
D. Carbon monoxide

25. The occurrence of hyperthyroidism following administration of supplemental iodine to subjects with endemic iodine deficiency goitre is known as
A. Jod Basedow effect
B. Wolf-Chairkoff effect
C. Thyrotoxicosis fadcitia
D. De quervains thyroiditis

26. A post operative patient developed septicemia and was empirically started on combination chemotherapy by a new resident doctor. However, when the patient did not respond even after 10 days of antibiotics treatment, the review of the charts was done. It was found that the resident doctor had started the combination of antibiotics which was mutually antagonistic in action. Which one of the following is the most likely combination that was given?
A. Vancomycin and Amikacin
B. Cephelexin and Gentamicin
C. Ampicillin and Chloramphenicol
D. Ciprofloxacin and Piperacillin

27. HBAlc level in blood explains
A. Acute rise of sugar
B. Long-term status of blood sugar
C. Hepatorenal syndrome
D. Chronic pancreatitis

28. To which of the following family of chemical mediators of inflammations the lipoxins belong?
A. Kinin system
B. Cytokines
C. Chemokines
D. Arachidonic acid metabolites

29. Which of the following is a procoagulation protein?
A. Thrombomodulin
B. Protein C
C. Protein S
D. Thrombin

30. All of the following anticancer agents cause bone marrow depression *except*
A. Chlorambucil
B. Daunorbubicin
C. Doxorubicin
D. Flutamide

31. Clinically significant drug interaction occurs between pyridoxine and all of the following drugs except
A. Isoniazid
B. Cyclosporine
C. Levodopa
D. Hydralazine

32. What is the lethal dose of flouride?
A. 4 gm B. 2 gm
C. 6 gm D. 100 mgm

33. Thiopentone has lower duration of action, can be because of
A. High inherent property
B. Lipid solubility
C. Greater extracellular distribution
D. It is a high ionizing potential

34. Which of the following is most preferred for asthmatics?
A. N_2O B. Ether
C. Halothane D. Alcohol

35. Nitrous oxide is best used with which agent in general anaesthesia
A. Ether
B. Halothane
C. Thiopentone
D. Diazepam

36. MMR vaccine is recommended at which age
A. 6 months B. 15 months
C. 24 months D. 20 months

37. In an acute emergency if blood has to be given immediately without full laboratory cross-matching it is best to give blood which is
A. Group O RhD – ve
B. Group O RhD + ve
C. Group AB RhD – ve
D. Group AB RhD + ve

38. Total body sodium amounts to
A. 2500 mmol B. 5000 mmol
C. 7500 mmol D. 10000 mmol

39. There is a danger in giving saline intravenously when it is made up as
A. Chemically normal saline
B. Isotonic saline
C. 0.9%
D. 0.18% with dextrose 4.3%

40. Minimum urine output for 24 hours required to excrete endproducts of protein metabolism is
A. 200 ml B. 300 ml
C. 400 ml D. 500 ml

41. The standard bicarbonate level in the plasma is normally
A. 12-15 mEq/l B. 16-21 mEq/l
C. 22-25 mEq/l D. 26-31 mEq/l

42. In health the ratio of bicarbonate to carbonic acid is normally
A. 10 : 1 B. 15 : 1
C. 20 : 1 D. 30 : 1

43. The daily minimum protein intake necessary to keep a healthy adult in positive nitrogen balance is
A. 25-30 g B. 34-40 g
C. 45-50 g D. 55-60 g

44. Eusol is a
A. Solution of Eugenol
B. Solution derived from boric acid and bleaching powder
C. Saline intravenous solution designed for the Indian common market
D. A type of carbolic acid

45. Mannitol is
A. Type of sugar
B. A type of dextran
C. A type of lipid for I.V. feeding
D. Contraindicated in the treatment of shock

46. Which of the following veins should be avoided in adults, if possible for intravenous infusion?
A. Median vein of the forearm
B. Cephalic
C. Long saphenous
D. External jugular

47. Potassium deficiency is present if the plasma-potassium level is less than
A. 5.0 mmol/l
B. 4.5 mmol/l
C. 4.0 mmol/l
D. 3.5 mmol/l

48. Adreno corticosteroids in excess cause
A. Osteoporosis
B. Osteosclerosis
C. Osteochondritis
D. Endochondral ossification

49. In head injuries which substance is not included in therapy?
A. Urea
B. Mannitol
C. Dexamethazone
D. Hyaluronidose

50. Long acting thyroid stimulator is
A. A glycoprotein
B. Di-iodothyromine
C. An IgM immunoglobulin
D. An IgG immunoglobulin

51. Which of the following is not an antithyroid drug?
A. Carbimazole
B. Propranolol
C. Propyl-thiouracil
D. Potassium perborate

52. Regarding the parathyroid glands, they ____
- A. Are normally two in number
- B. Lie inside the capsule of the thyroid
- C. Are reddish-blue in colour
- D. Are not the secretors of calcitonin

53. Cytotoxic agents used in the treatment of malignant disease include
- A. Nitrogen mustard
- B. Epoxyresins
- C. Methotrexate
- D. Vinka alkaloids

54. Regarding the Waterhouse-Friderichsen syndrome
- A. Most cases occur in adults
- B. Treatment should await the result of blood culture
- C. Adrenalectomy is indicated
- D. It is a complication of meningitis

55. In Cushing's syndrome
- A. There is chronic hypocorticism
- B. There is an excessive production of glucocorticoids
- C. There is a malignant adrenal neoplasm present in about 50% of cases
- D. One fluid of the patients have a basophil tumor of the adrenal

56. Regarding phaeochromocytoma
- A. It is bilateral in about 15% of cases
- B. It produces noradrenaline
- C. All patients under 60 years who present with sustained arterial hypertension deserve a routine test to confirm or exclude the condition
- D. Treatment should depend upon antihypertensive drugs

57. Factors leading to cardiac arrest include
- A. Obstruction to the airway
- B. Inhalation of fresh water
- C. Excess of potassium
- D. Excess of calcium

58. The functions of the spleen are
- A. To provide 500 ml of blood to add to the circulation in case of haemorrhage
- B. To destroy effect erythrocytes
- C. To produce antibodies
- D. To form erythrocytes and lymphocytes

59. Regarding sodium depletion
- A. It can be caused by increased secretion of aldosterone
- B. It occurs during the first 48 hours after operation
- C. It can follow prolonged gestric aspiration combined with unlimited ingestion of water
- D. The subcutaneous tissues feel lax
- E. The urine contains little or no chloride

60. Regarding potassium depletion
- A. After trauma there is increased excretion of potassium for about 3-4 days
- B. Hypokalemia follows prolonged gastroduodenal aspiration
- C. Muscular spasms are caused by hypokalemia
- D. Intravenous potassium is safe and can be administered freely

61. Tetracycline absorption is not influenced by
- A. Calcium
- B. Phosphorous
- C. Iron
- D. Antacids

62. Bioavailability of drug is maximum in which mode of administration
- A. Oral
- B. Intravenous
- C. Intramuscular
- D. Subcutaneous

63. Give the antidote of fluoride
- A. Banana
- B. Tea
- C. Biscuits
- D. Chocolates

64. Which of the local anaesthetics have the longest duration of action?
- A. Dibucaine
- B. Lidocaine
- C. Benzocaine
- D. Procaine

65. Which of the following drugs is excreted in bile?
- A. Ampicillin
- B. Erythromycin
- C. Pencillin
- D. Cloxacillin

66. Normal calcium level in blood is

A. 9 gm/l B. 9 mg/l
C. 0.9 mg/l D. 0.09 mg/l

67. Patients on exclusive vegetarian diet are likely to suffer

A. Vitamin C deficiency
B. Folic acid deficiency
C. Vitamin B_{12} deficiency
D. Vitamin A deficiency

68. Which of the following is not excreted in bile?

A. Vitamin D
B. Ampicillin
C. Chloramphenicol
D. Minocycline

69. Which anaesthetic agent is administered by open drop method?

A. Ether B. Halothane
C. Nitrogen D. Enflurane

70. Oral use of which drug for treatment of diarrhoea is banned in India?

A. Streptomycin
B. Nalidixic acid
C. ORS
D. Amikacin

71. Which is not true of adrenaline production in the adrenal medulla?

A. Depends on high level of glucocorticoids
B. Can result from stimulation of the hypothalamus
C. Leads to its storage in chromaffin cells
D. Is essential to life

72. Which of the following statement is not correct for local anaesthetics?

A. Sensory and motor fibers are equally sensitive to LAs
B. Non myelinated and myelinated fibres are equally blocked by LAs
C. LAs interact with a receptor sensitive to Na^+ channel
D. Exposure of higher concentration of Ca^{++} lessens the effectiveness of LAs

73. Tumors of the pituitary body include those which are

A. Basophil
B. Acidophil
C. Chromophobe
D. Craninopharyngiomas

74. Myxoedema

A. Is an advanced form of juvenile hypothyroidism
B. Is related to thyroidectomy and ^{131}I therapy
C. Is a cause of carpal tunnel syndrome
D. Is treated by d-thyroxine

75. Regarding anti-thyroid drugs in the treatment of thyrotoxicosis

A. Thiouracil is commonly used
B. Potassium perchlorate is frequently used
C. Carbimazole is in common use
D. Propyl thioaracil has been given up

76. Regarding the parathyroid glands

A. Parathormone stimulate osteoblastic activity
B. Parathormone stimulate the renal tubular reabsorption of phosphate
C. Calcitonin is secreted by the oxyphil cells of parathyroid
D. Chief cells produce parathormone

77. In the haemolytic anaemias, which is not true

A. Spherocytosis is due to abnormal immunological responses
B. Chronic ulcers of the legs occur in congenital haemolytic anaemia
C. Liver may be palpable
D. Patients tend to suffer from gallstones

78. A patient with an insulinoma

A. Has an alpha-cell tumor of the pancreas
B. May be in a mental hospital
C. Displays Saint's triad and this establishes the diagnosis
D. Is likely to have Zollinger-Ellison, syndrome

79. Which of the following is not true for autonomic nervous system?

A. At the junction between two sympathetic pre- and post-gangliones neurones (nictonic acetylcholine is the neurotransmitter)
B. Noradrenaline is the sympathetic post-synaptic parasympathetic neurotransmitter
C. Muscarinic acetylcholine is the post-synaptic parasympathetic neurotransmitter
D. During fasting sympathetic nervous system discharges become more frequent

80. Minerals and vitamins

A. Niacin is a constituent of the flavoproteins
B. Hyper vitaminosis D causes weight loss and ectopic calcification
C. Vitamin K is required to γ-carboxylate protein residue in clotting factors
D. Daily requirement of folic acid is 10 mg

81. Regarding iron

A. Twenty percent of ingested iron is normally absorbed
B. Gastric pH reduces Fe^{2+} to Fe^{3+}
C. Cereals may inhibit iron absorption
D. It is stored in intestinal mucosal cells as mucosal transferin

82. With regard to carbohydrate

A. Glucose is absorbed primarily by active transport
B. Maximal intestinal glucose absorption is approximately 12 g/h
C. Maltose is absorbed after digestion to glucose and galactose
D. Fructose is absorbed by facilitated diffusion

83. Which is not a cholagogues (stimulate gallbladder secrelim)?

A. Fat
B. Secretin
C. $Mg\,SO_4$
D. CCK-Pz

84. The kidney as an endocrine organ

A. Erythopoietin is produced by glomerular epithelial cells
B. Erythropoietin stimulates aldosterone secretion
C. Renin secretion is inhibited by angiotensin II
D. Local hormone secretion includes prostaglandin E_2

85. Following complication is associated with rapid transfusion of large volumes of blood

A. Disseminated intravascular coagulation
B. ARDS
C. A fall in ionized Ca^{++}
D. Jaundice
E. All of the above

86. T_4

A. Is proportionally more protein-bound than T_3
B. Is converted to tri-iodotryptophan in peripheral tissues
C. Is more biologically active than T_3
D. Increases the number of LDL receptors

87. Which of the following is a relevant formula in calculation for drug dosage in children?

A. $\frac{\text{Weight of child in lbs}}{150} \times \text{adult dose}$
B. $\frac{\text{S.A.}}{17} \times \text{adult dose}$
C. S.A. of the child in $m^2 \times 60 = \%$ of adult dose
D. All of the above

88. Drugs not eliminated by the kidneys

A. Amino glycosides
B. Amphotericin B
C. Sulfonamides
D. Macrolide

89. Which drug is not eliminated by renal mechanisms?
- A. Chlortetracyline
- B. Chloramphenicol
- C. Nalidixic acid
- D. Cephalosporin

90. In use of anticoagulant Acenocoumarol
- A. 1 to 8 mg/day single dose oral is recommended
- B. Maintain prothrombin time 1.5 times of normal
- C. Maintain prothrombin time not more than normal
- D. All of the above are correct

91. The venom of a wasp sting
- A. Is acid
- B. Remains in the avulsed venom gland of the wasp
- C. Is alkaline
- D. Is never dangerous

92. The disadvantage of using radio iodine to treat thyrotoxicosis is
- A. Drug therapy is prolonged
- B. An indefinite follow up is essential
- C. There is a progressive incidence of thyroid insufficiency
- D. It should be avoided under the age of 45

93. Regarding the synthesis of proteins
- A. mRNA must be remanufactured constantly as it is used up during translation
- B. tRNA uses complementary base sequences to mRNA to locate the correct position on the mRNA to locate its amino acid
- C. Unlike mRNA molecules the tRNA molecules are released
- D. The first amino acid translated on the ribosome is isolencine because the ribosome commences translation when it recognises the triplet coding for isoleucine

94. The following term is incorrect
- A. Transcription: the conversion of mRNA bases to the correspponding amino acid sequence
- B. Translation: the polypeptide sequencing resulting from ribosomal processing of mRNA
- C. Exon: the base sequences of DNA responsible for amino acid translation
- D. Intron: the base sequences of DNA responsible for regulating polypeptide translation

95. The following are not associated with oedema
- A. Kwashiorkor
- B. α-1-Anti trypsin deficiency
- C. Filiarsis
- D. Lymphoma

96. DNA
- A. In the DNA chain the nucleotides adenine and gnamine are bound together
- B. In the DNA chain the nucleotides guanine and cytosine are bound together by hydrogen bonds
- C. Nucleotides are arranged in groups of three to code for each amino acid
- D. Genetic information in converted into amino acid chains by the process of transcription

97. Regarding the synthesis of protein
- A. The amino acid sequence translated represents the ultimate protein molecule
- B. Amino acid sequences for more than one protein are produced from mRNA chains
- C. Most proteins produced by cells contain the original mRNA sequence of amino acids
- D. Hormones are unusual examples of proteins as they are cleaved from precursor peptides

98. The synthesis of protein moleculues (Which is incorrect)

A. Is brought about by three distinct processes transcription, translation and post-translational modification

B. The DNA sequence is read from the S' end

C. tRNA is responsible for attaching the amino acids to the correct portion of mRNA on the ribosome

D. The protein molecule is built starting at its N-terminal end

99. Which of the following is not true for adrenaline?

A. Dilates the pupil by relaxing the circular smooth muscle of the iris

B. Derivatives are excreted in urine

C. Increases the basal metabolic rate

D. Is more potent dialator of bronchioles than nor adrenaline

100. Local anaesthesia used in dentistry

A. Alter the resting nerve membrane potential

B. Delay the rate of repolarization thus reducing the frequencies of action potentials

C. Reduce the permeability of the nerve cell membrane to sodium

D. Block the cellular metabolism of nerves

Answers

1 C All are anti retro virus, reverse transcriptase inhibitors.

2 C

3 D Ciprofloxacin, Norfloxacin and Lomefloxacin are excreted unchanged in urine. Hence, their doses need to be regulated.

4 A

5 C Euphoria is ascribed to μ receptors (mu opioid receptors) δ (delta) opoid receptors cause affective behaviour, reinforcing actions.

6 B

7 A

8 D Buspirone has a partial agonistic action on 5-HT receptors and does not modify GABAergic transmission.

9 C

10 B

11 D

12 A

13 A

14 A

15 C

16 D

17 C

18 C

19 B Unconsciousness after propofol injections occurs in 14-45 secs. and losts for is minutes only with a very less chance of post-operative nausea and vomitting.

20 C

21 A

22 C

23 A

24 A

25 B

26 C Ampicillin—bactericidal.
Chloramphenicol—bacteriostatic.

27 B

28 D

29 C

30 A

31 A

32 A

33 B

34 A

35 B Halothane deficiencies in terms of poor analgesia and muscle relaxation are compensated by concomitant use of N_2O.

36 B

37 A AB +ve, is a universal receptor and O –ve is a universal donor.

38 B

39 A

40 C

41 C

42 C

43 B 0.8-1 g/kg/day is the recommended value.

44 B Used for dressing of severe infected necrotic wounds.

45 A

46 C

47 D

48 A

49 D

50 D

51 B

52 D

53 B

54 D

55 B

56 D

57 D

58 A

59 D

60 C

61 C

62 B

63 B

64 B

65 A

66 C

67 C

68 C

69 A

70 A

71 D High concentrations of glucocorticoids stimulate a methyl-transferase enzymes which is required the methylation of noradrenaline to adrenaline. These are achieved by the arrangement of the blood supply to the medulla. Blood supply to the medulla. Blood enters sinusoids from capillaries on the outer capsule and permeates the cortical cells en route to the medulla.

Most stress stimuli act through the limbic system, hypothalamus and autonomic nervous system. The splanchnic nerves to the adrenal medulla are thus activated.

Catecholamines are synthesized and stored in chromaffin cells and are released into the circulation when the preganglionic sympathetic nerves which innervate the cells are stimulated. The chromaffin cells have been likened to specialized post ganglionic neurons. It is not only the release that is initiated by sympathetic activity, but also synthesis.

Animal subjected to adrenal demedullation survive of maintained under stable environmental conditions. The medulla amplifies the role of the sympathetic nervous system.

72 A

73 A

74 C

75 C

76 D Parathormone reduces renal tubular secretion of phosphate and do not stimulate osteoblastic activity.

77 A

78 B

79 B

80 B Riboflavin is a constituent of the flavoproteins; deficiency causes glossitis and chelitis. Niacin is a constituent of NAD and NADP deficiency causes pellagra (the four D's: Dermatitis, Diarrhoea, Dementia and Death). Vitamin D is converted in liver to 25-DHCC, then in kidney to 1, 25-DHCC which enhances gastrointestinal Ca^{2+} and phosphate absorption. Clotting factors II, VII, IX and X require vitamin K for γ-carboxylation of glutamate residues. Recommended folate intake is 0.4 mg daily. Although zinc is required for tissue healing, it is as carbolic acid (Vitamin C) which is needed to hydroxylate proline.

81 C Only 5% of ingested iron is absorbed. The majority is absorbed as Fe^{2+} but some is also absorbed as Fe^{3+} and haem itself. Gastric pH reduce Fe^{3+} to Fe^{2+}. Phytase in cereals reacts with iron to form insoluble compounds. Fe^{2+} is absorbed by binding to mucosal transferrin but is stored in mucosal cells bound to apoferritin as ferritin. The quantity of ferritin is inversely proportional to the amount of iron entering the blood stream. Concentrations are 20 mm μm in women with slightly higher levels in men.

82 D Glucose is absorbed by secondary active transport with a Na^+/glucose synport. Insulin has no significant effects on glucose uptake, which is maximal at around 120 g/h. Maltose is digested by brush border oligo saccharidases to glucose. Lactose is digested to glucose and galactose. Fructose is absorbed by facilitated diffusion and pentoses by simple diffusion.

83 C

84 A Proximal tubular cells are the site for 1-hydroxylation, and hence activation, of 25-cholecalciferol, required for maintenance of Ca^{2+} homeostasis and the normal mineralization of bone.

85 E Massive transfusion (>8 units over 4 hours or >15 units over 24 hrs) is complicated by DIC due to the reduction in coagulation factors and functioning platelets in stored blood and also to the activation of the coagulation cascade and complement by microaggregates. Microaggregates are also implicated in the pathogenesis of ARDS and a blood filter of 20-40 μm is recommended in addition to the transfusion of recently collected blood.

Citrate toxicity may produce a fall in ionized calcium and the infusion of calcium gluconate is occassionally required.

86 A T4 is 99.98% protein bound compared to 99.5%. (T3) and therefore has a longer half-life. Most of its action is via peripheral de-iodination of T3 which is 5-10 times as potent. It increases numbers of LDL receptors which lowers cholesterol levels.

87 A

88 D

89 B

90 A

91 C

92 A

93 B Transcription has no effect on the integrity of the mRNA and several copies of the mRNAs amino acid sequence are manufactured. tRNA is recycled similar to mRNA is protein synthesis. The first amino acid to be translated from the mRNA chain is methionine, as its coding triplet is recognized by the ribosome.

94 B Translation is the process in which mRNA bases are converted into amino acids transcription on the other hand, is the conversion of DNA bases to the corresponding mRNA bases. Exons are the portions of DNA which code for protein synthesis, whereas introns are regions of the DNA which are not translated.

95 D In Kwashiorkor an inadequate diet results in relative protein deficiency and hypoproteinaemia induced oedema, which is also the net result of hepatic cirrhosis of a cause including α-1-antitryps in deficiency. Anaphylactic reaction results in the release of vasoactive substances VV histamine which increase capillary permeability and produce consequent oedema. Filiarial infestation olytructs lymphatic flow with resultant oedema.

Oedema is defined as the accumulation of abnormal amounts of fluid in interstitial tissue. Factors affecting interstitial fluid volume are: (A) Oncotic pressure; (B) Interstitial fluid pressure; (C) Capillary pressure; (D) Lymph flow; (E) Total extracellular fluid volume; (F) Cepillary filtration coefficient.

96 C The pairing nucleotides in the DNA molecule are adenine with thymine and cyto sine with gnanine. The amino acid are coded for the three base-pair nucleotides called "triplet". Amino acid sequences are formed from the DNA code by the processes of translation and transcription.

97 B The amino acid sequence formed by translation of the mRNA chain is subjected to post-translational modification which may yield several polypeptides, as in the case of hormones. Modification of the mRNA leads to the removal of bases from the original mRNA sequence. All amino acid sequences derived from mRNA translation are modified before the ultimate protein is produced.

98 A There are four processes involved in protein synthesis; transcription, post-translational modification; translational modification. mRNA has the same triplet system of coding for amino acids as does DNA, however using complimentary bases and the substitution of the base uridine in place of the thymine.

99 A Adrenaline causes contraction of the radial fibres of the iris, thus dilating the pupil. End products of catecholamine-o-methyl transferase (COMT) breakdown are excreted in urine, mostly in a conjugated form.

The hormone exerts a stimulating action on oxygen consumption. It also causes arousal and increased pulmonary ventilation.

Both catecholamines relax smooth muscle of bronchi and bronchioles, but adrenaline is more active. β_2 effect > β_1 effects.

100 B
1. They alter the depolarization phase of action potential.
2. Rate of repolarization is not significantly changed. In therapeutic concentrations they do not cause metabolic inhibitory effects. Agents that have such effects can interfere with nerve conduction, but the nature of block is different.

Syllabus

1. Aims and objectives.
2. Developmental disturbances of dental, oral and para-oral structures, including hereditary disorders.
3. Dental Caries.
4. Pulpal and periapical pathosis and their sequelae.
5. Environmental lesions of the oral and para-oral structures.
6. Defence mechanism of oral tissues and healing following injuries.
7. Diseases of periodontal ligament, gingivae and cementum.
8. Effects of nutritional disturbances and normal disorders on the oral and para-oral structures.
9. Infections: Diseases of oral mucosa.
10. Bone disorders affecting jaws.
11. Cysts of oral cavity.
12. Pra-cancerous lesions—etiology and pathology.
13. Neoplasms of oral cavity.
14. Diseases of salivary and lymph glands.
15. Diseases of Temporo-Mandibular joint.
16. Diseases of nerves, skin, blood and their implications to oral tissues.
17. Effects of radiation on oral and para-oral tissues.
18. Oral Microbiology.

Chapter 7

Oral Pathology and Microbiology

1. Beckwith-Wiedemann syndrome shows
- **A.** Fusion
- **B.** Macroglossia
- **C.** Concrescence
- **D.** Aglossia

2. Lupus vulgaris is the
- **A.** Lepromatous changes in the skin
- **B.** Actinomycosis of skin
- **C.** Tuberclosis of skin
- **D.** Other name of verruca vulgaris

3. Pseudoepitheliomatous hyperplasia of a lesion seen mimics histologically
- **A.** Verrucous carcinoma
- **B.** Leukoedema
- **C.** Squamous cell carcinoma
- **D.** Carcinosarcoma

4. Caliber-persistant artery occurs more commonly in
- **A.** Lip mucosa
- **B.** Buccal mucosa
- **C.** Tongue mucosa
- **D.** Palate

5. The systemic disease correlated with dentin dysplasia like alterations is
- **A.** Osteoradionecrosis
- **B.** Hyperthyroidism
- **C.** Calcinosis universalis
- **D.** Osteomylitis

6. Haim Munk syndrome shows
- **A.** Periodontal disease
- **B.** Dyskeratosis
- **C.** Dysplasia
- **D.** Palmoplantar keratosis and periodontal disease

7. Mostly the electricity burns are of the type
- **A.** Contact
- **B.** Arc
- **C.** Thermal burns
- **D.** Oral burns

8. *Myospherulosis* is a foreign body reaction to
- **A.** Topical antibiotics
- **B.** Topical steroids
- **C.** Topical analgesics
- **D.** Topic anesthetic

9. Lateral facial clefts represent
- **A.** 10% of all facial clefts
- **B.** 0.3% of all facial clefts
- **C.** 2% of all facial clefts
- **D.** 9% of all facial clefts

10. Ankyloglossia can lead or contribute to
- **A.** Open bite
- **B.** Crossbite
- **C.** Deep bite
- **D.** None of the above

11. Delamination refers to caries process in the
- **A.** Enamel
- **B.** Coronal dentin
- **C.** Cementum
- **D.** Radicular dentin

12. Hemimaxillo facial dysplasia represents
- **A.** Unilateral enlargement of only zygomatic process
- **B.** Unilateral enlargement of mandible
- **C.** Unilateral enlargement of maxilla, hypoplastic teeth and missing premolars
- **D.** None of the above

13. In Gunther's disease the
- **A.** Affected teeth have reddish-brown discoloration and exhibit a red fluorescence when exposed to UV light
- **B.** The affected teeth show greenish black discolouration caused by chromogenic bacteria
- **C.** Affected teeth show brown pitting stains
- **D.** None of the above

14. Cervical enamel extension is seen mostly in
- **A.** Mandibular premolars
- **B.** Maxillary molars
- **C.** Mandibular molars
- **D.** Mandibular molars with a prevalance of 8.6-37%

15. Demastication refers to
- **A.** The accelerated tooth wear caused by chewing an abrasive substance between opposing teeth
- **B.** The Erosion caused by ingestion of acidic solutions
- **C.** Physiological attrition
- **D.** None of the above

16. Perimolysis refers to the
- **A.** Abrasion caused by a dentrifice or an overzealous toothbrush use
- **B.** Erosion from dental exposure to gastric secretions
- **C.** Erosion caused due to acidic beverages
- **D.** None of the above

17. Muco-epidermoid tumor arises from
- **A.** Striated duct cells
- **B.** Inter calated duct cells
- **C.** Excretory duct reserve cells
- **D.** Myoepithelial cells

18. The low grade Mucolpidermoid tumor histologically shows
- **A.** More of epidermoid cells
- **B.** More of mucous cells
- **C.** More of intermediate cells
- **D.** A and C both

19. Pleomorphic adenoma histopathologically shows
- **A.** Outer rows of epithelial cells and inner rows of myoepithelial cells
- **B.** Inner rows of epithelial cells and an outer rows of myo epithelial cells
- **C.** Two layers of Ductal epithelial cells
- **D.** None of the above

20. Low grade adenoid cystic carcinoma shows
- **A.** Solid pattern of cells
- **B.** Tubulo glandular
- **C.** Cribriform pattern
- **D.** Hyaline

21. Mucoepidermoid tumor histopathologically shows maternal cells which are stained by
- **A.** Sudan stain
- **B.** Mucicarmine
- **C.** PAS
- **D.** None of the above

22. High grade acinic cell carcinomas histologically show
- **A.** Acinar-lobular pattern
- **B.** Micro cystic
- **C.** Papillary cystic
- **D.** Primitive tubular

23. Undifferentiated carcinomas of salivary gland comprise
- **A.** 10% of all the tumors of salivary glands
- **B.** 10-20% of all the tumors of salivary glands
- **C.** 30-40% of all the tumors of salivary glands
- **D.** 3% of all the tumors of salivary glands

24. The granularity of cells seen in oncocytoma is due to
- **A.** Abundant golgibodies
- **B.** Abundant mitochondria
- **C.** Abundant ribosomes
- **D.** Abundant vacuoles

25. 'Canalicular form' of monomorphic adenoma is
- **A.** Most common type seen in minor salivary glands
- **B.** Least common type seen in minor salivary glands
- **C.** Most common type seen in major salivary glands
- **D.** Both are A and B

26. In which of the following disorders are oral manifestations more common?
- **A.** Junctional type of epidermolysis bullosa
- **B.** Dermolytic type of EB
- **C.** EB simplex
- **D.** Both are A and B

27. Tin-tack sign is seen in
- **A.** Erythema multiform
- **B.** SLE
- **C.** Scleroderma
- **D.** Elastosis

28. Michrochimerism is refferred to as
- **A.** Giant cells seen in the tissue
- **B.** Foreign cells present in the tissues
- **C.** Endothelial cells
- **D.** Small apoptotic cells

29. Malignant form of Acanthosis nigricans may be associated with
- **A.** Oral carcinoma
- **B.** Basal cell carcinoma
- **C.** Carcinoma of GIT
- **D.** None of the above

30. Mutations in gene that encodes for ectodysplasin causes
- **A.** Acanthosis nigricans
- **B.** Submucous fibroma
- **C.** Ectodermal dysplasia
- **D.** Psoriasis

31. Spinous layers of the cells directly abut into connective tissue stroma in
- **A.** Pemphigus **B.** Leukoplakia
- **C.** Lichen Planus **D.** Darriers disease

32. Carcinoma of gingiva occurs more frequently in
- **A.** Attached gingiva
- **B.** Free gingival
- **C.** Interdental gingiva
- **D.** None of the above

33. Microaperta is a clinical feature of
- **A.** Cellulitis
- **B.** Myositis ossificans
- **C.** Oral submucous fibrosis (severe type)
- **D.** None of the above

34. Fibrous dysplasia can be differentiated from ossifying fibroma on the basis of
- **A.** Clinical features alone
- **B.** Histological features alone
- **C.** Clinical, radiographic features and histological features
- **D.** Radiographic features only

35. Metastasis from intra oral carcinoma takes place by
- **A.** Blood stream
- **B.** By Invasion of lymph nodes
- **C.** By neural invasion
- **D.** Lymphatics

36. The other name for self-healing carcinoma is
- **A.** Carcinoma-in-situ
- **B.** Kerato acanthoma
- **C.** Leukoplakia
- **D.** Carcino sarcoma

37. The chondroma usually involves the
A. Anterior part of maxilla
B. Postero-lateral part of maxilla
C. Posterior part of maxilla
D. None of the above

38. The follicular type of ameloblastoma shows follicles lined with
A. Ameloblast-like cells with nucleus away from the basement membrane
B. Towards the basement membrane
C. Ameloblasts like cells with pyknotic nucleus
D. None of the above

39. AOT shows ducts lined with cells showing cells having their nucleus
A. Towards the basement membrane
B. Away from the b.m.z
C. Neither of the A and B
D. Undergoing karyohexis

40. Lichen planus specific antigen is seen in
A. Stratum granulosum layer
B. Spinous layer of cells
C. Basal layer
D. Stratum corneum

41. Sun-rays appearance is a radiographic feature of
A. Ewing sarcoma
B. Giant cell granuloma
C. Osteoblastoma
D. Osteoma

42. Neurofibroma when occurring more than 3 lesions it is referred to as
A. Nemofibromatosis
B. Neuroma
C. Schwanomma
D. None of the above

43. Peripheral ossyfying fibroma shows
A. More cellularity as compared to fibroma
B. Less cellularity as compared to fibroma
C. More collagen deposition as compared to fibroma
D. None of the above

44. "Juxta oral organ of Chievitz" is a cluster of cells seen near
A. Condyle of the mandible
B. Internal oblique ridge of mandible
C. Coronoid process of mandible
D. None of the above

45. Bumpy lips are the clinical features of
A. Traumatic fibroma
B. Cellulitis
C. MEN disease
D. Neurofibroma

46. Nonhodgkins lymphoma involves
A. Extra nodal sites and lymph nodes
B. Only nodes axial lymph nodes
C. Only muscles
D. Both A and C

47. Microscopically ghost cells are seen in
A. Pseudosarcoma
B. Ghost teeth
C. Calcifying odontogenic epithelial cyst (CEOC)
D. Pyogenic granuloma

48. Compound odontome is seen more commonly in
A. Anterior part of maxilla
B. Posterior part of jaws
C. Only in mandible
D. Both A and B

49. In TNM (PS) classification of Oral Cancers the P denotes
A. Pathology of tumour and etiology
B. Histopathology
C. Progression of disease
D. Both A and B

50. Necrosis is a characteristic h/f feature seen in
A. Ewings sarcoma
B. Reticulam cells sarcoma
C. Multiple myeloma
D. Hemangioma

51. Formal dehyde when compared to glutaraldehyde as fixatives manifests
- A. Good morphological picture of tissues
- B. Poor morphological picture of tissues
- C. A loss upto 30% of α-helix structure of protein
- D. A loss upto 50% of α-helix structure of protein

52. Mercuric chloride is used commonly as a
- A. Primary fixative
- B. Secondary fixative
- C. Tertiary fixative
- D. A and C both

53. The commonly employed mixture of fixatives used are
- A. Karnowsky's paraformaldehyde-glutaraldehyde
- B. Mercuric chloride-glutaraldehyde
- C. Potassium dichromate-formaldehyde
- D. Osmium tetraoxide and mercuric chloride

54. The oral lesions of tuberculosis are
- A. Primary lesions
- B. Secondary lesions
- C. Tertiary lesions
- D. A or C

55. Tuberculosis of hard palate
- A. Is less common that of soft palate
- B. Is the most common oral lesion
- C. Is more common as compared to that of soft palate
- D. None of the above

56. Tuberculosis shows more involvement of
- A. Upper lip and maxilla
- B. Mandible and lower lip
- C. Maxilla and lower lip
- D. Lower lip and mandible

57. Mycobacterium leprae after entry into the body
- A. Multiply in fibroblasts
- B. Multiply in Schwann cells
- C. Multiply in haematopoietic cells
- D. Multiply in squamous epithelial cells

58. The tuberculoid type of leprosy manifests lesions that are
- A. Sharply demarcated with dry and rough surface
- B. Diffused and shiny
- C. With sloping surface
- D. None of the above

59. Odonto dysplasia leprosy is manifested as
- A. Teeth with large dimensions
- B. Teeth with less dimension
- C. Hyperplasia of enamel and cementum
- D. A and B both

60. The salivary gland are involved in
- A. Primary syphilis
- B. Primary and secondary syphilis
- C. Secondary and tertiary
- D. Tertiary syphilis

61. Early congenital syphilis shows
- A. Terrace shaped nose
- B. Upper lip involvement
- C. Hutchinson's
- D. Frontal bossing

62. 'Ray fungus' that is characteristic feature of actinomycosis is a
- A. Radiological feature
- B. Microscopic feature
- C. Is clinical feature
- D. Clinical and radiological feature

63. The microscopic features of ANUG shows
- A. Bacterial zone and neutrophil zone
- B. Zone of spirochetes
- C. Bacterial, neutrophil, necrotic zone
- D. Bacterial, neutrophillic, necrotic and zone of spirochetes

64. Gangrenous stomatitis is a
- **A.** Primary disorder caused by an agent
- **B.** Multifactorial disorder secondary to local factors
- **C.** Multifactorial disorder secondary to local and systemic factors
- **D.** Secondary disorder or primary disorder

65. HIV infection is related with
- **A.** Hodgkins lymphoma
- **B.** Basal cell carcinoma
- **C.** Non Hodgkins lymphoma and squamous cell carcinoma and Kaposis Sarcoma
- **D.** Only Kaposis Sarcoma

66. Hecks disease shows Microscopically
- **A.** Focal epithelial hypoplasia
- **B.** Epithelial hyperplasia
- **C.** Vesicle formation
- **D.** Pseudo epitheliomatous hyperplasia

67. Recurrence of the nerve tumor Schwannoma
- **A.** Is equal to that of Neurofibroma
- **B.** Is lesser than Neurofibroma
- **C.** Is greater than Neurofibroma
- **D.** None of the above

68. Ameloblastomas show expansion of mandible affecting
- **A.** Lingual plate first
- **B.** Buccal plate first
- **C.** Lingual and buccal at the same time
- **D.** None of the above

69. The invading Neoplasm of jaws that frequently invades pulp is
- **A.** Burkitts lymphoma
- **B.** Squamous cell carcinoma
- **C.** Ameloblastoma
- **D.** Verrucous carcinoma

70. Malignant hemangio endothelioma show microscopically
- **A.** Plenty of blood vessels
- **B.** Plenty of endothelial cells with scanty blood vessels
- **C.** Plenty of endothelial cells with cellular pleomorphism and mitoses, and poor capillary formation
- **D.** None of the above

71. The Ewing sarcoma may histologically mimic
- **A.** Reticulo sarcoma and metastatic neuroblastoma
- **B.** Reticulo sarcoma or hemagioendo thelioma
- **C.** Hemangio pericytoma and neuroblastoma
- **D.** Only neuroblastoma

72. The addition of a buffer in fixative glutar adheyde causes
- **A.** Increase in its effective concentration
- **B.** Decrease in its effective concentration
- **C.** Increase or decrease in its concentration
- **D.** None of the above

73. For electron microscopy, the tissue fixed in glutaraldehyde should be kept for
- **A.** More time than normally
- **B.** Lesser time than normally
- **C.** Less than 2 hours a day
- **D.** None of the above

74. Tissue fixed in formalin and embedded in paraffin wax
- **A.** Shrink by 50%
- **B.** May shrink by 33%
- **C.** May shrink by 5%
- **D.** May shrink by 64%

75. Baker's formal-calcium is used to fix the
- **A.** Lipids
- **B.** Proteins
- **C.** Carbohydrate
- **D.** A or C

76. Rossmans fixative is used for fixing
- **A.** Glycogens
- **B.** Lipid
- **C.** Protein
- **D.** None of the above

77. The principle of processing are in order of
- **A.** Dehydration, impregnation, clearing, embedding
- **B.** Dehydration, embedding and clearing
- **C.** Clearing, embedding and dehydration
- **D.** Dehydration, clearing, impregnation and embedding

78. Acetone as a dehydrating agent in processing of tissue is
- **A.** Rapid in action but with poor penetration
- **B.** Slower in action and slower penetration
- **C.** Rapid in action with rapid penetration
- **D.** None of the above

79. The chloroform as a clearing agent during processing of tissues
- **A.** Is rapid than xylene
- **B.** Is slow acting than xylene
- **C.** Is slow acting than xylene but causes less brittleness
- **D.** None of the above

80. Xylene, during processing of tissue
- **A.** Removes the dehydrant
- **B.** Increases the concentration of dehydrant
- **C.** May remove or increase the uptake of dehydrant
- **D.** None of the above

81. For embedding the tissue sections the paraffin wax
- **A.** Should be heated at higher temperature
- **B.** Should not be heated at higher temperature
- **C.** Should be heated at 10-20°
- **D.** Should not be heated at higher temperature, the optimal being between 56-60°C

82. Muscles when stained with Hematoxylin and Eosin gives the following reactions
- **A.** Yellow colour
- **B.** Deep pink
- **C.** Blue colour
- **D.** Red colour

83. Fibrous Dysplasia expands in a
- **A.** Fusiform Pattern
- **B.** Centrifugal Pattern
- **C.** Linear Pattern
- **D.** None of the above

84. Monostotic form of F.D. displays
- **A.** More radiolucent lesion
- **B.** More radiopacity
- **C.** Radiolucent or radiopacity
- **D.** None of the above

85. Extragnathic margins of F.D. appear
- **A.** Well defined in jaws
- **B.** Poorly defined in jaws
- **C.** Poorly defined in axial skeleton
- **D.** None of the above

86. The nidus of osteoid osteoma shows
- **A.** Capillaries in nidus
- **B.** Nerves in nidus
- **C.** Blood in nidus
- **D.** None of the above

87. The typical "Bony Restoration" is a microscopic feature of
- **A.** Aneurysmal bone cyst
- **B.** Cherubism
- **C.** Pagets disease
- **D.** Stafnes cyst

88. Noonan-syndrome associated with cherubism is referred as
- **A.** Turner syndrome
- **B.** Pseudo turner syndrome
- **C.** Pierre robin syndrome
- **D.** None of the above

89. Cherubism is histologically indistinguishable from
- **A.** Giant cell granuloma
- **B.** Osteo sarcoma
- **C.** Pagets disease
- **D.** Ewings sarcoma

90. Cleidocranial dysplasia is a disorder showing mutations in gene located on
- A. Chromosome 6p22
- B. Chromosome 6p21
- C. Chromosome 7b22
- D. None of the above

91. "Quarter moon" physiognomy was referred to
- A. Cleido cranial dysplsia
- B. Fibrous dysplasia
- C. Pagets disease
- D. None of the above

92. "The Pagets disease microscopically shows
- A. A net gain in volume of affected bone
- B. A net loss in volume of affected bone
- C. Only resorption of bone
- D. All of the above

93. A Paget disease patient undergoes fractures because
- A. The new bone laid is brittle
- B. Marrow is replaced with fibro vascular tissue
- C. Abnormal bone is deposited
- D. None of the above

94. Cementoblastoma shows formed cementum that is
- A. Scanty reversal lines
- B. Numerous regular reversal line
- C. Numerous irregular reversal lines
- D. None of the above

95. Pyknodysotosis shows
- A. Beaked nose and acute mandibular gonial angle
- B. Beaked nose and obtuse mandibular gonial angle
- C. *Frontal bossing* open frontanelles, hypoplastic malar, obtuse mandibular gonial angle and beaked nose
- D. A and B both

96. Cemental ossifying fibromas
- A. Resorb and displace tooth root
- B. Do not displace tooth root
- C. Expand in a linear fashion
- D. None of the above

97. Beckwith Wiedemann's syndrome is characterised
- A. By overgrowth of tissues
- B. By under growth of tissues
- C. By only regional overgrowth
- D. By local or general overgrowth

98. Mutated gene TCOFI has been seen in
- A. Treacher collin syndrome
- B. Pierre robin syndrome
- C. Acrofacial dysostosis
- D. None of the above

99. Buccal bifurcation cyst mostly is seen
- A. On bucal aspect of mandibular molar
- B. On lingual aspect of mandibular molar
- C. Distal or mesial of mandibular bicuspid
- D. None of the above

100. Haemangioma can be distinguished microscopically (on basis of) form pyogenic granuloma
- A. By absence of inflammatory cells in former
- B. By large vascular spaces in latter
- C. By presence of inflammatory cells in hemangioma
- D. None of the above

Answers

1 B Backwiths Wiedemann's syndrome is a rare heriditary condition that includes: Visceromegaly, gigantism, Neonatal hypoglycemia and Omphalocele (i.e.,Protrusion of part of intestine through a defect in abdominal wall at the umblicus.

2 C

3 B The pseudoepitheliomatous hyperplasia refers to hyperplasia of benign epithelial cells and growing of epithelial cells into the underlying connective tissue. The epithelial cells show no ominous signs of malignancy. The basement membrane also remains intact.

4 A

5 C Osteoradionecrosis is the serious complication of the radiation to head and neck regions. The altered bone becomes hypoxic, hypocellular and hypovascular, and consequently necrotic. The risk of necrosis increases in presence of teeth, trauma to bone, periodontal disease and concurrent chemotherapy. Hyperthyroidism refers to endocrinal disturbance characterized by excess production of thyroid hormone, while osteomylitis is the infection of bone and bone marrow spaces. Calcinosis universalis refers to the widespread deposition of calcium in the dermis, muscles etc. Dentin dysplasia like alterations are seen in the disorder.

6 D

7 B

8 A Myospherulosis exhibits as a unique foreign-body reaction to placement of topical antibiotic in a petrolatum base into a surgical site.

9 B

10 A

11 C Refer Cariology by Ernest Newbrun.

12 C

13 A Gunthers disease is an autosomal recessive disorder of poryphysin metabolism that results in the increased synthesis and excretion of poryphyrins and their related precursors. Affected teeth show discolouration.

14 D

15 A

16 B Erosion is defined as loss of tooth structure caused by a chemical process beyond that associated with bacterial interaction.

17 C Salivary gland tumors arise from 2 reserve cells i.e.; intercalated duct reserve cells and excretory duct reserve cells.

18 B

19 B

20 C

21 D Refer Soft Tissue Tumours by Batsakis.

22 D —— Do ——

23 D —— Do ——

24 B —— Do ——

25 A —— Do ——

26 D

27 B

28 D

29 C

30 C

31 C Pemphigus shows histologically suprabasilar split. The typical histopathological features of lichen planus is the degeneration of basal cells with disruption of basement-membrane zone. The spinous layers therefore about directly in the underlying C/T stroma.

32 A

33 C Refer Oral Diseases in Tropics by Prabhu, Daftary and Jhonson.

34 C Due to this spinous layers of cells directly about in the underlying connective tissue.

35 B The metastasis from intraoral carcinoma involves mostly the submaxillary superficial and deep cervical nodes and submental, pre and post auricular and supraclavicular.

36 B

37 A

38 A

39 A

40 B

41 A

42 A

43 A

44 B These clusters of epithelial cells are seen at site where the inferior alveolar nerve block has to be given or a biopsy to be taken from the region medial to mandibular internal oblique ridge and pterygo-mandibular raphe. These epithelial cells are seen intimately associated with the myelinated nerve.

45 C The bumpy lips refer to the neuromas seen as a characteristic feature of MEN. The neuromas on lips manifest as nodules that are sessile and elevated. Also at times the lips are puffy and diffusely enlarged.

46 A

47 C

48 A

49 C

50 A This feature is distinguishing point for Ewings sarcoma and Reticulam cell sarcoma.

51 B

52 B

53 A

54 B The primary lesions are on genitals.

55 C

56 D

57 B The mycobacterium has the propensity to proliferate in nerve cell.

58 A

59 B

60 C

61 B

62 B Ray fungus is seen under the microscope and neither clinically or radiologically. It represents colonies of gram positive anaerobic bacteria in club-shaped filamentous pattern.

63 D

64 C

65 C

66 A

67 D

68 A

69 A

70 C

71 B

72 A

73 A

74 B

75 A

76 A

77 D

78 A

79 C

80 A

81 D

82 B

83 A

84 B

85 B

86 A

87 B

88 B

89 A

90 B

91 A

92 A

93 B

94 C

95 C

96 A

97 A

98 A

99 A

100 A The hemangioma microscopically shows vascular spaces lined with endothelial cells. There are not many inflammatory cells as are seen in pyogenic granuloma.

Reference Books

1. Textbook of Oral Pathology by Neville.
2. Textbook of Oral Pathology by Shafers.
3. Clinico-Pathological Correlations by Regezzi and Scuibba.

Syllabus

- Introduction:
  - Aims of Medicine.
  - Definition of diagnosis, prognosis and treatment.
  - History taking and physical examination of a medical case.
  - Medical emergencies in dental practice.
- GI Disorders:
  - Stomatitis, glossitis, gastritis, Diarrhoea, Amobiasis, Ascites, malabsorption syndrome.
  - Liver.
  - Jaundice, Viral hepatitis, cirrhosis liver. Tender hepatomegaly.
- Cardiovascular System:
  - Congenital heart disease, classification Rheumatic heart disease subacute bacterial endocarditis.
  - Congestive heart failure left ventricular failure.
  - Hypertension.
  - Coronary artery disease.
- Respiratory System:
  - Pneumonia, Bronchitis, Emphysema, Lung Abscess, Eosinophilia, Plumonary Embolism, Pulmonary Tuberculosis, Respiratory failure.
- Renal Disease:
  - Nephritis, nephrotic syndrome
- Hematology:
  - Anaemia, Coagulation defects, Bleeding disorders.
  - Agranulocytosis, Leukaemia, Oral manifestations of hematological disorders, Lymphadenopathy and splenomegaly.
- Central Nervous System:
  - Meningitis, Facial Palsy, Facial pain Epilepsy, Headache, Syncope.
- Nutritional and Metabolic:
  - Normal balanced diet daily.
  - Protein caloric malnutrition requirements.
  - Avitaminosis.
  - Diabetes melitus.
  - Calcium homestasis.
- Endocrine Disorders:
  - Thyroid-Hypo and hyper pituitary.
  - Hypo and hyper parathyroid.
- Infections:
  - Enteric fever.
  - Mumps.
  - Viral exanthemata.
  - Diphtheria.
  - Syphilis.
  - Gonorrhea.
- Miscellaneous:
  - Allergy.
  - Drug reactions.
  - Drug interactions.
  - Evaluation of a case for general anaesthesia.

Chapter 8

General Medicine

1. **Best diagnosis of pancreatic disease is by**
   A. USG B. CT scan
   C. ERCP D. X-ray (Plain)
2. **Dane particle refers to**
   A. HAV B. HBV
   C. HCV D. NANB
3. **The following is transmitted non-parentally**
   A. HBV B. HCV
   C. HDV D. HEV
4. **Barret's oesophagus is a type of**
   A. Squamous cell Ca
   B. A type of Adeno Ca
   C. Gastric type of epinelium in lower oesophagus
   D. None of the above
5. **In Plumner Wilson syndrome ____ all are true *except***
   A. Esophageal webs
   B. Common in elderly males
   C. Dysphagia
   D. Premalignant
6. **Most common site for peptic ulcer is**
   A. 2nd part of duodenum
   B. Antrum
   C. 1st part of duodenum
   D. Fundus
7. **Causes of chronic liver disease are all *except***
   A. Alcoholic liver disease
   B. HBV infection
   C. HAV infection
   D. HCV infection
8. **Transdutive ascites is seen in all *except***
   A. Cirrhosis of liver
   B. Tubercular ascites
   C. Congestive heart failure
   D. Non cirrhotic portal hypertension
9. **Most common presentation of carcinoma stomach is**
   A. Anaemia B. Lump in abdomen
   C. Dysphagia D. Abdominal pain
10. **Most common form of abdominal tuberculosis is**
    A. Ascites
    B. Mixed
    C. Ileocaecal
    D. Mesenteric lymphadenopathy
11. **Bence Jones proteins in the urine are characteristic of**
    A. Multiple myeloma
    B. Acute glomerular nephritis
    C. Chronic glomerular nephritis
    D. Nephrotic syndrome
12. **Alcoholic jaundice is caused by**
    A. Infectious hepatitis
    B. Obstructive jaundice
    C. Hemolytic jaundice
    D. Cholestatic jaundice

13. Oedema is seen in
A. Hyperthyroidism
B. Cushing's syndrome
C. Protein deficiency
D. Vitamin B_{12} deficiency

14. External cardiac massage is usually done in
A. Lower 1/3 of sternum
B. Xiphisternum
C. Middle of sternum
D. Cardiac Apex

15. Delirium may be present in
A. Alcoholism
B. Encephalitis
C. Typhoid fever
D. All of the above

16. In enteric fever, diagnosis in the first week is done by
A. Stool culture B. Blood culture
C. Urine culture D. Widal test

17. Temperature regulation is mostly controlled by
A. Thalamus B. Hypothalamus
C. Medulla D. Cerebellum

18. In Anaphylactic shock first line of treatment is
A. S/C Adrenaline
B. I/V corticosteroid
C. Anti-histaminic
D. Atropine

19. Fever is caused by
A. Leukotrienes B. Histamine
C. Interleukin D. Prostaglandin

20. Roth spots are seen in
A. Infective endaortitis
B. Rheumatic fever
C. Typhoid fever
D. Rheumatoid arthritis

21. Clubbing is not a feature of
A. Carcinoma Lung
B. Bronchiectasis
C. Tropical Eosinophilia
D. Interstitial lung disease

22. Perioral rash, gonadal atrophy, pigmentation of skin creases, neuritis are seen in deficiency of
A. Zn B. Mg
C. Selenium D. Cobalt

23. Diarrhoea, dementia and dermatitis is due to deficiency of
A. Riboflavin B. Niacin
C. Thiamine D. Cyanocobalamin

24. Petechiae in scurvy is due to
A. Thrombocytopenia
B. Platelet dysfunction
C. Clotting factor deficiency
D. Endothelial dysfunction

25. Oral anticoagulant therapy is monitored by
A. PT B. PTT
C. TT D. None of the above

26. Pernicious anaemia is caused by
A. B_{12} deficiency
B. Iron deficiency
C. B_6 deficiency
D. Cobalt deficiency

27. Tuberculosis is exacerbated by
A. Gastrectomy B. Alcoholism
C. Diabetes D. All of above

28. Risus-Sardonicus is present in
A. Tetanus
B. Arsenic poisoning
C. Ankylosing spondylitis
D. Leprosy

29. Most common cause of transfusion hepatitis is
A. Hepatitis A B. Hepatitis E
C. Hepatitis C D. Hepatitis B

30. Anaemia can manifest as all *except*
A. Tinnitus B. Fatigability
C. Delirium D. Vertigo

31. **Barr body is seen in**
   A. Buccal mucosa smear
   B. WBC
   C. RBC
   D. Saliva

32. **Most common tumour associated with AIDS is**
   A. Kaposi's sarcoma
   B. Brain tumor
   C. Ca lung
   D. None of the above

33. **Most common rheumatic valvular disease is**
   A. Mitral regurgitation
   B. Mitral stenosis
   C. Aortic regurgitation
   D. Aortic stenosis

34. **Most sensitive test in secondary syphilis is**
   A. VDRL B. TPH
   C. Culture D. Wassermann

35. **Osler's nodes are pathognomonic of**
   A. Infective endocarditis
   B. Rheumatic fever
   C. Pulmonary TB
   D. Leprosy

36. **Erythema marginatum is seen is**
   A. Typhoid fever
   B. Rheumatic fever
   C. Infective endocarditis
   D. Leprosy

37. **Factor deficient in hemophilia A is**
   A. V B. VII
   C. VIII D. X

38. **Bacteria implicated in Dental caries is**
   A. S. pyogenes B. S. mutans
   C. Staph aureus D. Pneumococcus

39. **Most common presentation of secondary syphilis is**
   A. Lymphadenopathy
   B. Rash
   C. Condylomata
   D. Snail track ulcer

40. **Hutchinson's teeth involves**
   A. Incisiors B. Molars
   C. Premolars D. Canine

41. **Scurvy buds are seen over**
   A. Bones
   B. Costochondral junction
   C. Gums
   D. Capillaries

42. **Tumor marker for a highly vascular tumor is**
   A. Desmin B. Keratin
   C. Sa 200 D. α Fetoprotein

43. **Microcytic anaemia is seen in case of**
   A. Pernicious anaemia
   B. Iron deficiency
   C. Tropical sprue
   D. Megaloblastic anemia

44. **Which of the following is not associated with streptococcus?**
   A. Rheumatic fever
   B. Scarlet fever
   C. Acute glomerular nephritis
   D. Scalded skin syndrome

45. **Bitot's spots are seen in**
   A. Vitamin D deficiency
   B. Vitamin A deficiency
   C. Zn deficiency
   D. Vitamin D deficiency

46. **Generalized anasarca is due to**
   A. Nephrotic syndrome
   B. Hypothyroidism
   C. Chronic renal failure
   D. All of the above

47. **White umbilicated lesions on the face in a 6-year-old boy are caused by**
   A. Lichen planus
   B. Acne vulgaris
   C. Molluscum contagiosum
   D. Verruca plana

48. Triad of glossitis, angular fissure and corneal vascularization is due to deficiency
A. Riboflavin B. Thiamine
C. Niacin D. Pantothenic acid

49. Still's disease is characterized by
A. RA factor positive
B. Neutropenia
C. Macro papular rash
D. Renal involvement

50. Most common organism causing infective endocarditis is
A. Streptococcus faecalis
B. Streptococcus viridans
C. C. burnetti
D. S. aureus

51. Herpes zoster occurs after an attack of
A. Measles B. Small pox
C. Chicken pox D. Rubella

52. Causes of loud S_1 are all *except*
A. Anaemia
B. Thyrotoxicosis
C. Pregnancy
D. Acute myocardial infarction

53. Sinus bradycardia is heart rate
A. < 80/min B. < 40 min
C. < 60 min D. None of the above

54. Jone's criteria is for
A. Congestive heart failure
B. Rheumatic fever
C. Infective endocarditis
D. Rheumatic heart disease

55. Valvular lesion seen in Marfan's syndrome is
A. Aortic regurgitation
B. Mitral valve prolapse
C. Mitral stenosis
D. Aortic stenosis

56. Causes of carpel tunnel syndrome are all *except*
A. Pregnancy
B. Rheumatoid arthritis
C. Thyrotoxicins
D. Gout

57. Most common cause of LMN facial nerve palsy is
A. Bell's palsy
B. Trauma
C. Sarcoidosis
D. Ramsay Hunt syndrome

58. Causes of haemoptysis are all *except*
A. Pulmonary TB
B. Ca lung
C. Bronchiectasis
D. Gastric ulcer

59. Rice water stools are seen in
A. Cholera
B. Salmonellae
C. Shigella
D. Campylobacter

60. Behect's syndrome comprises all *except*
A. Recurrent oral ulceration
B. Genital ulceration
C. Eyes lesions
D. Kidney involvement

61. Diagnostic test for infectious mononucleosis is
A. Paul Bunnel test
B. Aldehyde test
C. VDRL test
D. None of the above

62. Koplik spots are seen in
A. Small pox B. Measles
C. Rubella D. Typhoid fever

63. Drug of choice for syphilis is
A. Erythromycin
B. Penicillin
C. Fluorquinolones
D. Cephalosporins

64. Decreased platelets are seen in all *except*
A. Disseminated intravascular coagulation
B. Henoch-Schonlein purpura
C. Myelo fibrosis
D. All of the above

65. The antihypertensive which causes gingival hyperplasia is
A. Metoprolol
B. Nifedipine
C. Hydralazine
D. Sodium nitroprusside

66. First line drugs for treatment of tuberculosis are all *except*
A. Isoniozide B. Rifampicin
C. Ethambutol D. Oflaxacin

67. Diagnostic test for bronchiectases is
A. Bronchoscopy
B. X-ray chest
C. CT scan
D. Pulmonary function test

68. In Kaposi sarcoma, all are true *except*
A. Cutaneous vascular disease
B. Rarely invasive
C. Koebner phenomenon present
D. Lymph node involvement implies metastasis and poor prognosis

69. Antibody found in SLE is
A. AMA B. Anti ds DNA
C. Anti RNA D. Anti ss DNA

70. Treatment of choice in SLE is
A. Indomethacin
B. Steroids
C. Phenylbutamine
D. None of the above

71. Diagnostic of infective endocarditis is
A. Serial blood culture
B. Antistreptolysin
C. ASO titre
D. None of the above

72. Treatment of geographic tongue is
A. Vitamin B_1 B. Vitamin B_{12}
C. Nothing D. Scrapping

73. Cancrum oris is
A. Localised gangrene of cheek
B. Multiple oral ulceration
C. Ca cheek
D. Pus accumulation in floor of mouth

74. Oral hairy leukoplakia is one of the clinical manifestations seen in
A. Tertiary syphilis
B. Mucocutaneous candidiasis
C. HIV infection
D. Leukoedema

75. Macroglossia may be seen in
A. Prader-willi syndrome
B. Moon biedl syndrome
C. Down's syndrome
D. Turner's syndrome

76. Treatment of choice for Vincent's angina/ Trench mouth is
A. Penicillin + Metronidazole
B. Amphotercin B
C. Tetracyclines
D. Streptomycin

77. Macroglossia seen in
A. Down's syndrome
B. Acromegaly
C. Amyloidosis (Primary)
D. All of the above

78. Strawberry tongue seen in
A. Rheumatic fever
B. Scarlet fever
C. Infectious mono nucleosis
D. Infective endocarditits

79. Fordyce's disease is
A. Ectopic sebaceous glands
B. Ectopic sweat glands
C. Hypertrophied mucosa
D. None of the above

80. Large teeth are associated with all *except*
A. Maternal diabetes
B. Maternal hypothyroidism
C. Large birth size
D. Maternal hypoparathyroidism

81. Dental caries is associated with
A. Diabetes mellitus
B. Sjögren's syndrome
C. Increased fluoride
D. All of the above

82. Enamel hypoplasia is caused by
A. Tetracyclines use in childhood
B. Vit D resistant rickets
C. Hypoparathyroidism
D. All of the above

83. Gingival hyperplasia is seen with
A. Phenytoin use
B. Nifedipine use
C. Idiopathic familial gingival fibromatosis
D. All of the above

84. Chancre is seen in below mentioned stage of syphilis
A. Primary B. Secondary
C. Tertiary D. None of the above

85. Pathognomonic of erythema multiforme is
A. Bullae formation
B. Target lesions
C. Crust formation
D. Vesicular eruption

86. Sulphur granules are seen in
A. Candidiasis
B. Actinomycosis
C. Histoplasmosis
D. Blastomycosis

87. Pain in tongue, pharynx, soft palate triggered by swallowing
A. Post herpatic neuralgia
B. Glossopharyngeal neuralgia
C. Trigeminal neuralgia
D. None of the above

88. Treatment modalities for trigeminal neuralgia is
A. Carbamazepine
B. Phenytoin
C. Surgical intervention
D. All of the above

89. Treatment of choice for cervico facial actinomycosis
A. Steroids
B. Antifungal
C. Tetracycline or penicillins
D. Cephalosporin

90. Acute leukaemia in adults is usually
A. Lymphoblastic type
B. Myeloblastic type
C. Undifferentiated type
D. None of the above

91. The level of Neutrophil alkaline phosphatase in polycythemia is
A. Decreased
B. Increased
C. In normal range
D. None of the above

92. In diurnal variation of body temperature, highest temperature is at
A. 2 AM to 4 AM B. Midnight
C. 4 PM to 6 PM D. Noon

93. Drug of choice in acute migraine is
A. Methylsergide
B. Ergotamine
C. Sumatriptan
D. Clonidine

94. Rash of measles occurs on following day of illness
A. Fourth B. Seventh
C. Fifth D. Second

95. Skin manifestations in secondary syphilis are all *except*
A. Macular
B. Papular
C. Pustular syphilides
D. Vesicle

96. Most common cause for acute pharyngitis is
A. Viral B. Bacterial
C. Both D. Fungal

97. Treatment of choice for giant cell arteritis is
A. Steroids
B. Indomethacin
C. Methylsergide
D. None of the above

98. EBV is associated with all *except*

A. Bell's palsy
B. Infectious mononucleosis
C. Hepatitis
D. Lannec's cirrhosis

99. The vector of Dengue fever is

A. Tsetse fly
B. Sand fly
C. Aedes aegypti
D. Culex fatigues

100. Commonest opportunistic infection in AIDS in

A. Candidiasis
B. Tuberculosis
C. Cryptococcal
D. Toxoplasma

Answers

1 B (pg. 1791-H) CT scan is considered as the best diagnostic test of acute and chronic pancreatitis and pancreatic tumors.

2 B

3 D (pg. 1728) HAV and HEV are transmitted via oro-faecal route.

4 C (pg. 1647) It is a condition of lower oesophagus in which the squamous epithelium is replaced by columnar epithelium as it is more resistant to acid pepsin damage.

5 B (pg. 1648) Also known as Patterson Kelly syndrome is more common in middle aged females, hypopharyngeal webs cause dysphagia. Also associated is iron deficiency anaemia and angular stomatitis.

6 C (pg. 1651) > 95% of duodenal ulcer occur in first part of duodenum with 90% occurring within first 3 cm of pylorus.

7 C (pg. 1744) Both are enterically transmitted forms of viral hepatitis; A & E are self limiting and do not cause chronic hepatitis.

8 B (pg. 262) Transudative/High gradient ascitis is seen with:

- Cirrhosis of liver
- Portal hypertension
- Congestive heart failure
- Hypoalbuminemia

(Either due to nephrosis or protein loosing enteropathy).

9 A (pg. 580) Ca stomach commonly presents as anaemia, presents as lump in abdomen in long-standing cases only, predicts regional extension. Anaemia seen is of iron deficiency anaemia, 85% of Ca stomach is adeno carcinoma.

10 C (pg. 1028) Any portion of GIT may be effected. However, ileocaecal is the commonest site to be involved.

11 A

12 B

13 C (pg. 218) Generalized oedema/anasarca is seen in CCF, renal failure, hypothyroidism, cirrhosis of liver, beriberi, hyproteinemia, drug induced.

14 A Cardiac massage is done in case of cardiac arrest. It is done with sufficient force to depress the sternum by 3–5 cm at the rate of 80–100/min. Conventional ventilation is given at the rate of 10–12/min.

15 D (pg. 132) Delerium is state of confusion accompanied by agitation, tremor, hallucination and illusion seen in many conditions like—Head injury, seizures, drug toxicity, drug withdrawal, hepatic encephalopathy, uraemic encephalopathy, meningitis, systemic infections, encephalitis, chronic demyelinating disease, cardiac failure.

16 B (pg. 972) Diagnosis of enteric fever is by

Blood culture (single or serial)	–	1st week
Widal test	–	2nd week
Stool culture	–	3rd week
Urine culture	–	4th week

However, widal test is not much helpful.

17 B (pg. 90) Thermoregulatory centre is located in hypothalamus.

18 A

19 D (pg. 92) Fever is caused by increase levels of PGE_2 in hypothalamic tissue and V_3. PGE_2 are increased by pyrogenic cytokines like IL–1, IL–6, TNF which are released from cells.

20 A (pg. 170) Roth spots are white centered retinal haemorrhages seen in fundus. Also seen in cases of anaemia, leukemias. DM in typhoid fever—Rose spots are seen.

21 C (pg. 216) Selective bulbous enlargement of distal segment of finger and toes due to proliferation of connective tissue on dorsal surface results in clubbing. It is seen in affecting following systems and associated conditions:

For example:

• Cardiac	- Cyanotic CHD - Infective endocarditis
• Pulmonary	- Lung abscess, Metastatic Ca to lung
• Bronchiectasis	- ILD fibrosis
• Cystic	
• Mesothelioma	
• Ca Lung	
• Cirrhosis liver	
• IBD	
• Heriditary	
• Idiopathic	
• Regional enteritis	

22 A Mild def of Zn results in stunted growth, impaired immune function. Severe deficiency results in hypogonadism and hypopigmentation of skin.

23 B (pg. 463) B3 (Niacin) deficiency results in pellagra characterized by 4 D's—Dementia, Diarrhoea, Dermititis leading to death.

24 D (pg. 7501) Vitamin C is required for synthesis of hydroxy proline → an essential component of collagen synthesis deficiency of vitamin C leads ↓ synthesis of collagen and hence ↓ supportive connective tissue around vessels leading to bleeding.

25 A (pg. 758) Oral anticoagulant therapy patients are at an increased risk of bleeding and thus need monitoring by PT.

26 A (pg. 677) Pernicious anaemia is caused by Intrinsic factor (IF) deficiency leading to B_{12} deficiency.

27 D

28 A (pg. 919) Tetanus is caused by C tetani which is characterised by generalized increased muscle tone and spasms. Sustained contractions of facial muscles results in grimace-Risus sardonicus.

29 C (pg. 738) HCV is considered as most common cause of transfusion hepatitis followed by HBV.

30 C

31 A

32 A

33 B (pg. 1343) Commonest valve effected in RHD is mitral leading to MS in maximum cases.

34 A

35 A

36 B (pg. 1342) It is an evanescent muscular eruptions with rounded borders with concentrate on trunk uncommon manifestation. Seen in < 10% of cases one of major criteria for diagnosis of RF.

37 C (pg. 750) Haemophilia A is due to deficiency of factor VIII while Haemophilia B is due to deficiency of factor IX.

38 B (pg. 193) S. mutans is the causative organism for dental caries.

39 B (pg. 1046) Localized or diffused symmetric meno-cutaneous lesions in form of rash are the commonest presentation of 2° syphilis.

40 A (pg. 649) Seen in cases of syphilis, Hutchinson's teeth are centrally placed, widely notches, upper central incisors.

41 B

42 A

43 B

44 D

45 A (pg. 458) These are the corneal opacities seen with vitamin A deficiency.

46 D

47 C (pg. 1116) Pearly flesh coloured umbilicated skin lesions seen anywhere on body except palms and soles are due to molluscum contagium caused by HPV.

48 A (Riboflavin/pg. 462) deficiency is manifested as lesions of meuocutaneous and skin, corneal vascularization, anemia and personality changes.

49 B (Still's/pg. 97) disease is an auto immune disease characterised by high spiking fever, polyarthritis, splenomegaly neutropenia, erythematous papules, ESR > 100 mm FHR.

50 B

51 C (Herpes zoster/pg. 1107) is the sequence of reactivation of latent VZV from the dorsal root ganglia.

52 D (pg. 1258) S1 is loudened in cases of:

- if diastole is shortened because of tachycardia
- high cardiac output state like anaemia, pregnancy
- short PR interval
- prolonged AV flow as in MS.

53 C (pg. 1284) Sinus bradycardia is < 60/min and Sinus tachycardia is > 100/ min.

54 B Jone's criteria is for RF and Dukes criteria for infective endocarditis.

55 A (pg. 2299) MVP occurs at an early age but the commonest valvular lesion seen in AR.

56 C Median nerve entrapment is called as carpel tunnel syndrome. It is seen in case of:

- Pregnancy
- Trauma
- Hypothyroidism
- Oedema
- Osteoarthritis
- Inflammatory arthritis
- Infiltrative disorders like amyloidosis.

57 A Idiopathic is the most common from of facial paralysis. Other causes include:

- Acoustic neuroma
- Lyme Disease
- Diabetes Mellitus
- Leprosy
- Guilliane Barré syndrome
- Ramsay hunt syndrome
- Multiple sclerosis

58 D

59 A

60 D (pg. 1956) Behcet's syndrome comprises recurrent oral and genital ulceration, eye lesions and skin involvement in form of folliculitis, erythema nodosum.

Superficial or DVT is seen arthritis seen does not cause any deformity.

Diagnosed on basis of Pathergy test.

61 A (pg. 1110) Paul Bunnd test is used for IM diagnosis. It is a test in which the antibodies (heterophile) are detected in the serum.

It is +ve in 40% of patient during first week of illness and in 80-90% during 3rd week.

Tests remain +ve for 3 months.

62 B (pg. 324, 1143) Seen in measles in which symptoms there are prodromal of covyza, cough, conjunctivitis followed by koplik spots on buccal mucosa which are 1-2 mm blue-white spots on a bright red background. Typically located on the buccal mucosa along side the second molars, may be extensive not associated with any other infectious disease. Spots disappear after the onset of rash.

63 B (pg. 1050) Penicillin is the drug of choice for all stages of syphilis. Other antibiotics effects are Tc, Erythromycin and Cephalosporins.

64 D (pg. 745) Causes of Myeloproliferative include:

1. Narrow aplasia/hypoplasia
2. Fibrous of marrow
3. Infiltration of BM by malignant cells in lymphoma myeloproliferative, disorders
4. Drugs like Heparin, penicillins
5. Congenital hypoplasia
6. Splenomegaly
7. Vasculitis
8. HUS
9. TTP, DIC
10. ITP
11. Non-immunologic thrombocytopenia
12. Intravascular prosthesis.

65 B (pg. 194) Phenytoxin and Nifedipine causes fibrous hyperplasia of the gingiva. Also seen in idiopathic familial gingival fibromatosis.

66 D First line of drugs for treatment of TB are Isoniozid, Rifampin, Pyrazinamide, Ethambutol and Streptomycin.

Second line of drugs are:

Capreomycin	Viomycin
Amikain	Etkionamide
Kanamycin	Cydoserive

Para aminosalicylic acid

Thiacetazone

Newer antituberculous drugs are:

Rifabutin, Rifapentive, Quinolones

67 C (pg. 1486) High resolution CT scan of chest is the diagnostic of Bronchiectasis. Others include: Bronchiectasis, chest X-ray.

68 B

69 B (pg. 1925, Table 311.1) ANA is the screening tests in SLE. >95% of the patients will have ANA. However, a positive test is not diagnostic for SLE.

Ab to dSDNA is most specific for D/g of SLE. It is seen is 70%. It is disease specific.

70 B (pg. 1927) Glucocorticoids are the DOC for treatment of SLE. Other cytotoxic drugs like AZP, cyclophosphamide, chlorambucil, are also used.

71 A (pg. 812) A total of 3 blood culture sets, separated by 1 hour. Should be obtained over 24 hours from different venipuncture sites.

It is the Major Duke's criteria for D/g of IE.

72 C (pg. 198) Also known as benign migratomy glostitis. It is asymptomatic inflammatory condition of tongue, which requires only diagnosis and no treatment.

73 A (pg. 191) Cancrum oris is a fulminant gangrenous infection of the oral and facial tissues that occurs in severely malnourished and debilitated patients.

Begins as a necrotic ulcer in gingiva of the mandible and is caused by oral anaerobes. Treatment—High dose penicillin, debridement.

74 C (pg. 197) Whitish areas ranging from small and flat to extensive and heavy, found in HIV carriers, rarely causes discomfort. Recurrences high.

75 C (pg. 198)

- Down's syndrome
- Tumour (Hemangioma or lymphangioma)
- 1° Anyloidosis
- Acromegaly
- Cretinism

76 A (pg. 191) Also c/o as acute neurotizing ulcerative gingivilis or trench mouth is caused by oral anaerobes and treatment is with oral penicillin + Metronidazole or with clindamycin alone.

77 D *Refer* Question No. 75.

78 B (pg. 198) "Strawberry" and "Raspberry" tongue is seen in scarlet fever due to hypertrophy of fungiform papillae and changes in filliform papillae.

79 A (pg. 197) These are small yellowish spots seen just beneath the surface of buccal and labial mucosa which is due to ectopic sebaclous glands.

80 D (pg. 194) Large teeth are associated with

- Maternal diabetes
- Maternal hypothyroidism
- Large birth size

81 D (pg. 193) Dental caries are associated with:

- Any
- Medications
- Cancer therapy patients
- Increased flouride.

82 D (pg. 194) Enamel hypoplasia of the primary and/or permanent teeth may be caused by disturbances of calcium and phosphate metabolism such as:

- Vit D resistance rickets
- Hypoparathyroidism
- Tc use in childhood
- Celiac disease
- Gastroenteritis

83 D *Refer* Question No. 65.

84 A (pg. 195) Lesions appear as small papule on lips, tongue or tonsillar area developing rapidly into large, painless ulcer with indicated border, unilateral lymphadenopathy.

Serological tests are +ve by 3rd/4th week. Healing of chancre virus in 1-2 months followed by 2° syphilis in 6-8 weeks.

85 B (pg. 196)
- Onset of lesions is very rapid.
- Intraoral bullae which rupture are lesion.
- Lesions also appear on skin of hands and feet.
- Ruptured bullae are surrounded by inflammatory area with appearance of iris or target lesions.

Treatment—Steroids.

86 B Sulphur granules area due to gm +ve mycelia and their hyphae.

87 B (pg. 199) Symptoms triggered by swallowing along the distribution of IXth cranial nerve is c/o as glossopharyngeal neuralgia.

88 D (pg. 199)

89 C (pg. 196)
- Prognosis is excellant
- Treatment—Tc or penicillins
- No antifungals.

90 A Acute leukaemia in children is usually lymphoblastic type.

91 B A raised neutrophil alkaline phosphatase strongly suggests the diagnosis of polycythemia versa provided the infection or other causes of phosphatase increase are absent.

92 C (pg. 90) In diurnal variation; low temperature is at 6.00 a.m. and highest temperature at 4.00-6.00 p.m.

93 C (pg. 76) Triptans which are selective. $5HT_1$ receptors agonists are treatment of choice in acute attack with β blockers in prophylactic treatment.

94 C

95 D (pg. 1046) Skin rash in 2° typhyllis is macular, papular, papillosquamous and occasionally pustular syphilides.

96 A (pg. 191) Of viral the commonest is by Rhinovirus, influenza and parainfluenza virus.

97 A (pg. 1964)

98 D (pg. 1109)

EBV causes
- Infectious mononucleosis
- Nasopharyngeal Ca
- Burkitt's lymphoma
- Infectious hepatitis
- Hodgkin's disease
- B cell lymphoma in immunodeficiencies.

99 C (pg. 1154)

100 A (pg. 194)

Reference: **Harrison's Principles of Internal Medicine (14th Edition).**

Notes

Syllabus

1. Introduction to surgery, surgery especially related to Oro-dental surgery, Classification of diseases.
2. Inflammation: Soft-tissue, hard tissue-Cause, varieties sequelae and treatment.
3. Infections—Acute and Chronic Abscess, Carbuncle Sinus, Fistula, Ulceration, Gangrene, Cellulitis, Erysipelas, Septicaemia, Pyaemia, Toxaemia, Cancrum Oris, Tuberculosis, Syphilis, Gonorrhea, Actinomycosis, Anthrax, Tetanus.
4. Wounds—Complications, Treatment, Repairs Asepsis and Antiseptic measures and procedure with particular reference to the Oral cavity. Haemorrhage and its treatment Haemophillia, Syncope, Shock, Collapse, Head Injury—Introduction.
5. Cysts and new growths—Their general consideration with special reference to those occurring in the Buccal Cavity.
6. Diseases of the Lymphatic glands, especially of the neck.
7. Outline of diseases of the mouth, lips, tongue, palate, tonsils and salivary glands.
8. Infections and diseases of the Larynx, Tracheostomy.
9. Nervous system—Injury to Facial nerves, Paralysis, Trigeminal Neuralgia.
10. Principles of surgical treatment, diathermy and radium treatment.
11. Fracture—General principles of treatment, Diathermy and healing.
12. Cleft lip and cleft palate.
13. Thyroid and Parathyroid.
14. Swellings of Jaws.

Chapter 9

General Surgery

1. 'Cold abscess' is found in

A. Syphilis **B.** Tuberculosis

C. Leprosy **D.** Typhoid

2. The place where one should look for icterus in jaundice is

A. Forehead

B. Palms of hands

C. Sclera of eyeball

D. None of the above

3. Vesicles are

A. Elevations of horny layer of the epidermis by collection of transparent or milky fluid within

B. Those which blanch on pressure

C. Flat edematous elevations of skin accompanied by itching

D. Alterations in colour of skin

4. The symptomless and symmetrical synovitis with boggy fluid distension of both knee joints in congenital syphilis is known as

A. Charcot's joint

B. Pseudo joint

C. Clutton's joint

D. Osteochondritis

5. The syndrome of acute appendicitis where pain comes first vomiting, and fever comes last of all is

A. Murphy's syndrome

B. Paget's syndrome

C. Greenspan's syndrome

D. Milian's sign

6. Neurilemmoma is otherwise known as

A. Local neurofibroma

B. Plexiform neurofibromatosis

C. Naevolipoma

D. Schwannoma

7. Ulcers seen in postoperative wounds with undermined margins and lot of granulation tissue in the floor are

A. Varicose ulcers

B. Meleney's ulcers

C. Martorel's ulcers

D. Infective ulcers

8. Pulsation of popliteal artery is felt

A. Behind the medial malleolus

B. At the wrist

C. Behind the knees

D. At the groin

9. Gordon's biological test in which an emulsion of affected human lymphnodes is injected into a rabbit intracerebrally that will initiate encephalitis is specific of

A. Hodgkin's disease

B. Syphilis

C. Tuberculosis

D. Filariasis

10. "Endolymphatic therapy" is done for
A. Secondary carcinoma
B. Acute lymphadenitis
C. Malignant melanoma
D. Filariasis

11. Which of the following lesion arises from the reticulum cells of diaphysial medullar cavity?
A. Ewing's tumour
B. Fibrosarcoma
C. Osteoclastoma
D. Chondromyxoid fibroma

12. 'Rotator Cuff' comprises how many muscles?
A. Three B. Four
C. Two D. Five

13. A 'Proctoscope' is used to inspect
A. The interior of bile ducts
B. Anal canal and lower rectum
C. The duodenum
D. Entire length of large bowel

14. Thiersch's grafts are
A. Full thickness grafts
B. Medium thickness grafts
C. Dermis only
D. Epidermis only

15. When there is division of a nerve with loss of cutaneous sensation and flaccid paralysis, it is called
A. Neuropraxia B. Neurotmesis
C. Axonotmesis D. Neuralgia

16. 'Cytokines' are secretions of
A. Proteins or peptides
B. Fatty tissues
C. Carbohydrates
D. Adrenaline

17. Implantation dermoid cysts are found at the sites of
A. Injury
B. Embryonic fusion
C. Junction of outer and upper margins of orbit
D. Tumors

18. Pain, redness and swelling at the side and base of a nail which may spread and involve the underlying pulp space is called
A. Onychogryphosis
B. Koilonychia
C. Paronychia
D. Septonychia

19. Excess secretion of growth hormone results in
A. Cushing's syndrome
B. Hypoparathyroidism
C. Acromegaly
D. Nelson's syndrome

20. Sodium retention results in
A. Hypertension with headaches and visual disturbances
B. Hypotension and tinnitus
C. Hyperkalemia
D. Bilateral adrenal hyperplasia

21. Which of the following is not a part of Fallot's tetralogy?
A. Obstruction of right ventricular outflow
B. Ventricular septal defect
C. Right ventricular hypertrophy
D. Pulmonary artery hyperplasia

22. Occlusion of subclavian artery (Subclavean steal") leads to
A. ↑ed blood pressure in the arm
B. ↓ed blood pressure in the arm
C. No change in blood pressure of arm
D. Claudication and tiredness in lower limb

23. The five 'Ps' of acute ischaemia are
A. Pallor, pressure, pain, paraesthesia, paralysis
B. Parotitis, Pallor, Paralysis, Pain, Poikilothermia
C. Pallor, Pain, Paraesthesia, Paralysis, Poikilothermia
D. Pallor, Paraesthesia, Pain, Papillomas, Peptic ulcer

24. A red-blue discolouration of skin on exposure to cold that turns bright pink when warm is known as
A. Acrocyanosis
B. Takayasu's arteritis
C. Cold injury
D. Raynaud' phenomenon

25. Irreducibility, obstruction, strangulation are complications of
A. Acute mesenteric adenitis
B. Hernias
C. Hematoma of rectus sheath
D. Ascites

26. Hypoglossal nerve involvement leads to
A. Paralysis of soft palate
B. Paralysis of tongue
C. Numbness over cheeks
D. Anaesthesia of tongue

27. 'Bronze diabetes" is a term used for
A. Hereditary neuropathic amyloidosis
B. Diabetes mellitus and pigmentary liver cirrhosis
C. Skin pigmentation and diabetes mellitus
D. Insulin dependent diabetes

28. The classical view of the metabolic response to injury has
A. Ebb and flow phases
B. Only flow phase
C. Septic phase
D. Diuresis phase

29. The principal intracellular cation is
A. Sodium B. Chloride
C. Potassium D. Nitrogen

30. In Acidosis
A. Hydrogen ions in ECF move out of the cells and potassium ions move into the cells from ECF
B. ↓ serum potassium concentration with ↓ excretion in urine
C. ↑ Serum sodium concentration in ECF
D. Hydrogen ions in the ECF move into the cells and equal amount of potassium ions move out of the cells into ECF.

31. If production of urine is less than 400 ml in 24 hours the condition is known as
A. Anuria B. Nocturea
C. Oliguria D. Polyurea

32. α Fetoprotein is a specific tumor marker which originates likely from
A. Bronchus and pancreas
B. Prostate and testis
C. Liver and testis
D. Ovary and chorion

33. 'Melanotic whitlow' is
A. Chronic inflammation beneath the nail
B. Carcinoma of nail bed
C. Pigmentation behind the ear
D. Pigmentation of palms and soles

34. "Cirsoid aneurysm" is a variant of
A. Portwine stain
B. Capillary hemangioma
C. Cavernous hemangioma
D. Strawberry angioma

35. In 'Carpal Tunnel' syndrome the following nerve is compressed
A. Ulnar nerve
B. Median nerve
C. Radial nerve
D. None of the above

36. Cardiac arrhythmias are more common with
A. Non-toxic goitre
B. Adenomas
C. Toxic multinodular goitre
D. Hypothyroidism

37. Sites of action of parathormone are
A. Renal and skeletal systems
B. Muscular and renal systems
C. Skeletal and vascular systems
D. Vascular and nervous system

38. 'Mineralocorticoids' are secreted from
A. Zona glomerulosa
B. Zona reticularis
C. Zona fasciculata
D. Zona spinosa

39. 'Aldosterone' secretion is controlled by
- **A.** Adrenal medulla
- **B.** Adrenal cortex
- **C.** Anterior pituitary
- **D.** Pancreas

40. 'Pheochromocytomas' are tumors that secrete
- **A.** Adrenaline and calcitonin
- **B.** Adrenaline and noradrenaline
- **C.** Cortisol and corticosterone
- **D.** Glucocorticoids

41. Cardiopulmonary bypass is a means of
- **A.** Removing arterial blood from the body, deoxygenating it and returning it to the systemic arterial system.
- **B.** Hyperoxygenating the myocardium and cooling it with high potassium content
- **C.** Removing systemic venous blood from the body, oxygenating it and returning it to systemic arterial system
- **D.** Resection of aortic coarctation to avoid hypertension and its complications

42. Rheumatic fever most commonly affects
- **A.** Mitral valve
- **B.** Aortic valve
- **C.** Pulmonary valve
- **D.** Tricuspid valve

43. Arterial septal defects result in
- **A.** Shunting of blood from lt. to rt. atrium
- **B.** Shunting of blood from right to left atrium
- **C.** Pulmonary artery blood bypassing the lungs
- **D.** Shunting of blood from left to right ventricle

44. 'Sunset foot' results from
- **A.** Reddening of the limbs on elevation
- **B.** Reddening on dependency
- **C.** Cyanosed (bluish) discolouration of limbs
- **D.** Hypertension

45. High protein oedema is due to
- **A.** Failure of lymphatics to remove interstitial protein
- **B.** Failure of lymphatics to remove dead cells
- **C.** Abnormally high net fluid filtration
- **D.** Abnormally high net nitrogen diffusion

46. Branchial cysts arise from failure of fusion of
- **A.** 1st and 2nd branchial arches
- **B.** 2nd and 3rd branchial arches
- **C.** 3rd and 4th branchial pouches
- **D.** 4th and 5th branchial arches

47. Cystic hygroma is a form of
- **A.** Lymphangio-endothelioma
- **B.** Lymphangiosarcoma
- **C.** Benign lymphangioma
- **D.** Teratoma

48. Secretions of submandibular salivary gland is predominantly
- **A.** Serous and rich in fluoride
- **B.** Mucous and rich is sodium
- **C.** Mucous and rich in calcium
- **D.** Serous and rich in phosphorus

49. Mumps affects
- **A.** Parotid glands (Unilateral)
- **B.** Submandibular glands (Unilateral)
- **C.** Submandibular glands (Bilateral)
- **D.** Parotid glands (Bilateral)

50. 'Chemodectoma' arises from
- **A.** Chemoreceptor cells within the carotid body
- **B.** Chemoreceptor cells within the carotid sinus
- **C.** Baroreceptor cells within the carotid sinus
- **D.** Baroreceptor cells within the carotid body

51. Concave and spoon shaped nail is peculiar to
- **A.** Achalasia
- **B.** Squamous cell carcinoma
- **C.** Pott's disease
- **D.** Paterson-Kelly syndrome

52. The pain of acute appendicitis usually starts in

A. Early morning **B.** Afternoon
C. Night **D.** Any time

53. Lines joining the umbilicus, right anterior superior iliac spine and symphysis pubis form

A. Cordman's triangle
B. Sherren's triangle
C. Cullen's sign
D. Boa's sign

54. "Coffee ground" vomiting is seen in cases of

A. Cholecystitis and intestinal obstruction
B. Duodenal ulcer
C. Carcinoma and gastric ulcers
D. Pyloric stenosis and pancreatitis

55. Gall bladder disease characterized by a dislike for fatty foods is called

A. Quantitative dyspepsia
B. Quantitative dysphagia
C. Qualitative hunger
D. Qualitative dyspepsia

56. If superficial veins are engorged on the sides of the abdomen, it implies

A. Obstruction of portal system
B. Obstruction of superior vena cava
C. Obstruction of inferior vena cava
D. Abdominal distension

57. Enlargement of which of the following group of lymphnodes in carcinoma of stomach is known as Troisier's sign?

A. Jugulo diagastric
B. Jugulo-omohyoid
C. Facial
D. Left supraclavicular

58. A bruit may be heard over

A. Aneurysm
B. Giant cell granuloma
C. Venous angioma
D. Sarcoma

59. The carcinoma of tongue which results in the tongue being transformed into an indurated mass is known as

A. Nodular type tongue
B. Warty type tongue
C. Cracked type tongue
D. Frozen type tongue

60. In Joffroy's sign there is

A. A fine tremor of hands on writing
B. Lagging behind of the upper eyelid when the patient looks downwards
C. Absence of wrinkling of the forehead on looking upwards with the face inclined downwards
D. Tachycardia or ↑ed pulse rate without rise of temperature

61. In renal ricket, the kidneys are unable to excrete

A. Phosphorus
B. Nitrogen
C. Calcium
D. Sodium

62. The X-ray appearance of a mixture of 'bubbles and strips' can be seen in

A. Solitary cyst
B. Von Reckling Hausen's disease
C. Monostotic fibrous dysplasia
D. Rickets

63. Early mental retardation, absence of ligament laxity, cardiopulmonary complications and presence of dermatan sulphate and heparin sulphate in urine is seen in

A. Morquio-Brails ford disease
B. Hurler's disease
C. Ollier's disease
D. Cleido-cranial dysostosis

64. Marrow biopsy is helpful in diagnosing

A. Multiple myeloma
B. Multiple exostoses
C. Myositis ossificans
D. Basal cell carcinoma

65. The artery which is felt at the wrist on the medial side of its volar is
- **A.** Brachial artery
- **B.** Radial artery
- **C.** Femoral artery
- **D.** Ulnar artery

66. 'Adson test' is done to detect compression of
- **A.** Subclavian artery
- **B.** Femoral artery
- **C.** Brachial artery
- **D.** Superficial temporal artery

67. Swellings in connection with vessels and nerves
- **A.** Move along the line of the said vessel or nerve
- **B.** Do not move along the line of the said vessel or nerve
- **C.** Move along with the adjacent tendons
- **D.** Move parallel to the associated structure

68. Raised and pearly-white beaded edge is a feature of
- **A.** Deep trophic ulcer
- **B.** Squamous cell carcinoma
- **C.** Rodent ulcer
- **D.** Venous ulcer

69. In diabetic gangrene, the gangrenous part becomes
- **A.** Dry and mummified
- **B.** Wet and putrefying
- **C.** Putrefying with presence of crepitus
- **D.** Necrosed and infected with aerobic bacteria

70. Intermittent bouts of remittent fever is quite peculiar to
- **A.** Hodgkin's disease
- **B.** Non-Hodgkin's lymphoma
- **C.** Tuberculosis
- **D.** Actinomycosis

71. 'Lymphoedema'means
- **A.** Accumulation of lymph within the tissues
- **B.** Accumulation of lymph within blood vessels
- **C.** Accumulation of plasma within lymph-nodes
- **D.** Accumulation of serum within lymph-nodes

72. The muscle which swings the thumb across the palm to touch the tips of other fingers is
- **A.** Lateral half of profundus
- **B.** Abductor policies brevis
- **C.** Flexor pollicis longus
- **D.** Opponens pollicis

73. A very significant finding in Hodgkin's disease is
- **A.** Casseous and tender lymphadenitis
- **B.** Splenic enlargement
- **C.** Pain induced by chewing tobacco
- **D.** Weight gain

74. The lesion of Brachial plexus caused by injury which leads to forcible ↑ of the angle between the neck and shoulder thus stretching the upper trunk of the plexus is known as
- **A.** Klumpke's paralysis
- **B.** Erb-Duchenne paralysis
- **C.** Brachial causalgia
- **D.** Clawhand deformity

75. Paralysis of long thoracic nerve of bell results in
- **A.** Wrist drop
- **B.** Clawhand deformity
- **C.** Foot drop
- **D.** Winging of scapula

76. The deltoid, supra- and infraspinatus and Teres minor are
- **A.** Abductors and lateral rotators of shoulder
- **B.** Extensors and medial rotators of shoulder
- **C.** Flexors and supinators of elbow
- **D.** Adductors and extensors of wrist joint

77. The muscle which is tested by asking the patient to elevate the shoulder against gravity is
- **A.** Serratus anterior
- **B.** Platysma
- **C.** Sternomastoid
- **D.** Trapezius

78. The appreciation of gross touch is known as
- **A.** Epicritic sensation
- **B.** Protopathic sensation
- **C.** Asteriognosis
- **D.** Sensation of "Pins and needles"

79. The presence of sulphur granules in the discharge of a sinus suggests
- **A.** Tuberculosis
- **B.** Osteomyelitis
- **C.** Actinomycosis
- **D.** Crohn's disease

80. Raynaud's disease affects
- **A.** The muscles **B.** Circulation
- **C.** Sensation **D.** Skeletal system

81. Sympathetic effusion of the neighbouring joints is a common feature of
- **A.** Osteoclastoma
- **B.** Chondrosarcoma
- **C.** Acute osteomyelitis
- **D.** Multiple myeloma

82. A rise in the level of serum acid phosphatase is characteristic of
- **A.** Multiple myeloma
- **B.** Acute osteomyelitis
- **C.** Osteitis deformans
- **D.** Prostatic metastasis

83. Excess callus formation at the site of trauma may be seen in
- **A.** Myositis ossificans
- **B.** Syphilitic osteitis
- **C.** Osteogenesis imperfecta
- **D.** Fibrous dysplasia

84. Sometimes in osteosarcoma, the tumor may be pulsatile. This is called
- **A.** Codman's osteosarcoma
- **B.** Telangiectatic osteosarcoma
- **C.** Periosteal osteosarcoma
- **D.** Plasmacytoma osteosarcoma

85. The fracture which is seen most commonly in the neck of the 2nd metatarsal bone due to repeated stress is known as
- **A.** March fracture
- **B.** Spiral fracture
- **C.** Butterfly fracture
- **D.** Crushing fracture

86. In fracture non-union, there will be
- **A.** No gap between the fracture ends
- **B.** Gap between the bone ends with radiolucency of the bony edges
- **C.** Presence of sclerosis at the bone ends and a gap between them
- **D.** Moth eaten appearance of the newbone formed between fracture segments

87. Pain and stiffness of the fingers, hyperaesthesia and moistness of ankle and patchy rarefaction of bone in the region of fracture is diagnostic of
- **A.** Osteo-arthritis
- **B.** Myositis ossificans
- **C.** Tardy ulnar palsy
- **D.** Sudeck's osteodystrophy

88. 'Melon seed' bodies which are fibrinous loose bodies resulting from haemorrhagic or inflammatory effusion are found in
- **A.** Osteochondromatosis
- **B.** Acute arthritis
- **C.** Tuberculous joints
- **D.** Haemophilliac joint

89. Bleeding from the ear or mouth indicates fracture of
- **A.** Anterior cranial fossa
- **B.** Middle cranial fossa
- **C.** Posterior cranial fossa
- **D.** Orbital floor

90. In extra-dural haemorrhage, after a period of initial uncosciousness (stage of cerebral concussion) there will be a stage of consciousness which is known as
A. Cerebral irritation
B. Cerebral contusion
C. Flaccid interval
D. Lucid interval

91. In paralysis of which of the following nerves, the tip of the tongue points to the paralysed side?
A. Glossopharyngeal nerve
B. Facial nerve
C. Hypoglossal nerve
D. Chordatympani nerve

92. When scratching the skin at the upper and inner part of the thigh, the testis will be drawn upwards. This is known as
A. Plantar reflex
B. Ankle jerk
C. Cremasteric reflex
D. Bell's reflex

93. Basophil adenoma gives rise to
A. Cushing syndrome
B. Medulloblastoma
C. Gigantism in children
D. Acromegaly in adults

94. Which of the following produces a sessile swelling, purplish in colour?
A. Fibrous epulis
B. Carcinomatous epulis
C. Sarcomatous epulis
D. Myelomatous epulis

95. 'Median mental sinus' is produced by an apical abscess of
A. Upper incisors
B. Lower incisors
C. Upper canine
D. Lower canine

96. The organism which is responsible for black hairy tongue is a
A. Bacteria
B. Virus
C. Fungus
D. Algae

97. Post-pertusis ulcer which occurs only in children with whooping cough, is usually seen at
A. Labial frenum
B. Lingual frenum
C. Hard and soft palate
D. Floor of the mouth

98. Which of the following salivary gland ducts open in the cheek opposite the crown of the upper second molar tooth?
A. Stensen's duct
B. Wharton's duct
C. Bartholin's duct
D. Minor salivary gland duct

99. When Warthin's tumor becomes devoid of lymphoid element and is composed entirely of epithelium, it is called
A. Mucoepidermoid tumour
B. Adenoid cystic carcinoma
C. Oxyphil adenoma
D. Pleomorphic adenoma

100. 'Surgical emphysema' means
A. Air in the lungs
B. Fluid in muscles
C. Air in pleural cavity
D. Air in subcutaneous tissue

Answers

1 B This abscess is cold and non-reacting in nature. It does not produce hot and painful abscess as seen in pyogenic infections. It is almost always a sequal of tubercular infection commonly in lymphnodes and bone.

2 C In jaundice the pigment that gets deposited in tissues is bilirubin. As bilirubin has an affinity for elastic tissue, one should look for icterus in the sclera of the eyeball which is made of elastic tissue.

3 A (B) is erythema, (C) is wheel and (D) is macule.

4 C (A) Charcot's joint is characterised by little pain and marked bone destruction leading to abnormal mobility of the joint associated with coarse crepitus.

Osteochondritis includes 3 distinctive types—crushing, splitting and pulling osteochondritis.

5 A

6 D

7 B Varicose ulcers are usually seen in the upper part of the limb and eczema and pigmentation are seen around the ulcer with discharge. Martorell's ulcers are found mostly in calves of older individiuals suffering from hypertension and take months to heal. Infective ulcers may be that of tuberculous or syphilitic in origin. But nowadays these ulcers have become rare and rather staph. aureus ulcers are becoming common among the infective kind which take the form of multiple small, red, scabbed sores on the leg or ankle.

8 C Posterior tibial artery is felt behind medial malleolus. Radial and Ulnar arteries are at the wrist on the lateral and medial sides of the volar aspect respectively. Femoral artery is felt at the groin.

9 A

10 C In malignant melanoma, sometimes radioactive phosphorus is added to the radio-opaque dye for lymphangiography. This will destroy the malignant cells in the lymphnodes. This process is called 'endolymphatic therapy'.

11 A

12 B

13 B In proctoscopy, haemorrhoids can be injected or banded, while carcinomas can be biopsied. Proctoscopy is usually undertaken with the patient lying in the left lateral position with the knees drawn up into the chest. The instrument is passed upwards into the direction of the axis of anal canal.

14 D

15 B (A) is transient loss of physiological function after slight injury. There is no loss of continuity and no degeneration: recovery occurs within 6 weeks, (C) Follows compression or traction damage, continuity of the nerve sheath is maintained but there is wallerian degeneration of the nerve fibres beyond repair. Recovery occurs by regeneration and growht of the axons, and (D) is pain due to nerve involvement in a pathology or compression etc.

16 A Cytokines are proteins e.g. IL-1, IL-6 and TNF which act as inflammatory mediators and contribute to such manifestations as pyrexia and acute phase response.

17 A It is a traumatic swelling and results from the surface ectoderm being driven into the subjacent tissue. This is commonly seen in a finger or a hand from a needle prick or prick with a thorn.

18 C

19 C It results in overgrowth of soft tissues of hands, feet and face, giving the patient large extremities and a characteristically coarse face with bulging supraorbital ridges and protruding jaw. Endochondral ossification and periosteal new bone formation account for some of these changes. All viscera are enlarged and there is muscle hypertrophy along with other systemic malfunction, (A) is due to excess seirction of corticosteroids, (B) in hypo parathyroidism, there is a ↓ in ionized clacium levels and PTH levels, and (D) is due to compression of optic chiasma by an adenoma.

20 A

21 D

22 B The commonest site of occulsion is the 1st part of subclavian artery which results in ↓ed BP in the arm and compensatory reversal of flow down the vertebral artery to supply the limb.

23 C

24 A (B) is a rare inflammatory disease mainly affecting the aortic arch vessels in young Asian women where progressive ischaemia of the arms and brain may occur (C) this is frostbite mostly affecting the elderly and alcoholics, which is marked by swelling redness and blistering followed by infection and superficial gangrene (D) In Raynaud's phenomenon, there is digital artery constriction resulting in white, numb and painful fingers due to exposure to cold.

25 B

26 B

27 C

28 A The short 'Ebb' phase corresponds to the period of traumatic shock and the 'Flow' phase has two parts. Initial catabolic phase is characterised by protein and fat mobilization with an associated ↑ in urinary nitrogen excretion and weight loss and usually lasts for 3-8 days. This is followed by an anabolic phase lasting for some weeks during which protein and fat stores are replenished and weight is regained.

29 C Whereas (A) is the principal extracellular cation.

30 D (A) represents alkalosis.

31 C (A) is less than 20 ml urine production in 24 hrs; (B) is excess urination at night, and (C) is excessive urination.

32 C Other specific tumour markers are: Human chorionic gonadotropin from chorion and testis; carcinoembryonic antigen from Bronchus and pancreas; CA 125 from ovary; and acid phosphatase and prostate specific antigen from prostate.

33 A

34 C Here, the mass of vein like structures is fed directly by arterial blood and becomes tortuous, dilated and pulsating mostly in the scalp.

35 B The median nerve is compressed as it runs below the flexor retinaculum at the wrist leading usually to nocturnal pain in the thumb and lateral three fingers, disturbance of sensation, and wasting of the muscles supplied by the median nerve.

36 C

37 A Parathormone mobilizes calcium from bone by stimulating osteoclastic activity. It ↑es renal phosphate excretion and calcium reabsorption and promotes renal conversion of less active forms of vitamin D to the highly active form 1-25, dihydroxycholecalciferol.

38 A (B) and (C) secrete glucocorticoids and androgenic steroids and DHA-S.

39 B (A) Secretes the catecholamines (adrenaline 80% and noradrenaline 20%) along with dopamine which is a precursor of noradrenaline. (C) secretes growth hormone, prolactin, ACTH, Leuteinizing hormone, follicle stimulating hormone and thyroid stimulating hormone. (D) The pancreas has exocrine as well as endocrine functions. It secretes (exocrine) 1-2 liters of enzyme rich alkaline juice/24 hrs which contains enzymes like trypsin, lypase, amylase. Pancreas has 4 types (endocrine) of islet cells i.e. A, B, D and PP cells which produce glucagon, insulin, somatostatin and pancreatic polypeptide respectively.

40 B

41 C By this method, blood is returned to the systemic arterial system at reasonably physiological pressure, devoid of gas bubbles or solid particles at a controlled temperature and at a rate capable of maintaining normal tissue metabolism.

42 A (B) and (D) can also be due to Rheumatic fever but are less affected as compared to (A); (C) is due usually to congenital stenosis with commonly fusion or hypoplasia of the valve annulus.

43 A

44 B 'Sunset foot' is a sign of chronically ischemic limb where the skin is thin and dry; on elevation of the leg, there is marked pallor and on hanging it down, it becomes bright red (dependant rubor).

45 A (C) is low protein edema.

46 B

47 C It is usually present at birth and can cause problems during delivery. There are multilocular cysts containing clear lymphatic fluid and are lined by endothelium can be present any where in the head and neck region and most commonly in supraclavicular triangle which may extend into the axilla or mediastinum to cause pressure symptoms. It usually regresses as the child grows, but when the cyst causes pressure symptoms, it has to be surgically removed under general anaesthesia.

48 C

49 D Mumps is viral parotitis which usually subsides with symptomatic treatment.

50 A These tumors are relatively symptomless and present as swellings in the region of carotid-bifurcation. In younger individuals it should be excised surgically after a confirmed diagnosis by carotid angiography. In older individuals it should be left as such.

51 D Associated with Anaemia and a tongue which is smooth, pale and devoid of papillae.

52 A Sudden pain which occurs around afternoon is due to perforation of a peptic ulcer (B).

53 B Presence of hyperaesthesia in this area is a guide to diagnose gangrenous appendicitis. If the hyperaesthesia disappears during the process of illness, it indicates the bursting of the gangrenous appendix. (D) is an area of hyperaesthesia between 9th and 11th ribs posteriorly on the right side suggestive of acute cholecystitis.

54 C 'Coffee ground' vomitting occurs due to slow haemorrhage in the stomach.

55 D

56 C (A) leads to venous engorgement around the umbilicus.

57 D

58 A

59 D

60 C (A), (B), (C) and (D) all are primary toxic manifestations of goitres affecting young individuals.

61 A In this condition, the kidneys are unable to excrete phosphorus properly due to developmental defect of the renal tubules or some organic disease affecting the kidney. The blood phosphate level ↑es and is secreted in the gut to combine with calcium so the serum calcium level falls resulting in excess parathormone secretion leading to the rickety condition.

62 C The lamellar pattern of the affected bone is replaced by multiple cysts and fibrous bands which may be calcified to give the X-ray appearance of a mixture of bubbles and strips.

63 B In (A) the vertebae is too flat, hip is grossly distorted, ligaments are markedly lax and there is presence of keratan sulphate in urine. The main defect in (C) is ossification of cartilage at growth discs resulting in short limb which is affected. The fingers and toes frequently contain multiple endochondromata (D) mainly affects the membranous bones mostly the clavicles and skull. The patient is short with a large head and drooping shoulders. As the clavicles are absent partly, the two shoulders of the patient can be brought in front of the chest.

64 A Numerous plasma cells will be present in the marrow which is diagnostic of multiple myeloma.

65 D (B) is felt on the lateral side of its volar whereas (A) is felt in front of the elbow just medial to the biceps tendon and (C) is felt at the groin, just below the inguinal ligament midway between anterior superior iliac spine and symphysis pubis.

66 A The patient sits on a stool and is instructed to take a deep breath in and to turn the face to the affected side. His radial pulse is examined which is often obliterated due to compression of the subclavian artery.

67 B They usually move to a little extent at right angles to their axes.

68 C This type of edge develops in invasive cellular disease and becomes necrotic at the centre. Punched out edge is seen in (A); rolled out (everted) edges is characteristic of (B) and sloping edge is seen in (D).

69 B

70 A

71 A It mainly affects the subcutaneous tissues of limbs and is due to stagnation of lymph within the lymphatics.

72 D Patient with paralysis of this muscle will be unable to do this movement which is supplied by the median nerve.

73 B

74 B Where the arm hangs by the side of the body and internally rotated with forearm extended at the elbow and fully pronated. It is described as the "policeman receiving the tip" deformity.

75 D There is paralysis of extensors of wrist joint; (A) is seen in paralysis of radial nerve, (B) is due to paralysis of interossei and lumbricals in combined lesions of ulnar and median nerves, (C) is due to paralysis of lateral popliteal nerve.

76 A

77 D This is to know the extent of damage to the accessory nerve.

78 B

79 C Actinomycosis israeli is the organism responsible for this disease which for mycelae, that appear as sulphur granules under the microscope.

80 B

81 C

82 D

83 A This condition occurs when the haematoma under the stripped periosteum is invaded by osteoblasts and becomes ossified. It is mostly marked where periosteum is loosely attached to bone.

84 B

85 A This is also called stress injury which is due to unaccustomed overuse e.g. after long march past. The patient will complain of a tender limb palpable at the neck or at the midshaft of 2nd metatarsal bone.

86 C

87 D

88 C

89 B

90 D

91 C If (A) is paralyzed, there is loss of sensation of posterior one third of tongue and back of the phanynx; If (B) is paralyzed, the nasolabial fold and furrows of the brow are less marked on the affected side. The angle of mouth is drawn towards the sound side. Patient will be unable to close the eye on the affected side and if (D) is paralyzed, there is loss of special sensation from the anterior one-third of tongue.

92 C (A) is flexion of the great toe when the inner or outer border of the foot is scratched. (B) is tested by slight dorsiflexon of the foot followed by a gentle stroke on the back of the Achillis tendon resulting in contraction of the calf muscles and a sharp plantar flexion of the foot.

93 A Gigantism and acromegaly are due to hyperpituitarism meduloblastoma is an intracranial space occupying tumor of childhood.

94 D (A) is a slow growing firm mass, (B) is otherwise known as epitheliama, (C) grows more rapidly with a softer feel and bleeds more readily.

95 B

96 C

97 B

98 A (B) open on either side of frenulum linguae; (C) opens in the floor of the mouth and (D) can open anywhere in the mouth i.e. palate, lips, cheek, floor of the mouth and tongue etc.

99 C Majority of (A) which most commonly affect the parotid glands are slow growing and may be solid, cystic or semicystic there are cords or sheets of serous, mucous or intermediate cells, (B) are poorly encapsulated infiltrating tumors. The tumor cells which are small are arranged about the stromal elements in an adenoid pattern which is highly hyalinized, and (D) it is a mixed tumor which contains epithelial as well as cartilage cells.

100 D

Syllabus

1. Concept and philosophy of public health and dental public health.
2. Health care system in India.
3. Concept and levels of Prevention of Dentistry.
4. Principles and methods of epidemiology.
5. Indices used in oral epidemiology.
6. Basic principles of bio-statistics and presentation of data.
7. Health education.
8. Role of 'Fluoride' in human health.
9. Pit and fissure sealants.
10. Incremental and comprehensive dental care.
11. School dental health programmes.
12. Payment for dental care.
13. Epidemiology and prevention of common dental health problems, viz.
    a. Dental caries
    b. Periodontal diseases
    c. Oral cancer
    d. Dento-facial anomalies, etc.
14. Ethical code of conduct for dentists.
15. Prominent health agencies, viz.
    a. Dental Council of India
    b. Indian Dental Association
    c. World Health Organization, etc.
16. Environmental health issues, viz.
    a. Biomedical waste management
    b. Safe water and sanitation, etc.
17. Social sciences including behaviour management as applied to health.
18. Oral health survey.
19. Planning and evaluation.
20. Dental manpower including auxiliaries.

Chapter 10

Preventive and Community Dentistry

1. **The following is a "Treatment Index"**
   A. PMA index
   B. Oral Hygiene index
   C. Periodontal disease index
   D. DMFT index
2. **Armamentarium required to record Periodontal Index is**
   A. Mouth mirror
   B. Sufficient illumination
   C. Probe
   D. None of the above
3. **Shick-Ash modified one of the components of**
   A. Plaque index
   B. Periodontal disease index
   C. Fluorosis index
   D. Oral hygiene index
4. **Gingival Index score of "1" signifies**
   A. Mild gingivitis
   B. Severe gingivitis
   C. Simple gingivitis
   D. Moderate gingivitis
5. **Components of periodontal disease index do not include**
   A. Periodontal B. Gingival
   C. Plaque D. Alveolar
6. **The most important attribute of a confirmatory test is**
   A. Sensitivity
   B. Specificity
   C. Predictive value
   D. Reliability
7. **Clinical sign that is graded as 4 on a periodontal index is**
   A. Tooth mobility
   B. Loss of epithelial attachment
   C. Gingivitis
   D. None of the above
8. **Score given for a tooth having subgingival flecks of calculus according to Oral Hygiene Index-(S) is**
   A. 1 B. 2
   C. 3 D. 4
9. **Average probing force used in a CPITN recording is**
   A. 5 grams B. 15 grams
   C. 25 grams D. 50 grams
10. **Summative score of "2" for the periodontal index denotes**
    A. Beginning destructive periodontal disease
    B. Terminal disease
    C. Irreversible periodontal disease
    D. Simple gingivitis
11. **Feature(s) differentiating a clinical probe from an epidemiologic probe in a CPITN study is/are**
    A. Ball diameter
    B. Graduations of the probe
    C. Length of the black band
    D. All of the above

12. Number of tooth surfaces examined in an oral Hygiene Index (original) are

A. 6 B. 12
C. 24 D. 148

13. A potential cause of "Bias" in a clinical trial that aims to study the efficacy of different toothpastes could be

A. Calibrating
B. Blinding
C. Training
D. Confounding

14. A non-sampling error in a study can be limited by

A. Using different examiners
B. Selecting adequate number of subjects
C. Using calibrated instruments
D. All of the above

15. "Odds Ratio" is calculated in the following epidemiologic investigation

A. Descriptive study
B. Follow-up study
C. Retrospective study
D. Cohort study

16. Treatment need for a status code of 4 on the CPITN is

A. TN1 B. TN2
C. TN3 D. TN4

17. A study design that would not be appropriate to conduct an "Observational investigation" on Periodontitis is

A. Ecological study
B. Case-control study
C. Field trial
D. Cross-sectional study

18. Disclosing solution indicated for use in the original periodontal disease index is

A. Erythrosin B. Bismarck brown
C. Basic fuschin D. Gention violet

19. Total number of tooth surfaces examined in modified navy plaque index are

A. 4 B. 7
C. 9 D. 11

20. University of Michigan "O" Probe is recommended for use in

A. PMA Index
B. Navy plaque index
C. Periodontal disease index
D. Calculus surface index

21. Loe and Silness proposed their index in the year

A. 1953 B. 1958
C. 1963 D. 1964

22. "Incidence" of Oral submucous fibrosis can be best used for

A. Estimating disease magnitude
B. Planning and administrative purposes
C. Understanding etiology and pathogenesis
D. All of the above

23. Cases of Juvenile periodontitis are usually

A. Epidemic
B. Endemic
C. Exotic
D. Sporadic

24. Root caries is assuming epidemic proportions among

A. Tobacco chewers
B. Males
C. Alcoholics
D. Elderly

25. Periodontitis during pregnancy is associated with the following sign(s) in the newborn

A. Low birth weight
B. Cleft lip and palate
C. Geographic tongue
D. All of the above

26. CPITN cannot be used on

A. An individual
B. A community
C. Primary schoolchildren
D. None of the above

27. Periodontitis can be a potential causative factor for the following systemic ailment(s)
- **A.** Rheumatoid arthritis
- **B.** Diabetes mellitus
- **C.** Osteoarthritis
- **D.** All of the above

28. Development of oral thrush among HIV + ve patients can be calculated as
- **A.** Cumulative incidence
- **B.** Attack rate
- **C.** Episodic incidence
- **D.** All of the above

29. Relative risk of Leukoplakia among smokers as compared to non-smokers can be analyzed from
- **A.** Cross-sectional studies
- **B.** Retrospective studies
- **C.** Community trial
- **D.** Incidence studies

30. An investigator prefers using plaque index over DMFT index for assessing efficacy of tooth brushing because it is
- **A.** Valid **B.** Full mouth index
- **C.** Irreversible **D.** All of the above

31. Glass index is used to measure
- **A.** Debris **B.** Plaque
- **C.** Calculus **D.** Dental caries

32. Massler and Schour developed
- **A.** Modified Navy plaque index
- **B.** Plaque control record
- **C.** Patient hygiene performance index
- **D.** PMA index

33. Code of "X" in CPITN is used to denote
- **A.** Extracted **B.** Excavated
- **C.** Excluded **D.** Examined

34. Teeth that are popularly known as "Ramfjords' Teeth" are
- **A.** 16, 21, 24, 36, 41, 44
- **B.** 16, 11, 26, 36, 31, 46
- **C.** 16, 12, 24, 36, 32, 44
- **D.** 17, 16, 11, 26, 27, 37, 36, 31, 46, 47

35. Index/indices not used for assessing malocclusion is/are
- **A.** Occlusal index
- **B.** PAR index
- **C.** Eastman esthetic index
- **D.** None of the above

36. Highest prevalence of gingivitis is seen during
- **A.** Pregnancy
- **B.** Puberty
- **C.** Elderly age
- **D.** All of the above

37. Intra-examiner bias in a study of oral cancer would hamper the following aspect(s) of an otherwise ideal study
- **A.** Reliability
- **B.** Internal-validity
- **C.** External-validity
- **D.** All of the above

38. Sulcus bleeding index was given by
- **A.** Podshadly and Haley
- **B.** Muhleman et al
- **C.** Quietly and Hein
- **D.** Turesky-Gilmore-Glickman

39. Periodontitis would generally exhibits a correlation coefficient of -0.5 with
- **A.** Age **B.** Residence
- **C.** Education **D.** Sex

40. Primary factor in the etiology of periodontal disease is
- **A.** Adverse habits
- **B.** Bacteria
- **C.** Nutrition
- **D.** Professional dental care

41. Region(s) of the oral cavity most vulnerable to gingivitis is/are
- **A.** Palatal aspect of upper teeth
- **B.** Interproximal areas of all teeth
- **C.** Buccal aspect of lower teeth
- **D.** Labial aspect of upper front teeth

42. Intra-oral occurrence of gingivitis is usually higher in
- **A.** Left half of the arch
- **B.** Right half of the arch
- **C.** Front teeth
- **D.** All teeth simultaneously

43. Dental caries and periodontal diseases are both
- **A.** Infectious diseases
- **B.** Dependent on each other
- **C.** Having variable etiology
- **D.** None of the above

44. Risk factors for Malocclusion do not include
- **A.** Race
- **B.** Sex
- **C.** Age
- **D.** None of the above

45. Pin-point bleeding on palpation on the gingival index is given a score of
- **A.** 1
- **B.** 2
- **C.** 3
- **D.** 4

46. "M" component of PMA index denotes
- **A.** Mesial
- **B.** Missing
- **C.** Massler
- **D.** None of the above

47. When one of the index (molar) teeth in Patient Hygiene performance index is less than 3/4th erupted, the recording is made of
- **A.** The same tooth
- **B.** The adjacent molar
- **C.** The adjacent premolar
- **D.** None of the above

48. Index/indices similar to CPITN is/are
- **A.** Periodontal screening and recording index
- **B.** Community periodontal index
- **C.** Primary essential periodontal examination
- **D.** All of the above

49. Oral epidemiologic index/indices popularly known as clinicians modification of periodontal index is/are
- **A.** CPITN
- **B.** PI
- **C.** PDI
- **D.** All of the above

50. If an index tooth in periodontal disease index presents with 3 mm recession and a sulcus depth of 3 mm, the periodontal component score for that tooth is
- **A.** 4
- **B.** 5
- **C.** 6
- **D.** 7

51. A young lady patient reports to the Dental Operatory with opaque spots on her teeth that involve more than 50% of the exposed tooth surface. Based on Dean's index, the following statements best interpret this condition
- **A.** Questionable fluorosis
- **B.** Mild fluorosis
- **C.** Moderate fluorosis
- **D.** Severe fluorosis

52. Age-group ideally suited for a "deft index" study is
- **A.** 3-7 years
- **B.** < 6 years
- **C.** 7-11 years
- **D.** < 12 years

53. Following sign is not considered as indicative of tooth decay according to WHO
- **A.** Discolouration
- **B.** Cavitation
- **C.** Softened wall
- **D.** None of the above

54. Findings of a DMFS index study in which an upper right first molar tooth has been coded by a red colour is indicative of
- **A.** 5 decayed surfaces
- **B.** 4 filled surfaces
- **C.** 4 decayed surfaces
- **D.** 5 missing surfaces

55. A technique used to avoid selection bias in case-control studies is
- **A.** Matching
- **B.** Randomization
- **C.** Blinding
- **D.** All of the above

56. AIDS is best classified as
- **A.** Point source epidemic
- **B.** Multiple exposure epidemic
- **C.** Cyclic epidemic
- **D.** Propagated epidemic

57. A figure of choice for presenting discrete data is

A. Histogram
B. Bar chart
C. Frequency polygon
D. None of the above

58. A type of ratio is

A. Incidence B. Prevalence
C. Relative risk D. All of the above

59. An advantage of concurrent cohort studies over other observational studies is that they

A. Save time
B. Are less costly
C. Calculate attributable risk
D. Calculate Odd's ratio

60. Concepts of "Health" do not include

A. Health for all
B. Ecological
C. Psycho-social
D. Holistic

61. The popular definition of "Dental Public Health" has been adapted from

A. Last JM B. Winslow CEA
C. Dean TH D. Russell AL

62. Most statistically significant difference in the occurrence of oral cancer between two groups can be deduced by following

A. $p < 0.05$ B. $r = +1$
C. $p = 0.001$ D. $p < 0.01$

63. In order to compare whether prevalence of anterior tooth injuries is higher in males as compared to female subjects a test of choice would be

A. Chi-square test
B. Student's t-test
C. Paired t-test
D. ANOVA

64. Sampling technique recommended for National oral health survey is

A. Simple Random
B. Stratified cluster
C. Systematic random
D. Non-random

65. Teeth that are least susceptible to dental caries are

A. Upper second molars
B. Upper incisors
C. Lower second premolars
D. Lower canines

66. National oral health survey of India was conducted by Dental Council of India in

A. 1921 B. 1948
C. 1976 D. 2002

67. The most suitable method of conducting health education for a nuclear family is

A. Lecture
B. Workshop
C. Group discussion
D. Personal interview

68. Prevalence can be calculated by

A. Incidence/Duration
B. Duration X Incidence
C. Incidence X number of cases
D. Duration/number of cases

69. Disease rate is ideally calculated as

A. Cases/Population at risk/1,000
B. Cases/Total population/1,00,000
C. Cases/Total population
D. Cases/population at risk/Total population/10,000

70. A description of "Colorado brown stains" was first documented by

A. Louis Pasteur
B. Pierre Fauchard
C. Trendley H Dean
D. Fredrick Mckay

71. Following is an investigation done to assess the caries activity in an individual

A. Mantoux test
B. Alban's test
C. Paul Bunnell test
D. Widal test

72. Artificial community water fluoridation began in
A. 1857 B. 1878
C. 1912 D. 1945

73. A descriptive epidemiological study can be conducted in the form of
A. Clinical examination
B. Interview
C. Questionnaire
D. All of the above

74. Spectrum of health includes the following dimensions *except*
A. Social dimension
B. Vocational dimension
C. Emotional dimension
D. None of the above

75. Ideal requirements of an index do not include
A. Acceptability B. Sensitivity
C. Subjectivity D. Simplicity

76. Lactobacillus colony count of 500 signifies
A. Slight caries activity
B. Moderate caries activity
C. Marked caries activity
D. Caries activity is absent

77. Tuberculosis can be most appropriately classified as a disease that is
A. Contagious
B. Communicable
C. Exclusively zoonotic
D. All of the above

78. A distribution that is skewed towards the right side of the graph is known as
A. Positively skewed distribution
B. Negatively skewed distribution
C. Gaussian distribution
D. None of the above

79. Acceptable concentration of fluoride in commercially available dentifrices is
A. 1 ppm B. 10 mg in 1 gram
C. 100 ppm D. 0.7% w/w

80. "Disability limitation" is
A. Primary level of prevention
B. Secondary level of prevention
C. Tertiary level of prevention
D. Primordial prevention

81. Following are registered dental auxiliaries in India
A. Dental licentiates
B. Dental chairside assistants
C. Dental laboratory technicians
D. All of the above

82. An index used for recording a patient's plaque status on a nominal scale is
A. Plaque control record
B. Oral hygiene index
C. Plaque index
D. Plaque component of PDI

83. New dental auxiliary types include
A. Denturist
B. Dental secretary
C. Dental aid
D. Expanded function dental auxiliary

84. Dentist Act was introduced in
A. 1957 B. 1920
C. 1942 D. 1948

85. Measure most appropriate for calculating central tendency is
A. Mode
B. Mean Deviation
C. Median
D. All of the above

86. Communication is not influenced by
A. Physiological barriers
B. Psychological barriers
C. Pathological barriers
D. Environmental barriers

87. Most suitable statistical diagram to depict the trend of oral cancer in Indian subcontinent during the last decade is
A. Bar chart
B. Line diagram
C. Frequency polygon
D. Pie chart

88. Standard deviation is calculated by the formula

A. $(\bar{x}\text{-}x)/n$ B. $(\bar{x}\text{-}x)^2/\sqrt{n}$
C. $(\bar{x}\text{-}x)/\sqrt{n}$ D. $\sqrt{(\bar{x}\text{-}x)^2/n}$

89. Objectives of health education include

A. Conducting survey
B. Providing care to patients
C. Guiding people into action
D. All of the above

90. The UCR concept for reimbursing Dentist's professional fee has been adopted by

A. Budget payment plans
B. Medicare plans
C. Third party plans
D. All of the above

91. The following country is not a member of WHO South-East Asia Region

A. Thailand B. Maldives
C. Bhutan D. Mauritius

92. Test cities used to study benefits of artificial community water fluoridation were

A. Grand Rapids, Kingston, Sarnia, Oak Park
B. Muskegon, Newburgh, Brantford, Evanston
C. Muskegon, Grand Rapids, Kingston, Oak Park
D. Grand Rapids, Newburgh, Brantford, Evanston

93. A suitable method of recycling solid waste is

A. Dumping B. Incineration
C. Composting D. All of the above

94. Potable water should be

A. Soft
B. Hard
C. Moderately hard
D. Very hard

95. Principles of Primary Health Care include

A. Environmental sanitation
B. Community participation
C. Health education
D. All of the above

96. The following is a mismatch

A. 0.02%-NaF mouthrinse
B. 1.23%-Brudevold solution
C. 1000 ppm-monofluorophosphate in dentifrice
D. 250 ppm-NaF in salt

97. Important conclusion(s) of Hopewood house study was/were

A. Oral hygiene and dental caries are not inter-related
B. Clearance time of sugar correlates closely with caries activity
C. Fructose group was as cariogenic as sucrose group in the first year and became less so at the end of second year
D. All of the above

98. Following statement is not true about human behaviour

A. Culture influences behaviour
B. Behavior sciences include study of anthropology
C. Behaviour can be shaped pharmacologically
D. None of the above

99. Mumbai is the Head office of

A. Indian dental association
B. Indian association of public health dentistry
C. Dental council of India
D. All of the above

100. Revised national health policy 2002 does not prescribe

A. Eradication of polio by year 2005
B. Providing free services for all secondary and tertiary health care services
C. Participation of private sector in all areas of health activities
D. Free provision of essential drugs at primary health centres

Answers

1 D 'M' and 'T' components of DMFT index are measures of treatment.

2 C

3 B

4 A Scores between 0.1 to 1.0 on gingival index signify mild gingivitis.

5 D 'Calculus' is another component of periodontal disease index.

6 B The ability of the test to identify those not having the disease.

Condition of interest

Test Result	Present	Absent
Positive	a True Positive	b False Positive
Negative	c False Negative	d True Negative

Sensitivity : $\frac{a}{a + c}$

Specificity : $\frac{d}{b + d}$

7 D A score of 4 on periodontal index is given only when radiographs are used.

8 B

9 C

10 C Established destructive periodontal diseases.

11 B Additional graduations are present at 8.5 mm and 11.5 mm in a clinical probe.

12 B

13 D 'A', 'B', and 'C' limit bias.

14 C 'A' can increase the error while 'B' will reduce error in sampling.

15 C

16 C

17 C Field trials are interventional investigations.

18 B

19 C Modified Navy Plaque Index.

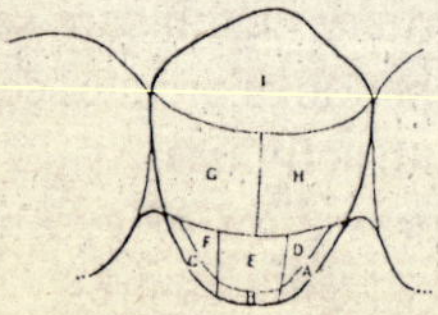

20 C

21 C Gingival index.

22 C Prevalence is an estimate of disease magnitide and can also be used for planning and administrative purposes.

23 D The word sporadic means scattered about. The cases occur irregularly, haphazardly and generally infrequently.

24 D

25 A

26 D

27 B

28 D

29 D Incidence studies are another name of cohort studies.

30 A Toothbrushing removes plaque that can be recorded by plaque index.

31 A

32 D

33 C

34 A

35 D

36 B

37 D 'A' is reproductility 'B' is the degree to which the results of an observation are correct and 'C' is the extent to which the results of a study apply to people not in it.

38 B

39 C Education is inversely correlated with periodontitis.

40 B Plaque is the chief etiological agent causing periodontal disease.

41 B

42 A

43 A Both the diseases are caused by bacteria derived from plaque, although of different strains.

44 B Malocclusion prevalence is not significantly distinct between males and females.

45 B

46 D PMA is abbreviated form of papillary-*marginal attached* (Gingiva) Index.

47 B

48 D

49 C

50 B CEJ to gingival margin – 3 mm. Gingival margin to crevice bottom = 3 mm. Loss of periodontal attachment = 3 – (– 3) = 6 mm

PDI score = 5

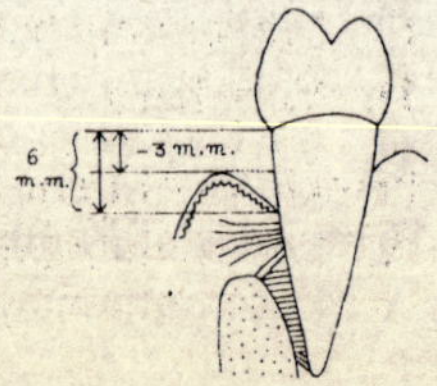

51 C Criteria for questionable fluorosis is presence of few white flecks, mild fluorosis is involvement of > 25% but < 50% of exposed tooth surfaces and severe fluorosis is corroded appearance of tooth.

52 C Mixed dentition period.

53 A

54 D Red colour is for missing tooth, black for decayed and silver for filled. A posterior tooth has 5 surfaces and an anterior tooth has 4.

55 A

56 D Propagated epidemics spread by person to person transmission.

57 B 'A' and 'C' figures are used for continuous data.

58 C

59 C 'A, B and D' are advantages of case-control studies.

60 A "Health for all" is the contemporary phase of public health.

61 B

62 C

63 A

64 B

65 D

66 D

67 D 'A, B and C' are means of group health education.

68 B

69 A 'B' is disease prevalence 'C' and 'D' are inadequate/inappropriate calculations.

70 D

71 B Alban's test is modified synder's test.

72 D

73 D

74 D 'A, B and C' are various dimensions of health.

75 C An index should be objective.

76 D Lactobacillus colony count upto 1000 signifies little or no caries activity.

77 B Tuberculosis does not spread by mere contact with man or animal.

78 A

79 D 1000 ppm (approximately).

80 C

81 C Dental laboratory technicians are known as dental mechanics in India.

82 A 'B, C and D' are interval scales.

83 C

84 D

85 C

86 C 'C' is an inappropriate term.

87 B

88 D 'A' is the formula for calculating mean deviation. B and C' are inappropriate formulae.

89 C

90 C 'A' is post-payment plan and 'B' is a public program.

91 D Mauritius is a member of WHO-African region.

92 D

93 C 'A and B' methods cannot recycle waste.

94 C

95 B 'A and C' are elements of primary health care.

96 A Mouthrinse contains 0.2% NaF.

97 A

98 C Behaviour shaping is a psychologic process.

99 A

100 B

Notes

Syllabus

I. Course outline for complete denture prosthetics:

1. Introduction to Prosthodontics.
2. Diagnosis and treatment planning.
3. Improving patient's denture foundation and ridge relations.
4. Objective of impression making with special emphasis on retention stability and support.
5. Biologic considerations—Maxillary impression and Maxillary impression procedure.
6. Biologic consideration—Mandibular impression.
7. Mandibular impression procedure.
8. Occlusal rims, recording and transfer of jaw relations.
9. Biologic consideration of jaw relation and jaw movements.
10. Articulators.
11. Biologic consideration of vertical jaw relation.
12. Biologic consideration of horizontal jaw relation (centric and ecentric).
13. Relating patient to articulator.
14. Selection of artificial teeth.
15. Occlusion.
16. Arrangement of teeth.
17. Appearance and functional harmony of denture bases.
18. Completion of try in and perfection of posterior palatal seal.
19. Processing of denture-remount procedure-occlusal equilibration finishing and polishing.
20. Completion of rehabilitation of patient.
21. Maintaining comfort and health of oral cavity of rehabilitated patients.
22. Immediate denture treatment.
23. Single complete denture.
24. Rebasing and relining CD.

II. Course outline for removable partial denture prosthodontics:

1. Introduction to removable partial denture prosthesis.
2. Terminology.
3. Classification.
4. Components of removable partial dentures.
5. Support for removable partial denture.
6. Impression registration (Impression materials) and procedures.
7. The diagnostic cast and its uses.
8. The surveyor and its uses.
9. The oral examination to precede prosthodontics.
10. Treatment planning and mouth preparation removable partial denture service (RPD).
11. Units of RPD—Functions and requisites of earth.
12. Stresses induced by RPD and practical measures for their control.
13. Designing of RPD.
14. Instruction for the patient receiving RPD service.

III. Course outline for fixed partial prosthodontics:

1. Introduction to fixed partial dental prosthodontics.
2. Diagnosis and treatment planning to fixed partial.
3. Classification of fixed partial dentures.
4. Indication and Contra-indication for FPD.
5. Bioengineering consideration in FPD.
6. Individual Restorations:
   a. Jacket Crown.
   b. Partial Veneer Crown.
   c. Complete Veneer Crown.
   d. Complete Veneer Crown with facing.
   e. Post and Core Preparation.
7. Component parts of fixed partial denture (bridge).
8. Impression procedure—Materials and technique.
9. Casts and Dies preparation.
10. Wax pattern.
11. Sprueing and Investing.
12. Casting, Finishing and Polishing.
13. Soldering.
14. Cementation.
15. Failure in FPD prosthetics—Actiology and Remedy.

IV. Miscellaneous:

1. Implant dentures.
2. Obturators.
3. Splints.
4. Overdentures.

Chapter 11

Prosthodontics and Crown and Bridge

1. Minimum temperature at which Benzoyl peroxide decomposes to free radical is
A. 50°C B. 65°C
C. 60°C D. 75°C

2. For a custom tray what is not true
A. It increases the accuracy of rubber base impression material
B. Reduces stresses during tray removal
C. Reduces the thermal contraction
D. Increases surface area/volume ratio, thereby reduces the dimension changes

3. The temperature of the storage bath for agar is
A. 40°C B. 100°C
C. 65°C D. 85°C

4. What is the Knoop hardness value of enamel?
A. 250 B. 150
C. 350 D. 450

5. If the wet liner in the casting ring is placed too lightly against the inner walls of the casting ring, the expansion will be
A. Increased
B. Decreased
C. Remains the same
D. Can either decrease or increase

6. Major noble metal in dental alloys are all *except*
A. Platinum B. Silver
C. Palladium D. Gold

7. The visible part of electromagnetic spectrum has a wavelength in the range of
A. 380-750 nm B. 380-570 nm
C. 450-750 nm D. 200-650 nm

8. Cast partial denture framework is made of gold alloys should be cast from
A. Type I alloy B. Type II alloy
C. Type III alloy D. Type IV alloy

9. Which is the most favorable site for implant placement?
A. Anterior mandible
B. Posterior mandible
C. Anterior maxilla
D. Posterior maxilla

10. Which of the following are micro-hardness used tests to measure?
A. Knoop–Brinell
B. Brinell–Rockwell
C. Vicker–Knoop
D. Rockwell–Vicker

11. In comparison to normal centrifugal casting machine, in air pressure casting machine the sprue diameter is
A. Larger
B. Smaller
C. Same
D. It makes no difference

12. All can alter normal setting expansion in gypsum-bonded investment, *except*
A. Water powder ratio
B. Ring liner
C. Increased mixing time
D. Length of casting ring

13. Which of the following pontic designs does not touch the mucosa?
A. Ridge lap B. Sanitary
C. Ovate D. Conical

14. To reduce the risk of failure in provisional restoration the connector
A. Must be of bigger size
B. Must be of smaller size
C. Must be placed buccally
D. Must be placed lingually

15. -¾ three quarter crowns, the preparation derives its name from
A. The number of surfaces involved
B. Number of axial walls involved
C. Number of axial walls covered with ceramics
D. Due to the specific rotation of bur in handpiece

16. Most metal ceramic alloys fuse at around
A. 600°C B. 800°C
C. 1000°C D. 1200°C

17. How many grams of high-density noble metal alloy is required for casting of a molar?
A. 3 gms B. 6 gms
C. 9 gms D. 12 gms

18. In CIELAB color system, L is comparable to which component in munsell system
A. Hue B. Chroma
C. Value D. None of the above

19. The floor of the occlusal rest seat should be inclined slightly towards
A. The marginal ridge
B. The center of the tooth
C. The buccal surface
D. The lingual surface

20. Hygroscopic setting expansion is accomplished by submerging the casting ring in a water bath at
A. 80° F B. 100° F
C. 120° F D. 140° F

21. For an upper IInd premolar, what should be the diameter of a wax sprue?
A. 1.5 mm B. 2.0 mm
C. 2.5 mm D. 3.0 mm

22. What factors determine the path of placement and removal of removable partial denture?
A. Retentive areas B. Guiding planes
C. Age of the patient D. Esthetics

23. Partial veneer crown are indicated in which of the following condition?
A. Short span FPD
B. Short clinical crown
C. Posterior teeth with buccal wall intact
D. Posterior teeth with lingual wall intact

24. In gypsum bonded investment, which component is responsible for thermal expansion at 300°C?
A. Gypsum B. Quartz
C. Cristobalite D. Silica

25. In metal ceramic restoration, to avoid fracture ceramic veneer must not exceed the thickness of
A. 1 mm B. 1.5 mm
C. 2 mm D. 0.5 mm

26. What gauge wax relief should be provided prior to duplication of the master cast beneath framework extensions onto ridge areas for attachment of resin bases?
A. 28 gauge B. 20 gauge
C. 10 gauge D. 32 gauge

27. In seven-eight-crown preparation which surface remains intact?
A. Distal half of the buccal surface
B. Mesial half of buccal surface
C. Buccal half of mesial surface
D. Buccal of distal surface

28. Permissible residual ash in inlay wax should be
A. 0.01% B. 0.1%
C. 0.4% D. 0.04%

29. Volumetric shrinkage in porcelain after firing is
A. 0-10% B. 10-20%
C. 20-30% D. 30-40%

30. Flexion of a long span bridge is proportional to
A. The length
B. Square of length
C. Cube of length
D. Square root of length

31. All of the following may be the cause of suck back porosity *except*
A. Too long sprue
B. Too short sprue
C. Too narrow sprue
D. Incorrectly placed sprue

32. Material of choice for tissue surface of pontic is
A. Polished gold
B. Glazed ceramic
C. Smooth resin
D. Metal ceramic restoration

33. Functional impression of class I partially edentulous arches may be made by
A. Reline method
B. Holmes technique
C. Hindel method
D. All of the above

34. Which of the following muscle do not take part in establishing centric relation?
A. Temporalis
B. Masseter
C. Lateral pterygoid
D. Medial pterygoid

35. Partial veneer crown generally includes all tooth surfaces *except*
A. Lingual B. Occlusal
C. Buccal D. Mesial

36. In natural dentition, Cusp–fossa, occlusal scheme is seen most commonly in
A. Class I occlusion
B. Class II malocclusion
C. Class III malocclusion
D. Not seen in natural dentition

37. Centric relation is recorded accurately so that
A. Vertical dimension of occlusion can be determined
B. Facebow transfer can be verified
C. Centric occlusion can be developed in harmony with centric relation
D. Condylar guidance can be measured

38. Backpressure porosity can be prevented by all of the following *except*
A. More porous investment
B. Locating the pattern near the end of the casting ring (6-8 mm)
C. Casting with vacuum technique
D. Increased water powder ratio

39. What is the minimum thickness of metal in metal ceramic restoration to avoid distortion during firing?
A. 0.1 mm B. 0.3 mm
C. 0.5 mm D. 0.7 mm

40. Resistance to horizontal forces is an attribute of complete denture, which is known as
A. Support B. Stability
C. Retention D. Buccal corridor

41. Magnitude of dislodging forces working on crown depends upon all of the following *except*
A. Sticky food
B. Surface area
C. Position of crown in the arch
D. Texture of restoration

42. All can achieve termination of the process of polymerization, *except*
A. Oxygen B. Hydrogen
C. Eugenol D. Hydroquinone

43. **Which of the following is not an objective of bevelling?**
A. To allow cast metal margin to be burnished against the prepared tooth
B. To protect unprepared tooth structure from chipping
C. To minimize marginal discrepancy
D. To increase the surface area and thereby increase the retentive form

44. **In a two-stage endosseous implant, the usual healing time for mandible is**
A. 1 month B. 3 months
C. 6 months D. 9 months

45. **Which of them is an antiflux?**
A. Borax B. Rouge
C. Boric acid D. Silica oxide

46. **For a cylindrical implant to be placed, what is the ideal dimension of horizontal bone available?**
A. 4 mm B. 6 mm
C. 8 mm D. 10 mm

47. **What is the minimum recommended distance between two adjacent implants?**
A. 1 mm B. 2 mm
C. 3 mm D. 4 mm

48. **Which is the most favorable site for implant placement?**
A. Anterior mandible
B. Posterior mandible
C. Anterior maxilla
D. Posterior maxilla

49. **All elastomeric impression materials are hydrophobic, *except***
A. Polysulfide
B. Additional polysilicone
C. Condensation polysilicone
D. Polyether

50. **Gingival retraction cord may have the following chemicals *except***
A. Epinephrine
B. Methyl cellulose
C. Aluminum chloride
D. Ferric sulfate

51. **If the impression has to be poured in epoxy, which of the impression materials cannot be used?**
A. Condensation silicone
B. Reversible hydrocolloids
C. Polyether
D. Additional polysilicone

52. **Outermost part of a gas, air torch is**
A. Reducing B. Combustion
C. Oxidizing D. Mixing

53. **Usually the vertical relation of occlusion on natural dentition**
A. Remain constant
B. Increase with time
C. Decrease with time
D. All of the above

54. **While doing jaw relation what is correct?**
A. First to adjust the fullness of the upper occlusal rim and then visibility of the occlusal rim is adjusted
B. First the visibility of the occlusal rim is adjusted and then to adjust the fullness of the upper occlusal rim
C. It can be done in either ways it makes no difference
D. Both the fullness and the visibility is checked simultaneously

55. **Interocclusal distance is important for**
A. Speech
B. Comfort
C. Denture efficiency
D. All of the above

56. **How much of upper occlusal rim should be visible below the relaxed upper lip?**
A. 0 mm B. 1-2 mm
C. 2-4 mm D. 4-6 mm

57. **Ideally how much of unprepared tooth structure cervical to finish line be discernible on the die**
A. 0-0.5 mm B. 0.5-1 mm
C. 1-1.5 mm D. 1.5-2 mm

58. As per ADA specification number 19 for type IV gypsum material should be able to reproduce ____ wide line
A. 10 µm B. 20 µm
C. 40 µm D. 80 µm

59. Anatomic posterior teeth have ____ cusp
A. 41° B. 33°
C. 22° D. 11°

60. If interocclusal distance is increased, what is true?
A. It will cause increased resorption
B. It causes discomfort in ears
C. It produces clicking sound
D. It produces difficulty in phonation

61. Stoichiometric amount of water needed for setting reaction of gypsum is
A. 18.6 ml B. 22 ml
C. 35 ml D. 48 ml

62. Rotational movement of condyle takes place in
A. Upper compartment
B. Lower compartment
C. Both of them
D. None of them

63. Which of the following is not a cause of wrinkling?
A. Decreased vertical dimension of occlusion
B. Ageing
C. Class II jaw relations
D. Poor lip support

64. Centric relation refers to relation of mandible to maxilla in
A. Anterior-posterior direction
B. Medio-lateral direction
C. Anterior-posterior and medio-lateral direction
D. None of the above

65. Pure rotational movement (without translation) is limited to
A. 6 mm of incisor separation
B. 12 mm of incisor separation
C. 18 mm of incisor separation
D. 24 mm of incisor separation

66. The stability of a complete denture is determined by
A. Arch form of residual ridge
B. Height of the residual ridge
C. Depth of the sulcus
D. Width of the residual ridge

67. Which of the following is not a relief area in maxilla?
A. Incisive papilla B. Rugae
C. Labial frenum D. Buccal frenum

68. Usually the mesio-distal width of upper central incisor is ____ of total bizygomatic measurement
A. 1/6 B. 1/16
C. 1/18 D. 1/20

69. The thickness of the complete denture in the buccal vestibule is determined by
A. Zygomatic process
B. Size of maxillary tuberosity
C. Condylar process
D. Coronoid process

70. Facebow record is used to
A. Orient maxillary cast to the centric relation record
B. Relates mandible to maxilla
C. Orients maxilla to transverse axis of mandible and transfer this orientation to the articulator
D. It facilitates mounting of mandibular cast

71. Which of the following is ideal for retention and stability of maxillary denture?
A. High, V shaped palatal vault
B. Broad flat palate
C. U-shaped palate
D. V-shaped with poorly developed rugae

72. Position of the labial surface of natural maxillary central incisor is ____ anterior to incisive papilla
A. 2-4 B. 4-5
C. 10-14 D. 8-10

73. Which component of circumferential clasp is placed below the survey line?

A. Reciprocal line B. Retentive arm
C. Rest D. Shoulder

74. All of the following factors are responsible for retention of maxillary complete denture *except*

A. Peripheral seal
B. Intimate contact between tissue and denture
C. Oral and facial muscles
D. Quality of soft tissue

75. Retromylohyoid curtain is bounded posteriorly by

A. Superior constrictor
B. Lingual tubercle
C. Mylohyoid muscle
D. Alveolingual sulcus

76. Korecta or Iowa waxes are called physiological waxes because

A. They do not disturb the physiology of the oral cavity
B. They are used during physiological functions of oral cavity
C. They soften at mouth temperature
D. All of the above

77. Vertical dimension of rest

A. Can be more than vertical dimension of occlusion
B. Is less than vertical dimension of occlusion
C. Is same as vertical dimension of occlusion
D. Is variable

78. Mandible is an example of

A. Class I B. Class II
C. Class III D. Class IV

79. Difference between occlusion and articulation is

A. Articulation is static and occlusion is dynamic
B. Arrangement of teeth on articulator is articulation and in mouth is occlusion
C. Articulation is dynamic and occlusion is static
D. Articulation is artificial and occlusion is natural

80. Massetric notch in mandibular complete denture is recorded by the action of masseter muscle upon

A. Buccinator
B. Orbicularis oris
C. Temporalis
D. Pterygo mandibular raphe

81. As an anterior determinant of occlusal form what will be the effect of increased vertical overlap of anterior teeth on posterior cusps?

A. Taller B. Short
C. Flat D. No effect

82. Border movement of mandible were first described by

A. Bennett B. Posselt
C. Schuyler D. Ramfjord

83. Which tooth provides maximum root surface area as an abutment?

A. First maxillary molar
B. First mandibular molar
C. Second maxillary molar
D. Second mandibular molar

84. Gypsum bonded investments are unstable above

A. 550°C B. 600°C
C. 650°C D. 750°C

85. For a crown to seat and have optimum retention all axial walls should have a taper (from cervical to occlusal) of

A. 2° B. 4°
C. 6° D. 8°

86. Opening and closing movement of mandible take place in

A. Sagittal plane
B. Horizontal plane
C. Frontal plane
D. None of the above

87. Food is more easily crushed when it is placed

A. Further back
B. In front
C. In the middle
D. It has no effect

88. One Pascal is equal to

A. 14 psi B. 145 psi
C. 1400 psi D. 14500 psi

89. Which is the best material for the surface hardening of dies?

A. Colloidal silica
B. Cynoacrylates
C. Gum Arabic and calcium hydroxide
D. Resins

90. Unilateral removable partial dentures are contraindicated because of all of the following, *except*

A. Aspiration
B. Lack of cross arch stabilization
C. It causes imbalance of masticatory forces
D. Excessive stress on abutment teeth

91. What type of flux must be used when chromium-cobalt alloys are soldered?

A. Borax
B. Boric acid
C. Graphite
D. Fluoride

92. While using wrought wire for retentive arm, what degree of undercut is desirable?

A. 0.01 inch B. 0.02 inch
C. 0.03 inch D. 0.001 inch

93. Which of the following is a disadvantage of combination clasp?

A. It may be distorted by careless handling
B. They bare more flexible
C. More esthetic
D. More adjustable

94. Flexibility of a clasp depends on all of the following *except*

A. Length of clasp B. Diameter
C. Location D. Material

95. All of the following provide retention to CPD *except*

A. Clasp
B. Accurate adaptation of denture base to tissue
C. Indirect retainer
D. Adaptation of major connector to tissue

96. During lateral movement the orbiting condyle travels

A. Backwards-medially
B. Forward-medially
C. Forward-laterally
D. Backwards-laterally

97. Class II deformity of residual ridges (in pontic selection in a fixed partial denture) is described as

A. Loss of ridge height
B. Loss of facio-lingual space
C. Loss of anterior-posterior space
D. Combination of all three

98. In Kennedy class III CPD; the rest should be able to transfer what percentage of occlusal load to the abutment teeth?

A. 25% B. 50%
C. 75% D. 100%

99. Which of the following is an example of fricative sound?

A. Ch B. J
C. F D. K

100. Minimum thickness of a master cast should be

A. 10-12 mm at the thinnest area
B. 10-12 mm at the thickest area
C. 14-16 mm at the thinnest area
D. 14-16 mm at the thickest area

Answers

1 A Free radical polymerization begins with the formation of free radical and subsequent combination of this free radical with a monomer. Free radicals are formed by the decomposition of a chemical (initiator). Possible initiator includes benzyl peroxide and camphoroquinone. Benzoyl peroxide decomposes to free radicals at approximately 50°C or higher in a process called as thermal activation. Excessive temperatures should be avoided during the early stages of thermal activation because some monomers vaporize as the temperatures nears 100°C.

2 D A custom tray improves the accuracy of an elastomeric impression by limiting the volume of the material, thus reducing two sources of error. Stresses during removal and thermal contraction.

Reverse is true for hydrocolloid impression material for which biggest size of stock tray is selected to reduce the surface area/ volume ratio to reduce the dimensional change due to water loss.

3 C Agar can be liquefied by immersing in boiling water, usually for 8-12 hours depending upon the bulk of the material. When the material is liquefied it can be stored for several hours and kept ready for use by immersing the container in water at 63°C-66°C. When needed the material is taken from the storage bath and placed immediately in a warmed tray. The loaded tray is tempered at 46°C for 2 minutes before it is inserted in the mouth.

4 C The Knoop hardness number of enamel is 343, dentin 68, cementum 40, porcelain 460, cobalt-chromium 390 and denture acrylic 20.

5 B The casting ring holds the investment in place during setting and restricts the expansion of the mold. Normally a liner is placed inside the ring to allow more expansion. Wetting the liner increases the hygroscopic expansion of the mold, but because an absorbent dry liner removes water from the investment and makes a thicker mix the total expansion increases. The liner should not be squeezed against the ring, as this prevents the scope of expansion of the liner and prevents the expansion of the mold.

6 B There are seven noble metals, which are used, in dental casting alloys. They are gold, platinum, palladium, osmium, iridium, rhodium and ruthenium. The noble metals along with silver are called as precious metals.

7 A Light is described as visible electro-magnetic energy whose wavelength is measured in nanometers (nm). The eye is sensitive only to the visible part of the electro-magnetic spectrum, a narrow band with wavelengths of 380-750 nm. At the shorter wavelengths lie ultraviolet, X-rays and gamma rays. At the longer wavelengths are infrared radiation, microwaves and radio and TV signals.

8 D Cast partial denture framework should be cast from type IV alloy, as they are known as extra hard alloys. The yield strength of type IV Gold is more than 340 MPa, therefore can be used in clinical situations where very high stresses are involved such as long span bridges or in cast partial denture. But they have low elongation value (less than 10%) therefore are difficult to burnish.

9 A With respect to anatomic limitations anterior mandible is the most straightforward area for treatment planning. It has adequate height and width for implant placement, and the bone quality is normally excellent, which makes it require the least amount of time for integration. When possible an implant in anterior mandible should be placed through the entire cancellous bone so the apex of the implant is engaged in the cortex of the inferior border of the mandible.

10 C The Vickers hardness number of dental alloy is generally measured using a symmetric diamond pyramidal indenter, although the Knoop hardness number obtained with different type of diamond indenter having long and short axes. Both the Vickers and Knoop tests measure the micro hardness number, in contrast to the older Brinell and Rockwell tests, which use larger indenters and measure the macro hardness number.

11 B In comparison to normal centrifugal casting machine, the air pressure-casting machine the sprue diameter is narrow. In air pressure machines the melt is made directly in the depression created by the crucible former and then forced into the mold by the sudden change in air pressure. With this technique a narrow sprue prevents the molten metal from flowing into the mold prematurely.

12 D Factors affecting the expansion of gypsum-bonded investment are:

Factors	*Normal setting expansion*
1. Water-powder ratio increased	decreased
2. Spatulation time increased	increased
3. Age of investment increased	decreased
4. Rate of spatulation increased	increased
5. Ring liner	increased
6. Particle size of silica decreased	increased

13 B Mucosal contact types of pontic are Ridge lap, modified ridge lap, ovate and conical. Sanitary (hygienic) and modified sanitary are non-mucosal contact type.

14 A The shape and position of connectors all influence the success of provisional prosthesis. Connectors must be sufficiently large to prevent distortion or fracture during function but not too large, otherwise they will interfere with effective plaque control. Adequate embrasure space must be present for oral hygiene aids cervical to connecter. If the connecter is too large inciso-cervically, hygiene is impeded.

15 B The three quarter crown preparation derives its name from the number of axial walls involved. Except a slight bevel or chamfer placed along the buccocclusal line angle, the buccal tooth surface remains intact. This kind of preparation is more conservative but demanding during preparation.

16 A High–fusing ceramics have a fusing temperature from 1315° to 1370°C, the medium fusing ceramics from 1090°-1260°C and low fusing ceramics from 870°-1070°C. The fusion temperature of feldspar varies from 1125°-1170°C depending upon its purity. The fusion temperature of the metal should be higher than that of porcelain, otherwise the metal substructure will melt and it will not be possible to put porcelain on the metal substructure.

17 C With high-density noble metal alloy 6 grams is adequate for premolar and anterior castings, 9 grams is adequate for molar casting and 12 grams is adequate for pontics.

18 C CIELAB color system is determined by the Commission Internationale de l'Eclairage in 1978. In both the munsell and the CIELAB color systems, the location in the color space of a particular shade is defined by three coordinates: value, hue and chroma for munsell; L, a and b for CIELAB. Value and L are proportional to each other and represent the lightness, brightness or black/white character of color.

19 B The floor of the occlusal rest should be apical to the marginal ridge and occlusal surface and should be concave or spoon shaped. This way the angle formed between the occlusal rest and the vertical minor connector from which it originates should be less than 90 degrees. This way (1) the occlusal forces are directed along the long axis of the abutment tooth. (2) It also prevents slippage of the prosthesis away from the abutment.

20 B If hygroscopic technique is used, the ring is placed in a 37° C (100° F) water bath for one hour.

21 B In general a relatively large diameter sprue is recommended because this improves the flow of the molten metal into the mold and ensures a reservoir during solidification. A 2.5 mm (10 gauge) sprue is recommended for molar and metal ceramic patterns. A smaller 2 mm (12 gauge) is adequate for premolars and partial coverage restorations.

22 C Factors that determine the path of placement are: guiding planes, retentive areas, interference and esthetics. While determining the path they should be assessed also in the same sequence.

23 C Partial veneer crowns are indicated to restore posterior teeth that have lost moderate amount of tooth structure, provided the buccal wall is intact. They are also commonly used as retainers for a fixed partial denture or where restoration or alteration of the occlusal surface is needed. Anterior partial veneers are rarely suitable for restoring damaged teeth but can be used as retainers to reestablish anterior guidance, and to splint teeth. They are contraindicated in short clinical crowns, as retainers in long span FPD's. They should not be used in endodontically treated posterior teeth.

24 C Three types of expansion can influence to obtain the desired size of casting: setting, hygroscopic and thermal. As the mold is heated to eliminate the wax, thermal expansion occurs. The silica refractory material is principally responsible for this because of solid–state phase transformation. Cristobalite changes from the α to β form between 200°C and 270°C. Quartz transforms at 575°C. These transitions involve a change in crystal form, an accompanying change in bond angles and axis dimensions, and a decreased density, producing a volume increase in refractory components.

25 C To avoid fracture the thickness of a ceramic veneer must not exceed 2 mm, however a minimum thickness of 1 mm is needed for an aesthetically pleasing restoration. The centric stop of any metal ceramic restoration can be located on either porcelain or metal. However they must be at least 1.5 mm away from the junction to prevent the porcelain fracture from the deformation of the metal.

26 B Beneath framework extensions onto ridge areas for attachment of resin bases 20-gauge wax is used. Beneath lingual bar connectors or the bar portion of linguoplates 32 gauge wax is used. It prevents impingement of lingual tissue on alveolar ridge when vertical forces fall on lingual bar. 28-gauge wax is used over the cingula and interproximal embrasure in a continous bar retainer.

27 B The seven-eights crown preparation includes, in addition to the surfaces covered by the three quarter crown, the distal half of the buccal surface. Therefore the mesial aspect of this preparation resembles that of a three quarter crown, the distal aspect resembles that of a complete crown. The mesial half of the buccal tooth surface remains intact and is protected by a narrow contrabevel or chamfer similar to the one used in the three quarter crown preparation.

28 B Specifications of ADA govern the important properties of residue, flow and expansion of inlay wax . Because the mold must burn out cleanly to allow the escape of gases and the complete entry of molten alloy, there can be no residual ash. However, the specifications allow a 0.1% residue, which apparently is effectively negligible.

29 C The amount of shrinkage in ceramic bodies depends upon average pore size, which is directly related to the particle size distribution. The linear firing shrinkage of feldspathic porcelain is around 14% in low fusing and 11.5% in high fusing porcelain. Low fusing porcelain has a volumetric shrinkage of 32 to 37% and high fusing porcelain shrink up to 28-34%. The greatest dimensional change will take place where the porcelain is thickest.

30 C Flexion under occlusal loads may cause failure of long span bridge. All FPD's flex slightly when subjected to a load. Longer the span, greater is the flexing. The relationship between deflection and the length of span is not simply linear but varies with cube of the length of the span.

31 B Porosity resulting from solidification shrinkage occurs if metal in the sprue solidifies before the metal in the mold, as may happen when a sprue is too narrow and long, or if it is incorrectly located or when a large casting is made in the absence of chill vent.

32 B The material used to fabricate pontic is based on two factors: biocompatibility and ease to maintain oral hygiene. Glazed porcelain is generally considered the most biocompatible of the available pontic material. Glazed porcelain is easier to clean than any other material. It also resists plaque accumulation. Nearest competitor is gold, well polished gold is smoother, less prone to corrosion, and less retentive of plaque than an unpolished casting. However even highly polished surface will accumulate plaque if oral hygiene measures are ignored.

33 D The objective of using the functional ridge form is to ensure that the prosthesis in function is supported. This cannot be achieved by a single impression procedure with irreversible hydrocolloid in a stock rim lock tray. The prescribed methods are: Hindel's double impression technique, Steffel's functional reline procedure and Holmes altered cast impression procedure.

34 C Rest position is always placed inferiorly and forward to centric position, therefore only elevators and retruders of mandible are required to obtain the centric position. Out of the given group of muscles lateral pterygoid is the only muscle, which belongs to the group of depressors of mandible. Lateral pterygoid is used mainly to open the jaw and move the mandible from side to side.

35 C An extra oral metal restoration that covers only part of the clinical crown is considered to be a partial veneer crown. Partial veneer crowns generally include all tooth surfaces except the buccal or labial wall in the preparation. It preserves tooth and is more demanding.

36 B Two occlusal schemes are generally recognized and should be understood. Cusp – marginal ridge and cusp – fossa. In the cusp fossa scheme mandibular centric cusp contact further distally into the mesial fossa of the maxillary tooth and contact only one tooth. The lingual (centric) cusps of the maxillary teeth contact the fossa of the mandibular teeth.

In cusp – marginal ridge scheme, the buccal cusps of the mandibular premolars and mesiobuccal cusp of molar contact the embrasures between the maxillary teeth.

Most adults with class I occlusion have cusp – marginal ridge scheme. In natural dentition, cusp fossa arrangement is found in class II malocclusion.

37 C As per the definition of centric relation, it is the most posterior-superior unstrained position of condyle in glenoid fossa at a given degree of jaw separation (vertical relation) from which lateral movement is possible. Therefore centric is always at a specific vertical or it changes with a change in vertical. Facebow is used for orientation of mandible to the true hinge axis and transferring the same relation to the articulator. Terminal hinge axis and centric are the same but the objective of centric relation is to develop occlusion at centric (which is called centric occlusion). Since edentulous patient loses all properioceptive sensation, deflective occlusal contact cannot be protected therefore it is advisable to develop occlusion in harmony with centric relation.

38 C Backpressure porosity may be caused by air pressure in the mold as the molten metal enters. Its occurrence is reduced by more porous investment, or by locating the pattern near the end of the ring (6-8 mm), and casting with a vacuum pump.

39 B The metal framework must be sufficiently thick to prevent distortion during firing. A minimum of 0.3 mm is advocated for the noble metal alloys, 0.2 mm is sufficient for base metal alloys, which can be finished thinner and still withstand distortion because of their higher melting range, modulus of elasticity and yields strength.

40 B Stability is a property by virtue of which a denture resists horizontal forces acting on it. A property by virtue of which it resists vertical forces acting towards the tissue is known as support. A property by virtue of which it resists vertical dislodging forces, acting away from the tissue, is known as retention.

41 C Forces that tend to remove a cemented restoration along its path of withdrawal are small compared to those that tend to seat or tilt it. A crown can be subjected to such forces by pulling with floss under the connectors, or when sticky food is eaten. The magnitude of dislodging forces depends on the stickiness of food and the surface area and the texture of the restoration being pulled.

42 B Due to the randomness of position of the growing chains, some of them may combine and terminate the growth process. Termination may also result from the reaction of the free radical with eugenol, hydroquinone or oxygen so contact with these substances must be avoided.

43 D The objective of bevelling is threefold: to allow the cast metal margin to be bent or burnished against the prepared tooth structure. To minimize the marginal discrepancy caused by complete crown that fails to seat completely. To protect the unprepared tooth structure from chipping.

44 B A two-stage implant requires two surgical procedures. First the implant is placed in the bone to the level of cortical plate and the oral mucosal is sutured over it, this is left for prescribed healing period of 3 months in the mandible and 6-9 months in the maxilla, depending on the quality of bone.

45 B Antiflux is used to limit the spreading of solder. It is placed on the casting before the flux application to limit the flow of molten solder. Graphite is often used as an Antiflux. However the carbon easily evaporates at higher temperature leaving the workplace unprotected. A more reliable antiflux is iron oxide (Rouge) in a suitable solvent such as turpentine.

46 B To maximize the chance of success the implant should be placed entirely in the bone and away from the significant anatomic structures. Ideally 10 mm of vertical bone dimension and 6 mm of horizontal bone should be available for implant placement. These dimensions will prevent encroachment on anatomic structures and allow 1 mm of bone on both facial and lingual aspects of implant.

47 C There should be adequate space between adjacent implants. The minimum recommended distance varies slightly among implant systems but is generally accepted as 3 mm. This space is needed to ensure bone viability between implants and allow adequate oral hygiene once the restorative dentistry is complete.

48 A The anterior mandible is the most straightforward site for the placement of implant. It has the adequate height and width for implant placement, and the bone quality is good enough to hold the implant. The bone quality is excellent which makes it require the least amount of time for integration. When possible an implant in anterior mandible should be placed through the entire cancellous bone so that apex of the implant is engaged in the cortex at the anterior border of the mandible.

49 D The patient's mouth is a challenging environment in which to make an accurate impression is a difficult task. Moisture control is probably one of the most important aspect of successful impression making. Except for polyethers, all elastomeric impression materials are hydrophobic (they do not tolerate or displace moisture). Any moisture will result in voids. Therefore saliva flow into the area must be reduced and diverted to obtain the necessary dry field of operation. This property of polyether is disadvantage also as if it is stored in wet or moist environment it may absorb moisture and undergo significant dimensional change.

50 B Better sulcus enlargement can be achieved with chemically impregnated cord or by dipping the cord in an astringent. These materials contain aluminum or iron salts and cause transient ischemia, shrinking the gingival tissue. Some of these medicaments also help in controlling the gingival fluid seepage. Aluminum chlóride and ferric sulfate are suitable because they cause minimal tissue damage. As an alternative, a sympathomimetic amine containing solution can also be used very effectively.

51 B Resins are used as a die material to overcome the low strength and abrasion resistance of the die stone. Most available resin die materials are epoxy resins or polyurethane. The amount of shrinkage upon polymerization is approximately equal to the expansion with shrinkage. Good results are obtained with silicones and polyether. Some impression materials such as polysulfide and hydrocolloids are not compatible with resin.

52 C Gas-air torch is used as the heat source to melt the alloy. Different zones of the flame from inside-outside are mixing zone, combustion zone, reducing zone and oxidizing zone. Usually the reducing flame is used to melt the alloy.

53 D Vertical dimension of occlusion decrease with time due to caries, attrition and trauma and total extraction. Sometimes it may increase also when the restoration placed in the mouth is high but it becomes too uncomfortable for the patient to tolerate for long time.

54 A It is always the fullness that is established before checking the visibility of the upper occlusal rim because the occlusal rim supports the upper lip and its fullness can alter the length of the lip or in other words the visibility of the occlusal rim.

55 D Interocclusal distance is important for the health of periodontal tissue, for the underlying tissues in denture wearer, speech and comfort of the patient.

56 B The anterior length of the maxillary rim is reduced to approximately 1 to 2 mm below the lower edge of the lip. This lip position is referred to as the low lip line.

57 B The remaining unprepared tooth structure immediately cervical to finish line should be easily discernible on the die, ideally 0.5 to 1 mm should be visible. It must be present to help the technician establish the correct cervical contour of the restoration to develop the emergence profile of the restoration.

58 B Surface detail reproduction is acceptable with type IV and type V gypsum products. The materials should be capable of reproducing a 20 μm wide line as prescribed by ADA specification No. 19.

59 B Anatomic posterior teeth have 33° cusps. It is the angle between the mesial slope of mesiobuccal cusp and the tangent drawn to cusp tip. The semi anatomic teeth have the angle of 22°. The non-anatomic teeth have 0° cusp. The anatomic teeth have this angle in unison with the condylar angle.

60 B If the interocclusal distance is increased it leads to the following: decreased nose chin distance, increased wrinkling on the face, discomfort at TMJ, reduced efficiency of the muscles of mastication, decreased tongue space, blockage of auditory canal and pain in the ears.

61 A 100 gms of plaster requires 45 to 50 ml of water, 100 gms of dental stone requires 30 to 35 ml and 100 gms of die stone requires 20 to 25 ml, depending upon particular brand. Theoretically, the stoichiometric amount of water needed for setting reaction of gypsum is 18.6 ml only. Only die stone has suitable physical properties for making cast restorations.

62 B The articular disk divides the glenoid fossa into two compartments upper and lower. Condyle with the articular disk moves in the upper compartment in translatory movement (downwards and forwards) and condyle alone rotates in the lower compartment. During initial mouth opening up to 14 to 16 mm the condyle purely rotates in the lower compartment but on further opening of the mouth the condyle rotates along with translatory movement in upper compartment.

63 C Wrinkling is commonly seen in natural ageing, decreased vertical dimension of occlusion, decreased fullness of the lip, poor lip support, loss of muscle tone and neuro muscular disorder.

64 C Centric relations are defined as horizontal jaw relations. It is the relation of mandible to maxilla in the horizontal plane that is both anterior-posterior and medio-lateral. By retruding the mandible patient establishes the horizontal position anteroposteriorly and mediolaterally.

65 B When the mandible opens and closes, rotation occurs around a transverse axis, which is more commonly called the hinge axis. The axis is called the terminal hinge axis when the mandible undergoes rotation while in centric relation. The mandible is capable of making a pure rotational movement while in centric relation. The maximum range of terminal hinge rotation averages about 12 degrees and creates arrange of 18-25 mm of interincisal opening. Although it is theoretically possible for the mandible to make pure rotation in locations other than centric relation, it is doubtful that it occurs actually.

66 B Stability of a complete denture is defined as that property by virtue of which it resists horizontal forces acting on it. These forces usually become active during normal tongue and cheek or lip movements. The height of residual ridge determines the support and resistance to lateral movement of the denture base. The arch form of the residual ridge is important in offsetting the rotational movement of the denture base. Width of the residual ridge is important to determine the amount of vertical support is offered by the ridge.

67 B All those structures, which cannot bear the masticatory load, should be relieved. It depends on the underlying structures (adipose tissue or glandular tissue), or any part where the nerves or the vessels are passing they should be relieved. All frenums which are just a fold of mucus membrane should also be relieved irrespective of whether they are active or passive.

68 B The average width of the maxillary central incisor is estimated to be one sixteenth of the width of the face measured between the zygoma. Trubyte tooth indicator determines this. The combined width of six maxillary anteriors is slightly less than one third of the bizygomatic breadth of face.

69 D The coronoid process of the mandible determines thickness of the denture in the buccal vestibule. Infact during impression patient is instructed to move the mandible sideways so that the thickness of the buccal flange of the maxillary impression is carved out. Various degrees of impingement of the coronoid process will be manifested upon compound border.

70 C Face bow is a caliper like device used to orient the maxillary cast on the articulator so that it has the same relationship to the opening axis that maxilla has to the opening axis of the jaws. It simply relates the maxilla to the transverse axis (terminal hinge axis) and transfers the face bow to the articulator such that the terminal hinge axis of the patient is superimposed on the opening axis of the articulator. Thereby the maxilla (or indirectly mandible) is oriented to the opening axis (transverse axis).

71 B Vertical support and retention for the maxillary denture is partially determined by the shape of the hard palate. Palate can be classified as flat, U, or V shaped. Out of all of these classes broad flat palate or class I offers the best vertical support and retention.

72 D Schiffman has shown that the maxillary incisors fall approximately 8 to 10 mm anterior to the point of intersection of a line that bisects the midline of the palate perpendicularly through the incisive papilla. This perpendicular bisecting line also extends outwards approximately through the midline of the maxillary canines. Labial incisal angle of the incisors should be placed so that the lip is supported by the plane of the labial two thirds of the surface of the incisors.

73 B Survey line divides the tooth into suprabulge and infrabulge area, all components of a cast partial denture should be placed above the suprabulge area except the terminal part of the retentive arm. The designing of cast partial denture should be done in this manner that desired amount of retention is gained by placing the terminal part of retentive arm in the undercut.

74 D Retention in complete denture is defined as the ability of denture to resist the vertical unseating forces which are produced by gravity, adhesiveness of food and forces during opening and closing of jaws. Retention is directly related to the relationship of the denture base to the underlying soft tissue. Factors responsible for it are adhesion, cohesion atmospheric pressure, quality of saliva, peripheral seal (border moulding), external surface of the denture (it is contoured in such a way that muscles in contact with these surfaces enhance the stability and retention).

75 A Retromylohyoid space, which lies distal of alveololingual sulcus. This space is bounded medially by anterior tonsillar pillar and posteriorly by retromylohyoid curtain. Superior constrictor forms Retromylohyoid curtain posteriorly, laterally it is formed by mandible and pterygomandibular raphe, anteriorly by lingual tuberosity and inferiorly by mylohyoid muscle.

76 C Both of these waxes are used to record the finer details of the oral cavity, like in case of posterior palatal seal. They are used to record the functional anatomy, as they soften at mouth temperature it is easy to handle them

and still record the details thereby they are called as physiological waxes.

77 A Vertical dimension/relation of rest (VRR) or rest is a postural position, which remains static and never changes throughout life, as muscles and ligaments rather than teeth determine it. VRR is always more than that of vertical relation of occlusion (VRO) by interocclusal distance or freeway space. Presence of freeway space is a must for the health of periodontal tissues. VRO can decrease with time in most of individuals because of caries, attrition and trauma. Interocclusal distance is the distance between the occluding surfaces of the maxillary and mandibular teeth when the mandible is in its physiological rest position.

Rest vertical dimension = occlusal vertical dimension + interocclusal distance.

78 C The mandible is a lever of class III type, which is the least efficient of the lever systems. An example of another class III lever would be a fishing pole. The longer the pole, the more effort it takes to pull a fish out of water. The same holds true for the muscles of mastication and the teeth. The farther anteriorly initial tooth-to-tooth contact occurs the less effective will be the forces exerted by the musculature and smaller the load to which the teeth are subjected.

79 C Occlusion is often confused with articulation. Occlusion is bringing the mandibular teeth up into contact with the maxillary teeth. This is a static (not moving or progressing, at rest) position when the jaws are centrically or eccentrically related. Articulation is defined as contacting of teeth as the mandible moved to and from centric relation and eccentric relation. This is a dynamic movement.

80 A The buccinator muscle joins the superior constrictor at the pterygomandibular raphe distal to the retromolar pad area. It is buccal to this area that the action of the masseter muscle pushes the buccinator muscle towards the retromolar pad. The impression will be reflected superiorly and medially forming a groove or a notch called as massetric notch.

81 A The characteristics of mandibular movement are established posteriorly by the morphology of the TMJ and anteriorly by the relationship of the anterior teeth. The anterior determinants are the vertical and horizontal overlaps and the maxillary lingual concavities of the anterior teeth. A greater vertical overlap causes the direction of mandibular opening to be more vertical during their early phase of protrusive movement and creates a more vertical pathway at the end of chewing stroke. Therefore if the vertical overlap of the anterior teeth is increased posterior cusps may be taller.

82 B Border movements were discovered by posselt, they are described as extremes of mandibular movement. His work helps in better understanding of how the determinants control the extent to which movement can occur. Posselt's diagram is a three dimensional representation of the extreme movements of mandible. All physiological movements of mandible take place under this envelop of motion. Posselt's diagram can be seen in both frontal (shield shaped) and sagittal plane.

83 A Root surface area is very important as per ante's law; it is unwise to provide a FPD when the root surface area of the abutment was less than the root surface area of the teeth being replaced. Maximum root surface area is provided by maxillary first molar (433 mm^2), maxillary second molar (431 mm^2), mandibular first molar (431 mm^2) and mandibular second molar (426 mm^2).

84 C Gypsum bonded investments are not stable above 650°C. The calcium sulfate bonded investment is usually limited to gold castings, and is not heated above 700°C. The calcium sulfate portion of the investment decomposes to sulfur dioxide and sulfur trioxide at temperature above 650°C, tending to embrittle the casting metal. Therefore calcium sulfate type of binder is usually not used in investments for making casting of palladium or base metal alloys.

85 C Selection of appropriate degree of taper for tooth preparation involves compromise. Too small a taper may lead to unwanted undercuts, too large a taper will decrease the taper. The recommended convergence between the opposing walls is 6 degrees. To create this angle there is no need to tilt the bur, as this will lead to over preparation rather it is achieved by rotary instrument of the desired taper held at a constant angulation.

86 A Mandible rotates in all three planes around an imaginary axis. Opening and closing movement of the mandible takes place in the sagittal plane around a horizontal axis.

Rotational movement in the horizontal plane takes place around an imaginary vertical axis and rotational movement in the frontal plane takes place around a horizontal sagittal axis.

87 A Food is more easily crushes as it is placed further back in the mouth because mandible is an example of class III lever. The farther anteriorly initial tooth-to-tooth contact occurs the less effective will be the forces exerted by the musculature and smaller the load to which the teeth are subjected.

88 B

89 B Gypsum has a disadvantage of poor resistance to abrasion. Colloidal silica has little effect on the surface hardness of the dental stone. Best results are obtained by impregnating the surface of the dies with a low viscosity resin such as cynoacrylates. Abrasion resistance is most improved by this technique. Mixture of gum Arabic and colloidal silica is used for the industrial purposes.

90 C Removable partial dentures are indicated in the following situations:

Distal extension situation, after recent extractions, long span edentulous space, need for bilateral stabilization, excessive loss of residual ridge, abutments with guarded prognosis and economic consideration.

91 D Use of a flux is essential to prevent oxidation of the parts being joined and the solder itself. A borax type flux is recommended for soldering gold alloys to gold alloys. Graphite is an antiflux and fluoride type flux is used when chromium-cobalt alloys are soldered to the alloys containing chromium.

92 B Theoretically the amount of undercut used may vary with the clasp to be used upto a full 0.03 inch. However undercuts of 0.01 inch are often adequate for the retention of cast retainers. If tapered wrought wire retention may safely use up to 0.02 inch without inducing undesirable torque on the abutment tooth. The use of 0.03 inch is rarely justified with any clasp. 0.001 inch is too little an undercut to be of any clinical significance.

93 A Combination clasp are used when maximum flexibility is desirable, such as on abutment tooth adjacent to distal extension base or a weak abutment. They are also used for its adjustability when precise retentive requirements are unpredictable and later adjustment to increase or decrease retention may be necessary. Being wrought in structure, it may be used in smaller diameter than may a cast clasp. They cover minimum of tooth surface. These clasps also have less fatigue failures in service. Combination clasp has several disadvantages such as it involves extra step in the fabrication, they may be less accurately adapted and provide less stabilization and they may be distorted easily.

94 C Flexibility of a clasp depends on length (directly proportional), diameter (inversely proportional), and cross-sectional form and material of clasp. It is not at all related to the location of the clasp.

95 C Retention in a cast partial denture depends on mechanical retention by means of clasps on abutment teeth and by the intimate relationship of denture base and major connectors with the underlying tissues. This type of retention is similar to retention in complete dentures. This retention is due to physical phenomenons like adhesion, cohesion, atmospheric pressure, effect of gravity and plastic molding of tissues around the polished surface. Indirect retainers help in preventing the lifting of the dentures away from the tissue in a distal extension base.

96 B Orbiting or balancing condyle moves in a forward and medial direction, it may take one of the four possible types of pathways during the lateral movement of mandible. These paths are; straight protrusion, progressive shift, precurrent shift and immediate shift. Muscle responsible for this movement is lateral pterygoid.

97 A

98 D Support for removable denture can be derived from teeth, residual alveolar tissue or both. In case of a complete denture support is derived from the underlying tissues. In case of distal extension base support is derived from both the teeth and the tissues and in Kennedy class III total support comes from abutments via rests placed on them.

99 C Typical examples of fricative sounds are f or v, while producing such sounds the vermilion border of the lower lip makes contact with the incisal edges of upper incisors. Such sounds are used to verify the position of upper anteriors.

100 C Thickness of a cast is always measured at the thinnest area that is in case of maxillary cast it is the palate and in case of mandibular cast it is the tongue area. Ideally it should be 14-16 mm if it is less than that it might fracture during fabrication of denture and if it is more than that it may create problem in flasking and closure.

Notes

Syllabus

- Introduction to the study of Operative Dentistry and background information on dental diseases.
- Classification of cavity and nomenclature.
- Hand cutting instruments for cavity preparation.
- Rotary cutting instruments for cavity preparation.
- Rotary cutting methods and use of high speed in operative procedures and biologic consideration.
- Steps and principles of cavity preparation in relation to pathology and clinical features of dental caries.
- Amalgam–technical consideration.
- Class I cavity preparation for amalgam.
- Class II cavity preparation for amalgam.
- Matrix.
- Wedge and separators.
- Cavity liners and bases.
- Silicate cement and composite resin.
- Glass inomer Technical considerations.
- Class III Cavity preparation for silicate cement, Glass Inomer and Composite.
- Class IV Cavity preparation for composite Resin and Sandwich technique.
- Class V cavity preparation for amalgam and composite.
- Temporary restorations.
- Inlay/onlay cavities indication, contra-indication advantages and disadvantages. Difference between Inlays and Amalgam.
- Preventive aspects of dental diseases, special reference to caries etc.
- Diagnosis in conservative dentistry and treatment plan.
- Biologic considerations—Restorative Materials.
- Features of inlay cavities.
- Pins in conservative dentistry.
- Failures of silver amalgam restoration.
- Control of pain during cavity preparation.
- Control of moisture during operative procedures.
- Hypersensitive dentin, attrition, abrasion and erosion–management.
- Gingival tissue management.
- Pit and Fissure sealants.
- Direct Gold restorations—Principles-Cavity preparation-Class III, Class V.
- Direct Gold restoration—Technical considerations and Manipulation.
- Restoration of contact point.
- Pulpal lesions.
- Periapical lesions.
- Diagnostic aids for endodontic treatment.
- Principles of Endodontics.
- Rationale of root canal treatment sterilization of root canal instruments and working length determination.
- Selection of cases for root canal treatment.
- Anatomy of pulp cavity.
- Anatomy of root apex.

- **Pulp capping, Pulpotomy, Pulp mummification.**
- **Pulpectomy and introduction to root canal treatment.**
- **Root canal instruments.**
- **Root canal preparation technique.**
- **Root canal obturation.**
- **Pulpotomy Apexogenesis and Apexification.**
- **Preparation of the root canal Biomechanical and chemical.**
- **Irrigation and Antiseptic medication of root canal.**
- **Bacteriologic Examination of root canal.**
- **Obturation of root canal.**
- **Procedural accidents and management.**
- **Healing after endodontic treatment, Post endodontic restoration.**
- **Inlays, Onlays Wax pattern direct and indirect techniques.**
- **Investing of Wax patterns.**
- **Casting, Finishing and Cementing on Inlay.**
- **Failures of cast restorations (casting defects).**
- **Discoloration of teeth and its management.**
- **Treatment of Fractured and Traumatized teeth.**
- **Dental Caries and prevention.**
- **Surgical endodontics.**
- **Surgical endodontics—Replantation, transplantation and implantation.**
- **Endo-Periodontal therapy radisectomy and Hemisection.**
- **Porcelain—Technical consideration and Inlays.**
- **Occlusion.**
- **Resorption.**
- **Lasers.**
- **Dentin bonding agents.**
- **Endodontic implants.**

Chapter 12

Conservative Dentistry including Endodontics

1. **The father of operative dentistry is**
   A. Pierre Fauchard
   B. GV Black
   C. Edward H Angle
   D. Samuel Hahnemann

2. **A popular modification of cavities occurring on both the proximal surfaces of posterior teeth is classified as**
   A. Class VI a
   B. Class VI b
   C. Class VII
   D. All of the above

3. **Cavity preparation in which 3 surfaces are involved is called**
   A. Simple cavity
   B. Multiple cavity
   C. Complex cavity
   D. Compound cavity

4. **Deepest part of a prepared cavity is**
   A. Axial wall B. Pulpal floor
   C. Isthmus D. Gingival seat

5. **If an instrument formula comprises three units, i.e. "A–B–C", then "A" denotes**
   A. Length of Blade
   B. Width of Blade
   C. Height of Blade
   D. Angle that blade makes

6. **A ring (indentation) on an instrument denotes**
   A. It is 'Right side' of instrument pair
   B. It is 'Mesial side' of instrument pair
   C. Both of the above
   D. None of the above

7. **A Bi-Bevelled instrument is**
   A. Straight Chiesel
   B. Ordinary Hatchet
   C. Spoon Excavator
   D. Angle former

8. **The following instrument(s) is not paired as 'Right' or 'Left'**
   A. Gingival marginal trimmer
   B. Binangle chiesel
   C. Spoon excavator
   D. Enamel hatchet

9. **A positive rake angle is utilised**
   A. To cut pathologic specimens
   B. To cut enamel and dentin
   C. Behind radial line
   D. All of the above

10. **Shape of smooth surface caries in enamel is**
    A. 'V' shaped
    B. Inverted 'V' shaped
    C. Lateral spread
    D. No particular shape

11. Matrix band(s) that cannot be used for silicate cement restorations is/are
A. Methyl Cellulose
B. Cellophane Paper
C. Mylar Strip
D. All of the above

12. Custom-made matrix do not include
A. Blacks matrix
B. Incisal corner matrix
C. Automatrix
D. T–Band

13. Following is not a function of 'Wedges'
A. Stabilization of band in place
B. Prevention of moisture contamination
C. Separation of teeth
D. None of the above

14. Following is not a function of 'Separators'
A. Diagnosis of proximal caries
B. Placement of restoration
C. Finishing of restoration
D. None of the above

15. Ultra speed rotary cutting instruments are indicated for all the following, *except*
A. Use at 1,50,000 RPM
B. Cavity preparation
C. Removal of old restorations
D. Gross crown cutting

16. Atraumatic restorative treatment technique
A. Is a substitute for conventional restorative procedures
B. Emphasizes excavation of infected rather than affected dentin
C. Is also known as manual restorative treatment
D. All of the above

17. Affected dentin has the following characteristic features, *except*
A. It is the outermost layer
B. It has a hard consistency
C. It can be stained by basic fuschin dye
D. It is capable of remineralization

18. Principle(s) of cavity preparation include
A. Restoration form
B. Conveyance form
C. Removal of remaining caries
D. All of the above

19. The following is/are feature(s) of resistance form in cavity preparation
A. Dovetail
B. Gingival seat groove
C. Reverse curve
D. All of the above

20. 'Liners' are usually distinguished from 'bases' by all of the following, *except*
A. Thickness
B. Chemical protection
C. Mechanical support
D. Thermal insulation

21. Calcium hydroxide when used in 5–10 microns thickness is referred to as
A. Liner
B. Sub-base
C. Base
D. All of the above

22. The advantage(s) of zinc oxide eugenol over zinc phosphate cement is/are
A. Antibacterial property
B. Chemical barrier
C. Reparative dentin formation
D. All of the above

23. The advantage(s) of zinc phosphate over polycarboxylate cement is/are
A. Chemical protection
B. Electric insulation
C. Varnish application is not contraindicated
D. All of the above

24. Dispensing of alloy and mercury should ideally be done by
A. Weight alone
B. Weight and volume, respectively
C. Volume alone
D. Volume and weight, respectively

25. Polishing of amalgam restorations is indicated 24 hours after placement in order to
- A. Improve its malleability and ductility
- B. Eradicate Galvanism
- C. Reduce its tarnish and corrosion
- D. All of the above

26. Trituration in amalgamator depends upon
- A. R.P.M.
- B. R.P.M. × seconds
- C. R.P.M. × seconds × Pestle size
- D. R.P.M. × seconds ÷ Pestle size

27. A prepared cavity with an underlying sub-base and base is classified as
- A. Type A
- B. Type B
- C. Type C
- D. Type D

28. Semi-Permanent restorative cements include the following, *except*
- A. Glass Ionomers
- B. Silicates
- C. Composites
- D. None of the above

29. Glass Ionomer cements were developed to overcome the following disadvantage(s) of silicate cement
- A. Lack of adhesion to tooth structure
- B. Inadequate esthetics
- C. Limited utility in mouth breathers
- D. All of the above

30. Strength is a limitation with
- A. Microfilled composites
- B. Hybrid composites
- C. Conventional composites
- D. None of the above

31. The following is/are disadvantage(s) of ultra-violet light cure as compared to visible light cure system for composite resins
- A. Depth of cure
- B. Time taken for curing
- C. Health hazard
- D. All of the above

32. Type IV glass ionomer cement is indicated for
- A. Deciduous tooth restoration
- B. Core build up
- C. Tunnel preparation and restoration
- D. All of the above

33. Abfraction occurs in relation to
- A. Occlusal, stress bearing cavities
- B. Non-occlusal, stress bearing cavities
- C. Occlusal, Non-stress bearing cavities
- D. Non-occlusal, Non-stress bearing cavities

34. When cavity access is gained lingually in direct gold restorations, it is referred to as
- A. Ferrier design
- B. Single moustache design
- C. Loma Linda design
- D. Pan handle design

35. Electralloy is
- A. Precipitated gold
- B. Mat gold
- C. Gold foil
- D. Modified silver amalgam

36. A cement that is generally not advocated for restoring class IV cavities is
- A. Glass Ionomer
- B. Silver Amalgam
- C. Composite
- D. None of the above

37. A sandwich restoration comprises following cements
- A. Calcium Hydroxide + Zinc Oxide Eugenol + Glass Ionomer
- B. Zinc Oxide Eugenol + Glass ionomer + Silver Amalgam
- C. Calcium Hydroxide + Glass ionomer + Composite Resin
- D. Zinc oxide Eugenol + Zinc phosphate + Glass Ionomer

38. Features of onlay cavity do not include
A. Occlusal divergence
B. Margin below suprabulge area
C. Restoration covers all the cusps
D. Lack of undercuts

39. A characteristic feature of cavity preparation for inlay restorations is
A. Butt-Joint
B. Lap-Slide-Joint
C. Internal outline > External outline
D. Width of Cavity < ½ Intercuspal distance

40. Following is not used for moisture control in operative dentistry
A. Gingival retraction cord
B. Rubber dam
C. Atropine sulphate
D. None of the above

41. Following does not minimize pain during cavity cutting
A. Sharp instruments
B. Rotation at a slow speed
C. Intraligamentary anesthesia
D. None of the above

42. Occlusal attrition includes
A. Reverse cusping on buccal aspect
B. Wearing of natural tooth opposing cast metal crown
C. Both of the above
D. None of the above

43. Light amplified stimulation of emitted radiation is not utilised in operative dentistry for management of
A. Abrasion cavities
B. Gingival tissue
C. Walking bleach
D. None of the above

44. Electrosurgery mechanism in gingival tissue management does not comprise
A. Dessication
B. Fulguration
C. Coagulation
D. None of the above

45. Cervical burnout refers to
A. Root surface caries
B. Erosion cavity
C. A physiologic entity
D. Toothbrush abrasion

46. Vital bleach utilizes
A. Hydrochloric acid + sodium hypochloride
B. Hydrochloric acid + sodium perborate
C. Hydrogen peroxide + sodium hypochloride
D. Hydrogen peroxide + sodium perborate

47. Hypersensitivity does not predispose to formation of
A. Dead tracts
B. Secondary dentin
C. Sclerotic dentin
D. None of the above

48. Following is/are not temporary restorative material(s)
A. Gutta percha stick
B. Chemically cured acrylic resin
C. Polycarbonate crowns
D. None of the above

49. Impression of an inlay cavity can be directly recorded by using
A. Platinum foil
B. Rubber base impression material
C. Zinc oxide eugenol
D. All of the above

50. All of the following are advantages of porcelain inlays, *except*
A. Tensile strength
B. Compressive strength
C. Abrasive resistance
D. Thermal conductivity

51. Pulpal tissues can withstand upto
A. 5°C
B. 15°C
C. 50°C
D. 55°C rise in temperature more than normal

52. All of the following will cause chemical pulpal injury, *except*
A. Silicate cement
B. GIC
C. Calcium Hydroxide
D. Monomer

53. The following chemical has the ability to dissolve pupal tissues
A. Hydrogen peroxide
B. Betadine
C. Sodium Hypochlorite
D. Chlorhexidine

54. The primary aim of debridement is
A. Removal of inflammed pulpal tissue
B. Removal of necrosed dentinal tissue
C. Removal of dental foci of infection
D. Bio-mechanical preparation of canal

55. Immobilisation of the tooth during RCT enables
A. The tooth to heal faster
B. The operator to have proper access
C. The tooth to withstand masticatory forces more efficiently
D. The patient to use the tooth during RCT

56. The rationale of RCT is
A. Removal of non vital pulp
B. Removal of vital pulp and obturation with an inert material
C. Removal of vital/non-vital pulp and obturation with an inert material
D. Removal of non vital pulp and obturation with a bio compatible material

57. The Bio mechanical preparation of the root canals is done to
A. Remove any necrotic pulp or dentine
B. Widen the root canal for better obturation
C. Make the irregularities in the root canal smooth
D. All of the above

58. The only absolute contraindication for RCT is
A. Horizontal fracture of the tooth
B. Vertical fracture of the tooth involving the entire length of the tooth
C. Prosthetic cardiac valves
D. Grossly destroyed crown

59. The primary objective of pulpotomy is to
A. Reduce the number of micro-organism invading the pulp
B. Gain access to the radicular pulp
C. Preserve the vitality of radicular pulp
D. Establish drainage of pus

60. The procedures of preserving pulp vitality are contraindicated in
A. Grossly carious teeth
B. Presence of severe inflammation
C. Presence of coronal pulp inflammation
D. All of the above

61. For apexogenesis to occur, the minimum amount of vital pulp tissue necessary is
A. 7 mm B. 5 mm
C. 3 mm D. 1.5 mm

62. All of the following are contraindications for pulpotomy, *except*
A. Abnormal sensitivity to heat and cold
B. Chronic pulpalgia
C. Inflammed pulp
D. Tenderness to percussion and palpation

63. Rotary burs are preferred for pulpotomy in
A. Anterior teeth
B. Premolars
C. Molars
D. All of the above

64. During pulpotomy procedure
A. As much pulp tissue as possible should be removed
B. As much pulp tissue as possible should be left in the root canal
C. Pulpal tissues beyond the cervical third of the tooth is removed
D. Fifty percent of coronal pulp should be removed

65. Apexification is a procedure to be applied on
A. Pulp-less teeth
B. Teeth with hyperemic pulp
C. Teeth with pulpotomy
D. All of the above

66. The objective(s) of apexification is/are
A. Closure of the open apical third of the root
B. Formation of an apical calcific barriers against which obturation can be done
C. Both A and B
D. None of the above

67. In young incompletely developed teeth the apical foramen is
A. Spherical
B. Tunnel shaped
C. Hour glass shaped
D. Oval

68. The pulp chamber of maxillary central incisor has
A. 2 pulp horns
B. 3 pulp horns
C. 4 pulp horns
D. No pulp horns

69. The periapical abscess most likely to drain in floor of nasal fossa is in relation to
A. Maxillary central incisor
B. Maxillary lateral incisor
C. Maxillary canine
D. Maxillary 2nd premolar

70. The floor of the pulp chamber of maxillary first molar is
A. Rhomboidal in cross section
B. Rectangular in cross section
C. Triangular in cross section
D. Square in cross section

71. The floor of the pulp chamber in maxillary first molar lies in
A. Middle of the crown
B. Cervical third of the crown
C. Cervical third of root
D. Apical third of the root

72. While preparing an access opening for maxillary first molar the bur is directed
A. Buccally
B. Mesially
C. Palatally
D. Distally

73. The access opening of maxillary first molar should not include
A. The mesiobuccal cusp tip
B. The marginal ridge
C. The oblique ridge
D. All of the above

74. The apical matrix is designed to
A. Drain the infection
B. Prevent the extrusion of obturating material into peri-apex
C. Both A and B
D. None of the above

75. The removal of food, debris and residual necrotic pulp is called
A. Pulpectomy
B. Debridement
C. Biomechanical preparation
D. Irrigation

76. Barbed broach is used for removal of
A. Entire pulp and necrotic debris
B. Absorbent points
C. Cotton pledgets and foreign materials
D. All of the above

77. The clearance of debris from the canal is proportional to
A. The type of irrigant used
B. The force at which the irrigant is used
C. The amount of irrigant used
D. None of the above

78. Disinfection with sodium hypochlorite is
A. Initially slow but increases progressively
B. Initially rapid and decreases later
C. Constant over a period of time
D. Reduced when combined with hydrogen peroxide

79. While combining NaOCH and H_2O_2 as irrigants
- **A.** H_2O_2 should be used last
- **B.** NaOCH should be used last
- **C.** First irrigation should be done by normal saline
- **D.** NaOCH and H_2O_2 should never be used simultaneously

80. The root canal can be dried after irrigation by all, *except*
- **A.** Aspiration with needle
- **B.** Absorbent points
- **C.** By sterile cotton pledgets
- **D.** Compressed air

81. The number on endodontic instruments represents
- **A.** Radius of the instrument in hundredths of a mm at the tip
- **B.** Diameter of the instrument in thousandth of a mm at the shank
- **C.** Diameter of the instrument in hundredth of a mm at the tip
- **D.** Radius of the instrument in hundredth of a mm at the shank

82. The diameter of the instrument at D_2 is
- **A.** 0.02 mm greater than D_1
- **B.** 0.20 mm greater than D_1
- **C.** 0.032 mm greater than D_1
- **D.** 0.32 mm greater than D_1

83. The constant increase in taper per mm in an endodontic instrument is
- **A.** 0.2 mm
- **B.** 0.02 mm
- **C.** 0.32 mm
- **D.** 0.032 mm

84. Smaller instruments are made from square blanks to
- **A.** Increase the resistance to torque forces
- **B.** Increase the resistance to compressive forces
- **C.** Increase the resistance to corrosion
- **D.** Increase the cutting efficiency

85. The most commonly used endodontic instrument length during RCT is
- **A.** 21 mm
- **B.** 25 mm
- **C.** 28 mm
- **D.** 40 mm

86. The reamers of length 40 mm are mainly used for
- **A.** Preparing molars root canals
- **B.** Preparing cuspid root canals
- **C.** Preparing root canals for endo-implants
- **D.** Draining peri apical abscess in posterior teeth

87. Reamer from Kerr Manufacturing Co. are used in a
- **A.** Rasping motion
- **B.** Pulling motion
- **C.** Pushing motion
- **D.** Pushing-rotating motion

88. The shape of blank used in K-flex file is
- **A.** Circular
- **B.** Diamond shaped
- **C.** Square shaped
- **D.** Triangular shaped

89. Which of the following statement is true?
- **A.** H files have higher cutting efficiency than K files but fracture easily
- **B.** H files have lower cutting efficiency than K files and fracture easily
- **C.** H files have higher cutting efficiency as well as more resistance to fracture
- **D.** K files have higher cutting efficiency than H files and don't fracture easily

90. Hedstroem files are manufactured from
- **A.** Round stainless steel wire that has been twisted to produce spiral flutes
- **B.** Round stainless steel wire that has been machined to produce spiral flutes resembling a cone
- **C.** Round stainless steel of different diameters and soldered together to form spiral flutes
- **D.** Diamond shaped blank twisted to produce spiral flutes in the shape of a screw

91. The widening of the root canal is done to
A. Remove micro-organisms
B. Remove pulp
C. Increase the capacity of root canal and shape the root canal to receive gutta-percha
D. All of the above

92. The most dependable criteria for adequate enlargement of root canal is
A. Enlargement upto three sizes larger than the instrument that bound
B. Clean dentinal shavings
C. Pain relief
D. Enlargement to at least size 30–40

93. All of the following are indications for endodontic implants, *except*
A. Periodontally involved teeth requiring stabilization
B. Transverse root fracture
C. Vertical root fracture
D. Internal resorption

94. For endodontic implants the root canal must be enlarged to at least the size of
A. No. 40 instrument
B. No. 50 instrument
C. No. 60 instrument
D. No. 90 instrument

95. The most important disadvantage of endodontic implant is
A. Poor apical seal
B. Extrusion of sealer into peri apex
C. Perforation of lateral root surface
D. Fracture during function

96. Replacement of a tooth in its socket when the tooth has been completely avulsed from its socket is referred to as
A. Implantation
B. Replantation
C. Transplantation
D. Endodontic implant

97. The least effective storage media for an avulsed tooth is
A. Tooth socket
B. Buccal vestibule
C. Under the tongue
D. Water

98. The following is not always required for treating an avulsed tooth
A. Tetanus consultation within 48 hours
B. Splinting of teeth
C. Radiographs
D. Antibiotics

99. The most important factor in the management of periodontal ligament of an avulsed tooth is to
A. Keep the ligament thoroughly clean
B. Prevent mechanical trauma
C. Prevent dehydration
D. Keep the extra oral time to minimum

100. The contraindication(s) for intentional replantation are
A. Periodontitis with extensive mobility of tooth
B. Missing septal bone
C. Inability to extract the tooth in one piece
D. All of the above

Answers

1 B 'A' is considered to be father of modern dentistry, 'C' of orthodontics and 'D' of homeopathy.

2 A 'B' is cavities on cusp tips and incisal edges of anterors and 'C' is a misnomer.

3 C 'A' is cavity preparation on single surface, 'B' is a misnomer and 'D' is on two surfaces.

4 D See diagram.

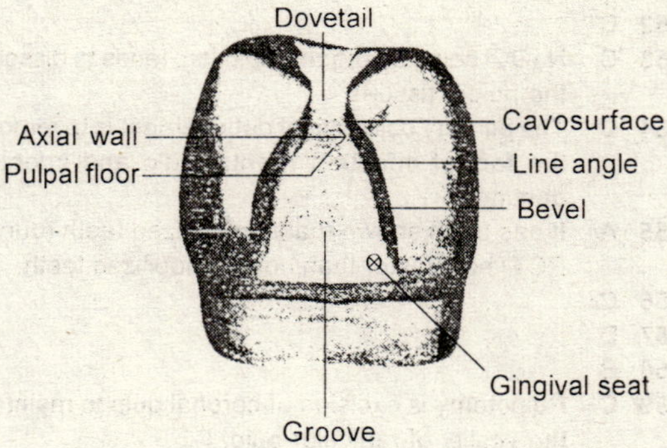

5 B A-B-C denote width, length and angle that blade makes, respectively.

6 C

7 B 'A' is monobevelled, 'C' is circumferential bevelled and 'D' is tri-bevelled instrument. 'B', unlike enamel hatchet (monobevelled), is mono bi-bevelled.

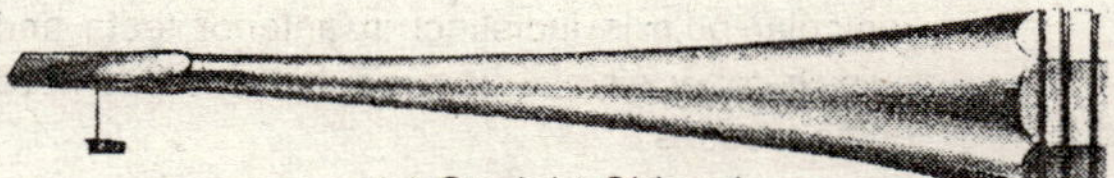

(a) Straight Chiesel

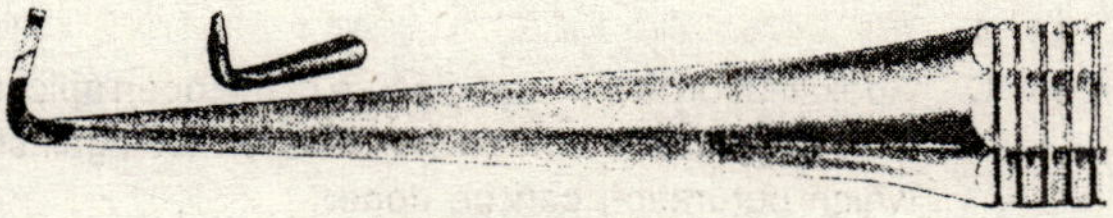

(b) Ordinary Hatchet

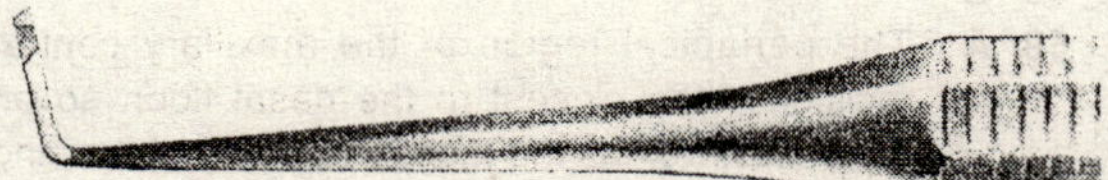

(c) Hoe

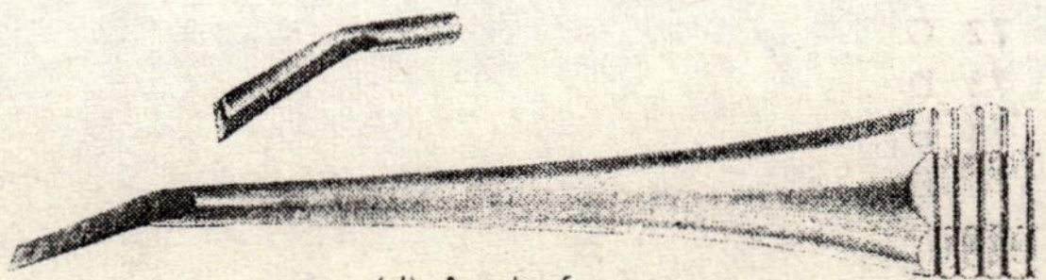

(d) Angle former

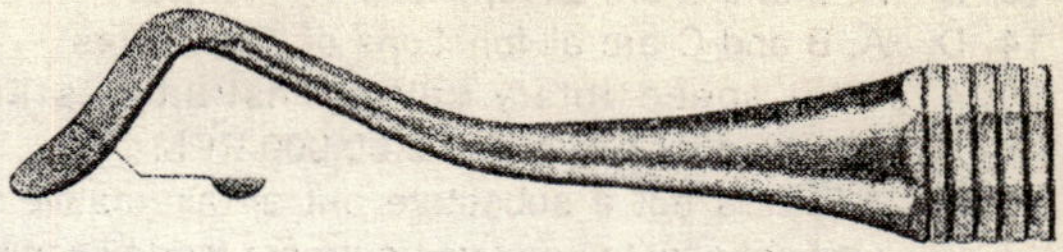

(e) Spoon Excavator

8 B Binangle chiesel is paired as 'Mesial' or 'Distal'.

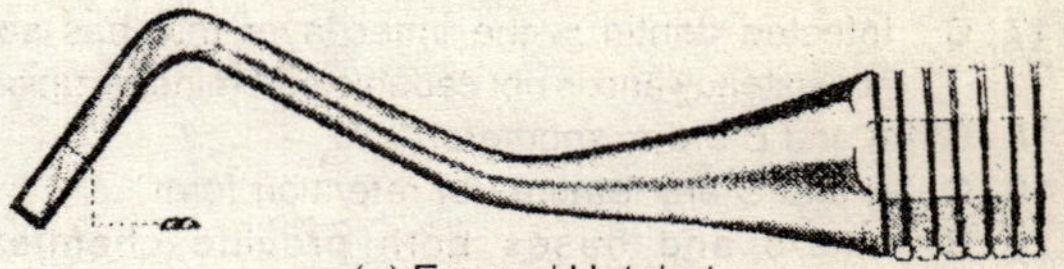

(a) Enamel Hatchet

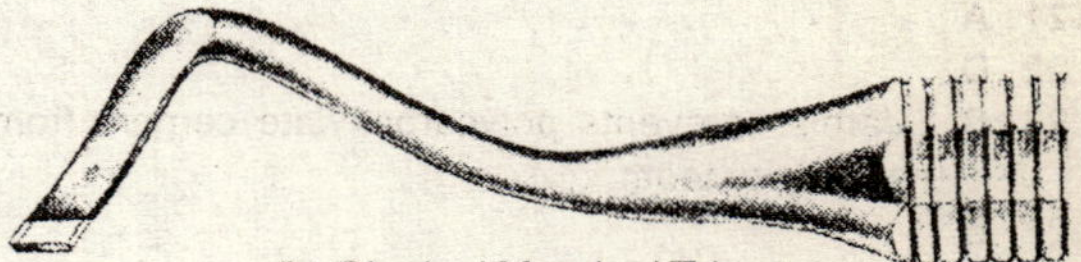

(b) Gingival Marginal Trimmer

9 A Negative rake angle lies behind radial line and is used to cut enamel and dentin.

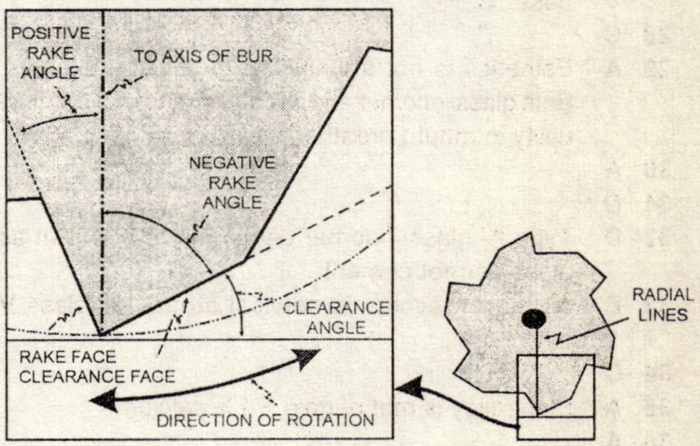

10 B See diagram

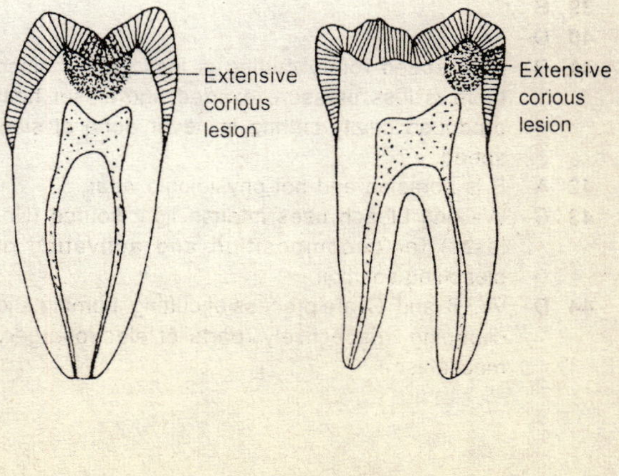

11 B Cellophane paper reacts with silicate cement.
12 C
13 D A, B and C are all functions of 'Wedges'.
14 D A, B and C are all functions of 'Separators'.
15 A Ultra speed rotary cutting instruments are indicated for use above 2,00,000 RPM.
16 B A.R.T. is not a substitute but an alternative to conventional restorative treatment for developing countries. Manual restorative treatment is different from ART since it utilizes silver amalgam as restorative material.
17 C Infected dentin is the inner layer that has soft consistency and is not capable of remineralization.
18 C A and B are misnomers.
19 C A and B are features of retention form.
20 B Liners and bases both provide chemical protection.
21 A
22 D
23 C Varnish prevents polycarboxylate cement from binding to tooth.
24 B
25 C
26 C
27 C 'A' is a cavity that has an underlying liner, 'B' has a base and 'D' has two sub-bases as well as a base.
28 C
29 A Esthetics is not a limitation of silicate cements. Both glass ionomer and silicate cement have limited utility in mouth breathers.
30 A
31 D
32 D Type IV glass ionomer cement is also known as glass cermet cement.
33 B Abfraction occurs in cervical areas, i.e. class V cavities.
34 C
35 A Electralloy is mat of gold + 1% calcium.
36 A
37 C
38 B
39 B
40 D
41 B High speed rotary cutting is less painful since there is less pressure exerted and lesser heat produced cavity cutting is never done at slow speed.
42 A B is abrasion and not physiologic wear.
43 C Walking bleach uses intense light source (Not laser) for decomposition and activation of bleaching solution.
44 D 'A', 'B' and 'C' are process of cutting, burning and clumping, respectively (parts of electrosurgery mechanism).
45 C
46 D
47 B Hypersensitivity predisposes to formation of tertiary (reparative) dentin, sclerotic dentin and dead tracts.
48 D
49 A B and C require custom made trays for making impression.
50 A Porcelain has poor tensile strength.
51 B
52 C
53 C NaOCl being an organic solution, tends to dissolve the pulpal tissues.
54 C The primary objective of debridement is to remove the foci of infection (dental pulp and infected dentine).
55 A It has been shown that immobilized teeth (during RCT) heal faster than non-immobilized teeth.
56 C
57 D
58 B
59 C Pulpotomy is excision of coronal pulp to maintain the vitality of radicular pulp.
60 B The formation of reparative dentine bridge is reduced in the presence of severe inflammation of the pulp. Hence pulpotomy procedures are contraindication in severe inflammation.
61 C
62 C Inflammed pulp is not a contraindication for pulpotomy as pulpitis can be a reversible phenomenon.
63 A As the distinction between the coronal and radicular pulp is indistinct in anterior teeth and pulp chamber is small, burs may be used to remove pulpal tissues.
64 B Pulpotomy being a conservative procedure aims at the preservation of maximum amount of vital pulpal tissues.
65 A
66 C Apexification is induced closure of the open apical third of the root so that a barrier is formed against which obturation can be done.
67 B
68 B
69 A The periapical region of the maxillary central incisior is the closest to the nasal floor, so an abscess here has the most probability of draining into it.
70 C
71 C
72 C
73 D
74 B
75 B
76 D
77 C

78 A
79 B Because residual H_2O_2 might react with debris and produce gas that can cause continuous pain.
80 D As compressed air may cause tissue emphysema
81 C
82 D
83 B
84 A
85 B
86 C
87 D
88 B
89 A
90 B
91 D
92 D
93 C
94 C
95 A
96 B
97 D
98 D Antibiotics are only prescribed if indicated e.g. medically compromised patient or a contaminated avulsion.
99 C
100 D

Notes

Syllabus

1. Introduction to Pedodontics:
   a. Definition.
   b. Scope.
   c. Main differences between pedodontics and other specialities.
   d. The child as a patient.
2. Growth and Development (in brief):
   a. Importance of study of growth and development in pedodontics.
   b. Definition and description.
   c. Prenatal and postnatal factors.
   d. Growth theories.
   e. Growth spurts.
3. Development of dentition with brief revision of chronology and its importance.
4. Outlines of principles of examination, diagnosis and treatment planning.
5. Radiology for the child patient.
6. Pediatric considerations in oral surgery.
7. Pediatric operative Dentistry:
   a. Morphology of Primary and Permanent dentition.
   b. Principles of Pediatric Operative Dentistry.
   c. Modifications required for cavity preparation.
   d. Isolation.
   e. Matrices.
   f. The stainless steel crown.
8. Child Psychology:
   a. Theories of Psychological development (in brief).
   b. Psychological development with age.
   c. Application of understanding of psychological growth and development to the practice of Pedodontics.
   d. Fear and its management.
   e. Factors affecting child's reaction to dental experience.
9. Behavioral Science:
   a. Definition.
   b. Types of behaviour encountered in the clinic.
   c. Procedures undertaken.
11. Pernicious oral habits in children and their Management.
12. Dental Caries:
   - Etiology and Pathogensis.
13. Periodontal disease in children.
14. Preventive Dentistry:
   a. Principles and scope.
   b. Types of Prevention.
   c. Different measures used in Preventive Dentistry.
   d. Modern trends in Preventive Dentistry.
   e. Prevention at a community level.
   f. Dental health education.
15. Fluorides:
   a. Historical background.
   b. Mechanism of action.
   c. Its role in preventive dentistry.
   d. Types and methods of fluoride therapy.
   e. Toxicity.
16. Trauma and its sequelae in children:
   a. Injuries to anterior teeth.
   b. Classification and importance.
   c. Management.
17. Pulp therapy for the primary and young permanent dentition.
18. Dental care of the handicapped child.

19. Epidemiology:
- **a. Definition and classification.**
- **b. Indices used for dental caries, periodontal disease and Malocclusion.**
- **c. The survey technique.**
- **d. Epidemiology of dental diseases in children.**

20. Oral manifestations of systemic disease in children.

21. Congenital Anomalies.

22. Chromosomal Aberrations.

23. Nutrition and Dental Health including nutritional disorders.

24. Adolescent Dentistry.

25. Dental Auxillaries in Pedodontics.

26. Prosthetics in Pediatric Dentistry.

Chapter 13

Pedodontics with Preventive Dentistry

1. **Ander's Formula for calculating drug dosage is**

   A. $Dose_{ADULT} = Dose_{CHILD} \times \left(\frac{\text{Weight of Child}}{\text{Weight of Adults}}\right)^{0.7}$

   B. $\frac{\text{Age}}{\text{Age} + 12} \times \text{Adult Dose}$

   C. $\frac{\text{Weight}}{70} \times \text{Adult Dose}$

   D. None of these

2. **Fluoride supplement indicated for a 5-year-old child residing in a community with negligible/No fluoride present in drinking water is**

   A. 0.25 mg B. 0.50 mg
   C. 1.0 mg D. Nil

3. **Management of intrusive luxation of a deciduous upper central incisor in a 3-year-old child should include**

   A. Repositioning alone
   B. Repositioning along with splinting
   C. Replacement by a space maintainer
   D. Observation only

4. **Physiologic thumb sucking should regress by age**

   A. 1 year B. 2 years
   C. 3 years D. 5 years

5. **Following teeth are not affected by nursing bottle caries**

   A. Lower molars B. Upper incisors
   C. Upper molars D. Lower incisors

6. **Pit and fissure sealants are not indicated in**

   A. Deciduous teeth
   B. Incipient caries lesion
   C. Permanent teeth that have erupted for more than four years
   D. None of the above

7. **Following natural sugar is least cariogenic**

   A. Glucose B. Sucrose
   C. Saccharine D. Starch

8. **GIC indicated for use as sealants in young permanent teeth is**

   A. Type I B. Type II
   C. Type III D. Type IV

9. **Ultrasonic scaling is not indicated in**

   A. Adolescent patients having extrinsic stains
   B. Children having gingivitis
   C. Postpubertal periodontitis
   D. All of the above

10. **A 16-year-old teenager who has caused injury (mobility) to an anterior teeth of another individual during a fist fight can be penalised by court of law as a case of**

    A. Criminal offence
    B. Juvenile delinquency
    C. Grievous hurt
    D. All of the above

11. Peak incidence of dental caries seen in deciduous teeth is at age

A. 1-3 years B. 3-4 years
C. 4-8 years D. 8-11 years

12. Safety of following drug(s) is not established for young children

A. Nimesulide
B. Rofecoxib
C. Omeprazole
D. All of the above

13. Children's day is celebrated on

A. 7th April
B. 1st July
C. 14th November
D. 1st December

14. Pulse polio programme is

A. A part of universal immunization schedule
B. Based on oral vaccination
C. Substitute to parenteral polio vaccine
D. All of the above

15. Handicapped child includes following, *except*

A. Diabetes
B. Cerebral palsy
C. Rheumatic heart disease
D. Juvenile periodontitis

16. A common syndrome associated with periodontal diseases in children is

A. Ramsay hunt syndrome
B. Greenspan syndrome
C. Papillon-lé-Fevre syndrome
D. Brittle bone syndrome

17. Following characteristic feature(s) of deciduous teeth differentiates them from permanent teeth

A. Less calcified
B. Bucco-lingual width of anterior teeth is less than mesio-distal width
C. Crown root ratio is 1: 1.3
D. All of the above

18. The following is not true about Down's syndrome

A. Macroglossia is a commonly associated
B. Brachycephaly is a characteristic feature sign
C. The condition is also called as trisomy 21
D. None of the above

19. A hemophiliac child aged 10 years reports to the dental operatory with a history of pain and swelling in relation to decayed deciduous lower canine with grade I mobility. The treatment of choice is

A. Medicate symptomatically
B. Perform incision and drainage followed by suturing
C. Institute pulp therapy under nerve block anaesthesia in the affected tooth
D. Extract the affected tooth after cryoprecipitate infusion

20. A 5-year-old feeble child reports for dental consultation along with his guardian. Upon examination the patient is found to have fever, tenderness in area of parotid gland and enlarged submandibular as well as sublingual lymph nodes. The dentist should suspect

A. Measles B. Parotitis
C. AIDS D. All of the above

21. School dental nurse and dental therapist can both

A. Make a diagnosis
B. Operate on children
C. Plan treatment
D. All of the above

22. Topical fluorides act in all the following ways, *except*

A. Exert bactericidal action
B. Alter tooth morphology
C. Remineralize incipient caries lesions
D. Inhibit production of extracellular polysaccharides

23. Preventive Resin Restorations are indicated in
- **A.** Deep and narrow pits and fissures of posterior teeth
- **B.** Incipient carious lesions on occlusal surfaces of molar teeth
- **C.** Interproximal carious lesions of premolar teeth
- **D.** None of the above

24. An asthmatic child needing restorative dental care has to be treated with following precautions, *except*
- **A.** Keeping bronchodilators available in the operatory
- **B.** Using micromotor hand piece for cavity preparation
- **C.** During morning appointment, preferably
- **D.** None of the above

25. A fearful child patient starts crying upon seeing the syringe and needle in the dental operatory. The following behaviour management technique will have to be used after parental consent
- **A.** Contigency management
- **B.** TSD
- **C.** Modelling
- **D.** HOME

26. The following reflex cannot be elicited in a child at birth
- **A.** Grasp reflex
- **B.** Asymmetric tonic neck reflex
- **C.** Cough reflex
- **D.** Babinski reflex

27. Children particularly vulnerable to anterior tooth injuries are
- **A.** Cerebral palsy patients
- **B.** Having class III malocclusion
- **C.** Females
- **D.** All of the above

28. The following type of cry seen in children is not a true cry
- **A.** Obstinate
- **B.** Frightened
- **C.** Hurt
- **D.** Compensatory

29. If a child gets afraid on seeing a dentist for the first time, it is a case of
- **A.** Xenophobia
- **B.** Nyclophobia
- **C.** Zoophobia
- **D.** Anthropophobia

30. Ephebodontics is practised in
- **A.** Fearful patients
- **B.** Mentally handicapped children
- **C.** Subjects who have attained puberty
- **D.** Medically compromised cases

31. Diet counselling is not indicated for
- **A.** Adolescents
- **B.** Children in whom first permanent molars have not erupted
- **C.** Parents
- **D.** None of the above

32. All of the following clinical features are suggestive of Dental Fluorosis, *except*
- **A.** Usually seen on tips of cusps or incisal edges of teeth
- **B.** Resembles line shading with glazed appearance that is not clearly differentiated from adjacent normal enamel
- **C.** Most frequently seen on permanent canines, premolars and second/third molars
- **D.** Seen most easily under strong light source focused on line of sight perpendicular to tooth surface

33. Pulpectomy procedure on a grossly decayed upper primary second molar of a 6-year-old should not be followed by
- **A.** Amalgam restoration
- **B.** Porcelain fused to metal crown
- **C.** Stainless steel crown
- **D.** None of the above

34. An international agency that works exclusively for the welfare of children is
- **A.** WHO
- **B.** UNIFEM
- **C.** UNDP
- **D.** UNICEF

35. A 9-year-old patient report with complaint of tenderness in decayed lower first permanent molar for last few days. Upon excavation, an area of bleeding is detected. IOPA reveals normal root length without any periapical changes. The treatment of choice is
 A. Pulpectomy **B.** Pulpotomy
 C. Pulp capping **D.** Extraction

36. Exarticulation refers to
 A. Tooth avulsion
 B. Peripheral dislocation of tooth
 C. Extrusive luxation of tooth
 D. Posterior malocclusion

37. Medicament of choice for pulpotomy in deciduous incisors is
 A. Calcium hydroxide
 B. Camphorated monochlorophenol
 C. Calcium hydroxide + Camphorated monochlorophenol
 D. Formacresol

38. The community periodontal index of treatment needs when used in children upto 15 years age, examines the following status codes
 A. 0, 1 **B.** 0, 1, 2
 C. 0, 1, 2, 3 **D.** 0, 1, 2, 3, 4

39. Most prevalent of the following malnutritions seen among Indian chidren is
 A. Beri-beri **B.** Obesity
 C. Marasmus **D.** Goitre

40. A young athlete complains of burning sensation in tongue. Upon examination of soft tissues the only finding is macerations at corners of lips. The likely diagnosis is
 A. Anorexia nervosa
 B. Protein energy malnutrition
 C. Vitamin deficiency
 D. Dehydration

41. Untreated occlusal caries lesion in decidous first molar can lead to
 A. Caries in erupting first premolar
 B. Turner's hypoplasia
 C. Caries in decidous second molar
 D. All of the above

42. Case of crown infarction in relation to upper left canine is usually indicated for
 A. Restoration alone
 B. Pulp therapy followed by fixed restoration
 C. Extraction followed by prosthetic replacement
 D. Periodontal splinting

43. While giving inferior alveolar nerve block for children below 5 years of age, the needle should be inserted
 A. Below the level of occlusal plane
 B. At the level of occlusal plane
 C. Above the level of occlusal plane
 D. Any of the above

44. Safest local anaesthesia that can be used in children is
 A. Chloroprocaine
 B. Lignocaine
 C. Bupivacaine
 D. Mepivocaine

45. Commonest complication related to extraction of mandibular 1st deciduous molar is
 A. Trismus **B.** Dry socket
 C. Lip biting **D.** Mandibular fracture

46. A child is considered mentally retarded, when his/her intelligence quotient is
 A. Below 59 **B.** Below 69
 C. Below 79 **D.** Below 89

47. Bird or fish like facies, hypoplasia of facial bones (Especially malar bone and mandible), macrostomia, cleft palate and blind fistulas at the angle of mouth in a child are associated with
 A. Cranio facial dysostosis
 B. Pierre Robin syndrome
 C. Treacher Collins syndrome
 D. Marfan syndrome

48. Juvenile periodontitis is
A. Associated with Down's syndrome
B. Characterized by mid-line diastema and localized angular bone defects in the 1st molar and incisor region
C. Associated with horizontal bone defect
D. All of the above

49. Koplik's spots are an oral manifestation of
A. Varicella B. Shingles
C. Rubella D. Rubeola

50. Cheiloscopy is a useful adjunct in
A. Extra oral radiography of pediatric patient
B. Thyroid function test among children
C. Investigating child abuse
D. None of the above

51. Operative modification(s) undertaken for a class II cavity preparation in a deciduous molar is/are
A. Depth of the cavity is 0.25 mm in dentin
B. Ginginval cavosurface margin is not bevelled
C. Isthmus does not exceed 1/3rd of intercuspal width
D. All of the above

52. A primary risk factor for dental caries is
A. Time B. Saliva
C. Oral hygiene D. Detergency of food

53. The child of an overprotective mother is likely to be
A. Lacking cooperation
B. Tensed cooperative
C. Hysterical
D. Timid

54. The following social scientist described psychologic development of a child on the basis of development tasks using terms related to human organs
A. Abraham Maslow
B. Ivan Pavlov
C. Erick Erickson
D. Sigmond Freud

55. An autosomal recessive trait is inherited in the ratio of
A. 1 : 3 B. 2 : 3
C. 1 : 1 D. None of the above

56. Relative to the lower primary incisors, the permanent incisors are
A. Superior and lingual
B. Superior and facial
C. Inferior and lingual
D. Inferior and facial

57. Correlation between the age and weight in a child is best represented by
A. Histogram
B. Line diagram
C. Scatter diagram
D. Bar diagram

58. Tooth buds which develop after birth are
A. All permanent teeth
B. All permanent teeth and some primary teeth
C. First premolar, second premolar, second molar and third molar
D. First molar

59. The primary germ layers develop during
A. Presomite period
B. Somite period
C. Post somite period
D. Fetal period

60. If both parents have cleft lip and palate, the probability of the first child having the same condition is
A. 1:50 (2%) B. 1:25 (4%)
C. 1:10 (10%) D. 3:5 (60%)

61. Which of the following is true about Catlans appliance?
A. It is used to treat cross bite of maxillary posterior teeth
B. It is constructed on the lower anterior teeth
C. If used for a long period it results in anterior deep bite
D. If constucted on the upper anterior teeth it has a 45 degree angulation

62. Which of the following shows a strong familial tendency?
- A. Proclined maxillary incisors
- B. Deep bite
- C. Open bite
- D. Unilateral cross bite

63. Dolicocephalic facial pattern is associated with
- A. Broad dental arch
- B. Long and narrow dental arch
- C. Paraboloid dental arch
- D. Square dental arch

64. First evidence of tooth formation is in
- A. 14th week intrauterine
- B. 11th week intrauterine
- C. 6th month intrauterine
- D. 4th month after birth

65. Generalized growth failure in first six months of an infant will show
- A. Enamel hypoplasia
- B. Maxillary retrusion
- C. Mandibular retrusion
- D. Dentinogenesis imperfecta

66. 14-year-old boy with thumb sucking habit will show on the cephalogram
- A. Increased posterior facial height
- B. Decreased posterior facial height
- C. Increased posterior and anterior facial height
- D. Increased anterior facial height

67. Dental analysis in the absence of radiographs can be done in all *except*
- A. Carey's and Nance analysis
- B. Moyer's analysis
- C. Huckaba's analysis
- D. Pont's analysis

68. 90 degree turn of expansion screw leads to movement of
- A. 0.1 mm
- B. 0.2 mm
- C. 0.36 mm
- D. 0.09 mm

69. Gemination and fusion are due to disturbance during
- A. Initiation and proliferation
- B. Morphodifferentiation
- C. Apposition
- D. Calcification

70. In serial extraction, after extraction of upper 1st premolar, canine will move
- A. Down and backward
- B. Down and forward
- C. Primarily backward
- D. Primarily downward

71. 1st evidence of wisdom teeth is at
- A. 6 months in
- B. At birth
- C. 1 month after birth
- D. 1 year after birth

72. In the treatment of anterior cross bite, which is not correct
- A. Should be attempted as soon as it is detected
- B. Deep bite is an advantage
- C. Should be corrected with an inclined plane
- D. Cross elastics have deleterious effect

73. Distal shoe space maintainers are indicated when
- A. 1st permanent molars are exfoliated
- B. 1st deciduous molars are exfoliated
- C. 2nd deciduous molars are exfoliated
- D. 1st permanent molars should have erupted

74. Which analysis is not applicable for mixed dentition
- A. Hixon old father
- B. Nances
- C. Moyers analysis
- D. Hold way ratio

75. Primate spaces are as
- A. Between lateral incisors and canines is the mandibular arch
- B. Between lateral incisors and canines in the maxillary arch
- C. Spaces spread out equally in the dental arches
- D. Between canines and 1st molars in the maxillary dental arch

76. The two blocks in the twin block functional appliance are angulated at

A. 75° B. 70°
C. 65° D. 80°

77. Negative growth is a characteristic of

A. Testis B. Brain
C. Mandible D. Thymus

78. Normal facial index is

A. 65-75% B. 75-80%
C. 80-90% D. 100%

79. The body tissue that grows rapidly but shows minimal growth after the age of 6-7 years is

A. Neural tissue
B. Lymphoid tissue
C. Skeletal tissue
D. Genital tissue

80. The implant method of studying growth was proposed by

A. S common B. Borg
C. Belchier D. Björk

81. Maxilla is "primarily" formed by

A. Intramembranous bone formation
B. From cartilage
C. Endochondral bone formation
D. Equally by intramembranous and endochondral bone formation

82. Which statement best describes tooth development during eruption

A. The crown pierces the alveolar crest when 2/3 root is complete.
B. The crown reaches the occlusal plane when 2/3 root is complete
C. The crown pierces the alveolar crest when 3/4 of root is complete
D. The crown does not emerge in the oral cavity until root formation is complete

83. The following statements about breast milk are true *except*

A. The maximum milk output is seen at 12 months
B. The coefficient of uptake of iron in breast milk is 70%
C. Calcium absorption of human milk is better than that of cow's milk
D. It provides about 65 Kcals per 100 ml

84. The current recommendation for breast feeding is that

A. Exclusive breast feeding should be continued till 6 months of age followed by supplementation with additional foods
B. Exclusive breast feeding should be continued till 4 months of age followed by supplementation with additional foods
C. Colostrum is the most suitable food for a new born baby but it best avoided in first 2 days
D. The baby should be allowed to breast-feed till one year of age

85. Anodontia affects the growth of

A. Maxilla
B. Mandible
C. Alveolar bone
D. Cranium

86. Large anterior fontanelles, open sutures, small slanting eyes, decresed sexual development, macroglossia and enamel hypolasia are seen in

A. Cranioacial dysostosis
B. Downs syndrome
C. Osteopetrosis
D. Treachers collins syndrome

87. Which of the following is most likely to have bifurcated roots?

A. Mandibular canine
B. Mandibular cental incisor
C. Maxillary incisor
D. Mandibular lateral incisor

88. Malocculsion which can be prevented

A. Loss of proximal contacts
B. Absence of teeth
C. Cleft palate
D. One due to growth disturbances

89. **Abnormal swallowing habit can result in**
A. Posterior crossbite
B. Anterior open bite
C. Class III malocclusion
D. Unilateral crossbite

90. **A 14-year-old boy has delayed eruption of the second molar. Radiography shows a dentigerous cyst surrounding the crown of tooth. The treatment of choice is**
A. Extraction of the molar
B. Aspiration of the cyst
C. Observe
D. Expose the crown and keep it exposed

91. **Delayed eruption of teeth may be seen most likely in which of these condition**
A. Downs syndrome
B. Mental retardation
C. Autism
D. Cerebral palsy

92. **Unilateral upper cleft lip occurs due to the failure of fusion of**
A. Medial nasal and maxillary process
B. Medial and lateral nasal
C. Maxillary processes
D. Maxillary process with the palatal process

93. **There are multiple supernumerary teeth, delayed eruption. These features are seen in**
A. Downs syndrome
B. Craniofacial dysostosis
C. Cleidocranial dysostosis
D. Ectodermal dysplasia

94. **Characteristics of Class II Div 2 malocclusion**
A. Deep over bite, retruded central incisor and protuded lateral incisor
B. Increased overjet
C. Open bite
D. Cross bite

95. **Carpal index refers to**
A. Accurate bone age
B. Dental development
C. Age of root
D. Mental development

96. **After six years growth mainly occurs**
A. Distal to molars
B. Between canines
C. Between premolars
D. Mesial to premolars

97. **Freeway space is utilised for**
A. Late mesial shift
B. Early mesial shift
C. Relieving crowding in deciduous teeth
D. Correction of mandibular diastema

98. **Palatal sutures are closed by**
A. 8-10 weeks B. 18 months
C. 1 year D. 2 years

99. **Adenoid facies are seen in**
A. Tongue thruster
B. Lip sucker
C. Mouth breather
D. Thumb sucker

100. **In permanent incisors, enamel formation is complete at**
A. Birth B. 3½ years
C. 5 years D. 7 years

Answers

1 B $\frac{\text{Age}}{\text{Age} + 12} \times \text{Adult Dose}$ 'B' is Young's formula.

C $\frac{\text{Weight}}{70} \times \text{Adult Dose}$ 'C' is Clark's formula.

2 B According to ADA, 0.25 mg is for children 6 months-3 years old, 0.5 mg for 3-6 years old and 1 mg for 6-16 years old in communities where concentration of fluoride in drinking water is < 0.3 mg.

3 D The tooth would generally re-erupt on its own.

4 C

5 D

6 D

7 D Saccharine, though not cariogenic, is not a natural sugar.

8 C 'A' is used for base, 'B' for restoration, and 'D' as Glass-cermet.

9 B Ultrasonic scaling is not indicated in children.

10 D

11 B

12 D

13 C 14th November is celebrated as Children's Day in India because it is Pandit Jawaharlal Nehru's birthday. 'A' is World Health Day, 'B' is Doctors' Day, and 'D' is AIDS Day.

14 B

15 D Handicap is any disadvantage which limits the fulfilment of a role that is normal for an individual in the long run.

16 C 'A' is associated with transient facial palsy and intra-extra oral vesicles while 'B' is associated with diabetes, hypertension and lichen planus, and 'D' is osteogenesis imperfecta.

17 A

18 D

19 A The deciduous canine is likely to shed soon in the given situation.

20 D Inflammation around salivary glands can be of a viral origin. Since lymphnodes are involved and patient appears weak and without parental escort (parents might have succumbed to HIV), a dentist cannot rule out AIDS either.

21 B However their dental therapist cannot diagnose or plan treatment (Unlike Dental nurse). Common target population is school children.

22 B Systemic fluorides can alter tooth morphology during early stages of tooth development.

23 B Sealants are indicated for 'A' and restorations for 'C'.

24 C Evening appointments are preferable for asthmatic patients since there is excess sputum production in morning.

25 D 'A', 'B' and 'C' are behaviour shaping techniques that do not require any parental consent.

26 B

27 B Children aged 1-3 years, especially males, are more vulnearble to anterior tooth injuries.

28 D

29 A 'B' is fear of night, 'C' is fear of animal, and 'D' is fear of people.

30 C Ephebodontics is also known as adolescent dentistry.

31 B

32 D

33 B 'B' is a permanent crown that is not indicated for deciduous teeth.

34 D United Nations International Children's Emergency Fund (UNICEF).

35 B Although direct pulp capping could be a rare option, the duration of carious exposure would be critical in that case.

36 A

37 D 'A' causes internal resorption in deciduous teeth and 'C' is used for apexification.

38 B

39 C Protein malnutrition.

40 D

41 B

42 A Crown infarction is tooth fracture limited to enamel or dentin.

43 A Inferior alveolar.

44 A

45 C

46 B I.Q classification guide:

IQ range	*Grade*
Above 140	Very superior
120-139	Superior
110-119	High average
90-109	Average
80-89	Low average
70-79	Borderline impaired
< 69	Mentally retarded

47 C 'A' is Crouzon syndrome associated with cranial synostosis, ocular proptosis and hypoplastic maxilla. 'B' is Robin anomalad characterized by U-shaped cleft palate, micrognathia, glossoptosis and hydro/microcephacy. 'D' is associated with craniofacial, skeletal, ocular and cardiovascular anomalies.

48 B

49 D Koplik's spots are an oral manifestation of measles.

50 C Study of lip prints in forensic odontology.

51 B Enamelrods in cervical areas of deciduous teeth do not taper apically.

52 A Risk factors in caries (Neuburn 1982) include.

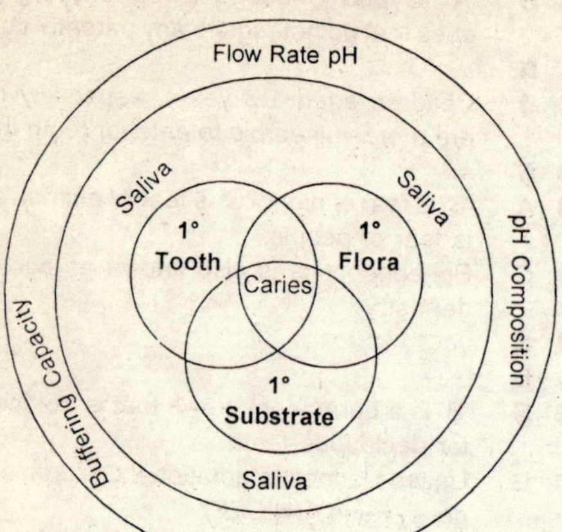

2° (Host) : Age
Fluorides
Morphology
Nutrition
Trace elements
Carbonate level

2° (Agent) : *Strep. mutans*
Oral hygiene
Fluoride in plaque

2° (Environment) : Oral clearance
Oral hygiene
Detergency of food
Frequency of eating
Carbohydrate (type, concentration).

53 D 'A' is for handicapped children, 'B' for battered child, 'C' for children of overindulgent mother.

54 C Comparison between Erickson's and Freud's psychological stages.

Age	Erickson's psychological stage	Freud's psychological stage
0-1	Basic trust versus	Oral stage
2-3	Autonomy versus shame doubt	Anal stage
4-5	Initiative versus guilt	Phallic stage
6-12	Industry versus inferiority	Latency stage
13-18	Identity versus role confusion	Genital stage

55 A

56 C All permanent tooth germs from the central incisor to the 2nd premolar are at firth located in the fibrous connective tissue overlying the incised or occlusal edge or the occlusal surface of the corresponding deciduous teeth. As a result of the combined action of bone growth and active eruption of the deciduous teeth, which brings about a gradual increase in the height of the alveolar process, the germs of the permanent teeth change their position downwards in a lingual direction.

57 B Bayley established growth curves based on height and weight in relation to physical maturity. Children who are accelerated will have growth and weight curves at about the 2 upper times. Those who mature slowly will show a curve at about the 2 lower times.

58 C
59 A
60 D
61 B
62 B
63 B
64 A
65 A
66 A

67 D Pont's analysis is a model/cast analysis and does not require radiographs. Inference is attribute to measurements on plaster casts. Rest other analyses involve radiographs.

68 B
69 B

70 A The relative position of the 1st premolar and the permanent canine must be ascertained before extractions are undertaken. When radiographic examination shows that the canines might erupt before the 1st premolars, Dewel advises extraction of the 1st decidous molars before extracting the decidous canines to prevent the canines from erupting before the 1st premolars. If the canines are permitted to erupt first, there may be impaction of the 1st premolars. However, early 1st decidous molar extraction. When the permanent canines are not erupting in advance of the 1st premolars and the deciduous cannines are in position they should be allowed to remain in place.

T weed suggests when 1st premolars are extracted 4 to 6 months prior to eruption of the permanent canines, the permanent canines usually shift posteriorly and erupt in the space left by the extracted premolars.

71 B

72 D Treatment of anterior crossibite should be done as soon as it is detected. Deep bite has an

advantage for the retention aspect is concerned. Besides inclined plane use of cross elastic is advocated for correction of cross bite in the literature.

73 C
74 D
75 B
76 C Refer Am Journal of Orthodontics 1989 by Clarke.
77 D
78 B
79 B
80 D
81 A
82 A
83 A The milk output depends on the "let-down" reflex which in turn depend on the sucking by the baby. As long as the baby sucks at breast there is stimulus sent to post pituitary and in turn to hypothalamus releasing oxytocin for release of milk and prolactin for production of milk (galactogoges of the stimulus that is baby is deprived from mother, this cycle stops.
84 A Weaning should be started at 6 months as breast milk is sufficient at this stage and teething appear by 6 months and physiological demand of baby correlates. This is widely recommended by WHO for developing countries.

Colostrum is rich in immunoglobins and vitamin A so it should be first food for new born for first two days. Breast feeding should be continued till or after 2 years of age as the baby demands, as it has an additional advantage of contraception.

85 C
86 B
87 D
88 D
89 B
90 D
91 A
92 C
93 D
94 D
95 A
96 A
97 A
98 D
99 C
100 D

Notes

Syllabus

1. Introduction to oral surgery: Aims, scope and objectives.
2. Neurology of facial pain.
3. Local anaesthesia definition, concept, types of local anaesthesia, indications and contraindications, advantages and disadvantages.
4. Ideal requirements of local anaesthetic solution, composition and mode of action.
5. Anaesthesia of mandible. Direct technique of ID nerve block.
6. Anaesthesia of maxilla.
   a. Infra-orbital block.
   b. Posterior superior alveolar nerve block.
   c. Maxillary nerve block.
7. Complications of local anaesthesia.
8. Exodontia—Indications, contraindications, principles, techniques, complications.
9. Impacted mandibular third molar, maxillary third molar and canine.
10. Post extraction bleeding.
11. Infections of the oral cavity:
    a. Anatomy of facial spaces above the Hyoid bone.
    b. Acute alveolar abscess.
    c. Ludwig's Angina.
    d. Osteomyelitis of the jaws.
12. Trigeminal neuralgia.
13. Benign cystic lesions of the jaws.
14. Preservation of infected teeth.
15. Maxillary sinus:
    a. Surgical anatomy.
    b. Surgical approach.
    c. Oro-antral fistula.
16. Facial pain clinical aspects.
17. Emergencies in oral surgery.
18. Antibiotics and analgesics.
19. Pre-prosthetic surgery.
20. TM joint:
    a. Surgical anatomy.
    b. Dislocation and pain dysfunction syndrome.
21. Fractures of the mandible introduction, surgical anatomy and classification.
22. Fractures of the middle third of face introduction, classification.
23. Complications of the jaws.
24. Odontogenic tumors.
25. Salivary glands.
26. Developmental deformities of the jaws.
27. Biopsy.
28. Premalignant lesions of the oral cavity.
29. Oral cancer.
30. General anaesthesia.

Chapter 14

Oral and Maxillofacial Surgery

1. When a maxillary tooth is being extracted, the chair should be adjusted so that the site of operation is about

A. 3 inch above shoulder level
B. 8 inch above shoulder level
C. 3 inch below shoulder level
D. 6 inch above elbow level

2. Read forceps are used for extraction of

A. Maxillary incisors
B. Maxillary premolars
C. Mandibular incisors
D. Mandibular premolars

3. When multiple lower incisor teeth are to be extracted, a straight elevator can be used in between them to loosen each one to fascilitate extraction. This technique is known as

A. Bryan technique
B. Valsalva technique
C. Stobie technique
D. Campbell technique

4. For a better blood supply, a flap should be designed in such a manner that

A. The base should be broader than the apex (free end)
B. The base should be narrower than the apex
C. Base should rest on the pathology
D. Edges of the flap rest on the pathology

5. Oblique facial clefts usually extend from

A. Upper lip to ear
B. Lower lip to chin
C. Upper lip to the eye
D. Upper lip to nose

6. Antimongoloid slanting, deficient malar bones, absence of zygomatic arches, middle ear abnormalities and hypoplastic rami and mandibular condyles are features of

A. Cleidocranial dysostosis
B. Pierre Robin syndrome
C. Marfan's syndrome
D. Treacher Collins syndrome

7. The 'midface' contains

A. Craminum and supra-orbital region
B. Supra-orbital and nasal region
C. Orbit, nose and cheeks
D. Nose, lips and chin

8. 'Satellite' cysts in the fibrous tissue capsule or at a distance in the marrow spaces of cancellous bone are common with

A. Keratocytes
B. Dentigerous cysts
C. Cystic ameloblastoma
D. Calcifying odontogenic cysts

9. Liquid nitrogen spray is used in

A. Chemical cautery **B.** Electro cautery
C. Cryosurgery **D.** Laparoscopy

10. Most radicular cysts are lined by
A. Keratinized squamous epithelium
B. Non Keratinized squamous epithelium
C. Keratinized columnar epithelium
D. Keratinized Cuboidal and respiratory epithelium

11. Sialogram of a normal parotid gland is described as
A. Branchless fruit laden tree
B. Tree in winter
C. Tree in summer
D. Bush in winter

12. In a severely burned patient, the surface area of the trunk and head represent ____ proportion of the body surface
A. 18 percent B. 29 percent
C. 36 percent D. 45 percent

13. Severe trismus resulting from acute dental infection indicates ____ involvement
A. Retropharyngeal space
B. Sublingual space
C. Masticator space
D. Mandibular space

14. The usual first clinical sign of mild lignocaine toxicity is
A. Lethargy B. Tachycardia
C. Convulsion D. Nervousness

15. The lingual nerve is more likely to be damaged during surgeries of
A. Parasymphysis area
B. Mylohyoid ridge
C. Vertical impactions
D. Mental region

16. History of allergy, Hyperactive bronchi, change in caliber of bronchi to various irritants, are all features of
A. Bronchitis
B. Bronchiectasis
C. Asthma
D. Pulmonary embolism

17. Incision lines in the neck should be
A. Parallel to platysma fibres
B. Perpendicular to platysma fibres
C. Parallel to natural skin creases
D. 45° to natural skin creases

18. Ideally what should be the interval between pre-irradiation extractions and the beginning of radiotherapy?
A. 2-14 days B. 3-6 days
C. 7-14 days D. 10-20 days

19. For maximal control, a scalpel is held in a
A. Pen grasp
B. Palm and thumb grasp
C. Finger and thumb grasp
D. Pen and paper grasp

20. Patients who have had a cerebrovascular accident are generally placed on
A. Anticonvulsant B. Antidepressants
C. Analgesics D. Anticoagulants

21. Fine brittle hair, hyperpigmentation of skin, excessive-sweating and tachycardia are all due to
A. Excessive insulin production
B. Deficient insulin production
C. Excessive parathormone production
D. Excessive thyroid hormone production

22. The final stage of wound repair or 'wound maturation' is known as
A. Inflammatory stage
B. Fibrinolytic stage
C. Remodelling stage
D. Fibroplastic stage

23. The beaks of the forceps during extraction of teeth should be placed
A. Parallel to the long axis of the tooth
B. Perpendicular to long axis of the tooth
C. At an angle of 45° to long axis of the tooth
D. At the crown of the tooth

24. The canine fossa approach is otherwise known as
A. Intranasal antrostomy
B. Burger's approach
C. Caldwell-LUC approach
D. Eilli's approach

25. In subcutaneous emphysema
A. Air is forced into blood vessels
B. Air is forced into connective tissue of intramuscular or facial spaces
C. Blood is forced into intramuscular spaces
D. Air is forced into joint spaces

26. Secondary haemorrhage is bleeding that develops
A. During surgery
B. 24-48 hours after surgery
C. Several days after surgery
D. Due to excessive physical activity

27. Birn's hypothesis is suggested to describe
A. Chronic osteomyelitis
B. Septic periostitis
C. Ecchymosis and haematoma
D. Acute alveolar osteitis

28. Third stage of healing of extraction wound shows
A. Replacement of granulation tissue by connective tissue and epithelialization of wound
B. Haemorrhage and clot formation
C. Organization of the clot by granulation tissue
D. Replacement of connective tissue by coarse fibrillar bone

29. The term used for removal of partly erupted/unerupted teeth or retained roots that cannot be extracted by forcep and therefore must be removed by surgical excision is
A. Odontotomy
B. Odontectomy
C. Apicoectomy
D. Odontoplasty

30. During 'lingual split bone technique' the chisel is positioned
A. At an angle of 80° to the alveolar bone
B. Parallel to internal oblique ridge
C. At an angle of 45° to the alveolar bone
D. Perpendicular to internal oblique ridge

31. In 'Field and Ackerman' classification of maxillary canine impactions, when the canine with its crown lies between the lateral incisor and 1st premolar roots it is known to be in
A. Palatal position
B. Intermediate position
C. Labial position
D. Unusual position

32. The 'Ochsenbein-luebke' flap is
A. A combination of horizontal and vertical incisions
B. A combination of semilunar and vertical incisions
C. A combination of semilunar and envelope incisions
D. A combination of vertical and envelope incisions

33. 'Periapical osteitis' is
A. When the infection is confined within the tooth
B. When the infection is confined within the alveolar bone
C. When the infection spreads into the surrounding soft tissues
D. When the infection localizes and suppuration starts

34. Clinically the 'Buccal space infection' appears to be
A. Dome shaped
B. Dumbell shaped
C. Triangular shaped
D. Spherical shaped

35. Initial symptoms of cavernous sinus thrombosis are
A. Edema of eyelids and lacrimation
B. Pain in the eye with tenderness to pressure
C. Chemosis and retinal haemorrhages
D. Signs of advanced toxemia and meningitis

36. Hyperbaric oxygen therapy is indicated in
A. Osteodystrophy and Paget's disease
B. Osteomyelitis and osteogenic imperfecta
C. Osteomyelitis and osteoradionecrosis
D. Osteoradionecrosis and pathological fractures

37. Augmentation of atrophic mandible can be done by all of the following *except*
A. Superior border augmentation with ribgrafts
B. Superior border augmentation with iliac-crest grafts
C. Inferior border augmentation with ribgrafts
D. Inferior border augmentation with humerus grafts

38. When resorption and deposition of subperiosteal bone results in only a thin layer of bone overlying a cyst, the surface can be indented with an examining finger fracturing the bone and producing the so called ____.
A. Fluctuation effect
B. Tennis ball effect
C. Ping pong ball effect
D. Elastic effect

39. A Toller's double lumen needle is used to
A. Deposit contrast medium into a cyst
B. Enucleate a cyst
C. Take a punch biopsy
D. Marsupialize a cyst

40. 'Phlebolith's are
A. Hemangiomas containing fatty tissue
B. Lymphangiomas containing glandular tissue
C. Hemangiomas containing calcified bodies
D. Vascular malformation with crepitus

41. Treatment of choice of amputation neuroma is
A. Cryosurgery
B. Electrocautery
C. Chemical cautery
D. Surgical resection

42. Hyperparathyroidism can be associated with
A. Osteomas
B. Giant cell lesions
C. Neurofibromatosis
D. Salivary neoplasms

43. 'Botryoid odontogenic cyst' is a variant of
A. Apical periodontal cyst
B. Circumferential dentigerous cyst
C. Lateral periodontal cyst
D. Residual cyst

44. Which of the following radiological picture is common to Ameloblastoma, myoxoma, Giant cell granuloma and aneurysmal bone cyst?
A. Soap bubble appearance
B. Onion peel appearance
C. Sunburst appearance
D. Tramline appearance

45. The surgical procedure where the entire tumor is removed intact with a rim of uninvolved bone while maintaining the continuity of the mandible is
A. Enbloc resection
B. Segmental resection
C. Hemimandibulectomy
D. Total mandibulectomy

46. A Weber-Fergusson incision is used for
A. Removal of a tumor in temporal region
B. Removal of a tumor in the maxilla
C. Removal of a tumor in mandible
D. Removal of a tumor in parotid gland

47. **In which of the following condition the clinical features of excessive tipping of lower incision, narrow maxillary arch and difficulty in speech will be encountered?**
A. Abnormally attached high lingual frenum
B. Abnormally attached high labial frenum
C. Hemifacial microsomia
D. Microglossia

48. **The extracellular supporting tissues, including extra cellular fluid and the mineral mass comprises ____% of the body weight**
A. 55% B. 30%
C. 15% D. 0%

49. **Mouth props are used to**
A. Keep the mouth firmly closed
B. Provide continuous suction
C. Keep the mouth open
D. To retract soft tissues

50. **Normal cells which are most affected by chemotherapy for malignant disease are**
A. Endothelial cells
B. Epithelium of GI tract and bone marrow cells
C. Mesenchymal cells and salivary glands
D. Epithelial lining of respiratory tract and cardiac tissue

51. **Necrotizing sialometaplasia usually affects**
A. Minor salivary glands
B. Submandibular gland
C. Stensen's duct
D. Mucous secreting glands of GI tract

52. **Chances of cerebrospinal fluid rhinorrhoea is maximum with**
A. Leforte I fracture
B. Leforte II fracture
C. Leforte III fracture
D. Zygomatic complex fracture

53. **Coalman's sign is a feature of**
A. Mandibular body fracture
B. Mandibular ramus fracture
C. Leforte I fracture
D. Condylar fracture

54. **'Hess chart' is maintained to record**
A. Activity of orbicularis oculi
B. Activity of extraoccular muscles
C. Neurological deficit
D. Intra occular pressure

55. **Which of the following zygomatic fracture is unstable after reduction (elevation) only?**
A. Arch fracture only (medially rotated)
B. Fracture rotated around a vertical axis
C. Orbital rim fracture
D. En bloc dislocation of zygomatic complex fracture

56. **A single incision by the help of which the frontal bone, zygomatic complex and nasoethmoidal complex fractures can be treated by reduction and fixation is**
A. Bicoronal
B. Alkyat Brahmley
C. Bird's wing ('W') incision
D. Blepharoplasty incision

57. **"Creeping substitution" is a process used in connection with**
A. Autologous bone grafting
B. Silastic/Teflon grafting
C. Allogenic freeze dried bone
D. Osseomyocutaneous flap

58. **'CT cisternography' is used to detect**
A. CSF leak
B. Sialolith
C. Presence of aeorcele
D. Intra-cranial haemorrhage

59. **Ideal time of reducing a displaced zygomatic arch fracture is within**
A. 1-2 weeks following trauma
B. 2-3 weeks following trauma
C. 3-4 weeks following trauma
D. 4-5 weeks following trauma

60. The gunning type splint is most commonly used to treat
A. Dentate mandibular fractures
B. Edentulous mandibular fractures
C. Leforte fractures
D. Zygomatic complex fractures

61. One of the most dangerous complications of spread of infection from retropharyngeal space is
A. Cavernous sinus thrombosis
B. Laryngeal edema
C. Mediastinitis
D. Pharyngitis

62. The greatest benefit of thrombolytic drugs in a patient with MI is observed if it is administered within
A. First 1-3 hours after infarction
B. Upto 12 hours after infarction
C. After 24 hours of infarction
D. Never used

63. If there is daily symptoms of wheezing (over a period of several days), exacerbations that affect activity and sleep and may last for days, nocturnal asthmatic attacks at least once a week, limited exercise tolerance, ER visit, FEV_1 60-80% predicted, 20-30% variability, then such type of asthma is classified as
A. Mild intermittent
B. Mild persistent
C. Moderate persistent
D. Severe persistent

64. Cancer patients who undergo whole body irradiation or high-dose chemotherapy or have bone marrow involvement due to disease are susceptible to
A. Thrombocytopenia
B. Neural and chemosensory changes in the form of diminished sense of taste, unpleasent odors and conditioned aversions to food
C. Sclerosis of bone
D. A and B

65. In a patient with hypertension, the local anaesthesia of choice is
A. Xylocaine with adrenaline
B. Xylocaine with noradrenaline
C. Prilocaine with ferlypressin
D. Prilocaine with levonordefrine

66. If a pregnant woman falls into syncope during pregnancy while undergoing dental treatment, she should be placed in
A. Right lateral position
B. Left lateral position
C. Sitting position with head bent in between two knees
D. 10° Trendelenberg position

67. Caprylhydrocuprienotoxin can be used in place of ____ in a local anaesthetic
A. Methyl paraben
B. Thymol
C. Adrenaline
D. Xylocaine

68. 'Vogelgeschit' deformity is found in
A. Bilateral TMJ ankylosis
B. Unilateral TMJ ankylosis
C. Bilateral condylar fracture
D. Bilateral angle fracture of mandibular

69. In thyrotoxicosis, which of the following agents is contraindicated?
A. Xylocaine
B. Adrenaline
C. Prilocaine
D. All of the above

70. Poswillo's skin hook is used to
A. Reduce symphysis fracture
B. Reduce nasal bone fracture
C. Reduce zygomatic complex fracture
D. Reduce edentulous mandibular fracture

71. Branchiogenic cyst arises from
A. 2nd branchial cleft
B. 2nd branchial arch
C. 3rd branchial cleft
D. 3rd branchial arch

72. In which of the following case there will be clicking, masticatory muscle tenderness and limitation of mandibular movement?
- A. U/L TMJ ankylosis
- B. Myofacial pain dysfunction syndrome
- C. Fracture parasymphysis
- D. All of the above

73. The temporomandibular joint is in close relation to
- A. 1st part of maxillary artery
- B. 2nd part of maxillary artery
- C. 3rd part of maxillary artery
- D. None of the above

74. Sodium psylliate is a
- A. Fibrinolytic agent
- B. Sclerosing agent
- C. Anticoagulant
- D. Contrast medium

75. After removal of a sialolith from the duct; it
- A. Should be sutured with catgut
- B. Should be sutured with silk
- C. Should not be sutured
- D. Should be resected

76. Oxyphilic adenoma is a ____ tumour of the salivary glands
- A. Epithelial
- B. Endothelial
- C. Mesenchymal
- D. Unclassified

77. Twitching of lower lip during surgery of the mandible on the same side indicates contact with
- A. Inferior alveolar neve
- B. Nerve to mylohyoid
- C. Marginal mandibular nerve
- D. Cervical branch of facial nerve

78. Complication of parotid gland surgery include
- A. Frey's syndrome
- B. Sjögren's syndrome
- C. Facial paralysis
- D. A and C

79. In vertical subsigmoid osteotomy
- A. The distal segments are moved backwards with the proximal segments overlapping laterally
- B. Proximal segments are moves backwards with the distal segments overlapping laterally
- C. There is no overlapping between segments
- D. Anterior segment of mandible is moved upwards

80. Costochondral (rib) grafts in girls are usually taken from
- A. 3rd and 4th ribs
- B. 4th and 5th ribs
- C. 5th and 6th ribs
- D. 2nd and 3rd ribs

81. Skin tension was first noted by
- A. Lister
- B. Dupuytren
- C. Langer
- D. Kocher

82. 'Catgut' is made from
- A. Cat's gut
- B. Dog's gut
- C. Synthetic material
- D. Sheep's gut

83. Sutures should be placed approximately
- A. 1-2 mm apart
- B. 2-3 mm apart
- C. 3-4 mm apart
- D. 8-10 mm apart

84. In 'Antral regime' which of the following is used as a mucolytic agent
- A. Diphenhydramine hydrochloride
- B. Menthol
- C. Pseudoephedrine
- D. Xylometazoline

85. The method of dry heat sterilization which uses glassbeads, molten metal and salt as the sterilizing medium is an example of
- A. Cold sterilization
- B. Heat transfer device
- C. Hot air oven
- D. Gas sterilization

86. With one rescuer, the ratio of chest compression to lung inflations should be
A. 15 : 2 B. 10 : 3
C. 20 : 4 D. 25 : 1

87. Curvilinear lines of McGregor and Campbell are viewed in a ____ X-ray plate
A. PA view of skull
B. Lateral oblique view of mandible
C. Occipetomenton view of skull
D. OPG of mandible

88. Towne's projection is a
A. Antero-posterior view
B. Postero-anterior view
C. Lateral view
D. Panoramic view

89. The estimation which gives the average amount of haemoglobin in 100 ml of packed red blood cells is
A. Mean corpuscular volume (MCV)
B. Mean corpuscular haemoglobin (MCH)
C. Mean corpuscular haemoglobin concentration (MCHC)
D. Packed cell volume (PCV)

90. A large barrel-shaped chest may be diagnostic of
A. Pulmonary emphysema
B. Asthma
C. Coronary artery disease
D. Hypertension

91. Raised intracranial pressure due to venous engorgement may be treated by
A. Intravenous barbiturate
B. Intravenous mannitol
C. Antihypertensive
D. Diuretics

92. Involucrum is
A. Perforations in the bone through which pus discharges
B. The new bone that is formed after the acute phase of osteomyelitis passes and encloses the sequestra
C. The sequestra which is extruded from the site of the lesion
D. The pus under tension in an apical abscess

93. The absorption of which of the following drugs is hampered if taken along with milk products and drugs containing magnesium, calcium or aluminium
A. Penicillin
B. Pentaprazole
C. Enalapril
D. Tetracycline

94. 'Paracetamol' which is a very commonly used drug for analgesia and antipyresis may invariably lead to
A. Nephrotoxicity
B. Hepatotoxicity
C. Anaemia
D. Dyspepsia

95. If there is any doubt about the nature of comatous state in a diabetic patient in a dental chair, one should inject into the patient
A. 20 ml of 9% normal saline
B. 10 ml of Dextrose normal saline
C. 10 ml of 20% Dextrose solution
D. All of the above

96. In the technique of surgical repositioning, the displaced tooth is rotated through an angle which must be ____ to avoid injury to the apical vessels
A. < 90°
B. > 90°
C. > 90° but < 180°
D. 360°

97. Which of the following tooth is the most frequent cause of palatal infection?
A. Upper central incisor
B. Upper lateral incisor
C. Upper canine
D. Upper 3rd molar

98. Rebound thrombosis following sudden discontinuation of Dicoumarol group of anticoagulants is due to

A. Excessive concentration of factor VIII
B. Diminished concentration of factor VIII
C. Excessive concentration of factor II
D. Diminished concentration of factor XII

99. Which of the following is a Obwegeser's instrument?

A. Chin retractor
B. Ramus retractor
C. Bone Awl
D. All of the above

100. The wasmund, wundrer and cupar methods are for

A. Posterior maxillary alveolar osteotomy
B. Anterior maxillary alveolar osteotomy
C. Total maxillary osteotomy
D. Mandibular body osteotomies

Answers

1 C
2 B
3 C
4 A
5 B
6 D
7 C
8 A
9 C
10 B
11 B
12 D
13 C
14 D
15 B
16 C
17 C
18 C 7-14 days. This period is sufficient for soft tissue healing and re-epithelialization has occurred in this period. The sooner the radiotherapy is begun, the more beneficial it will be.
19 A
20 D
21 D
22 C
23 A This will facilitate extraction without breakage of the tooth. All other options lead to tooth breakage during extraction.
24 C In canine fossa approach, the maxilla is exposed by making an opening in the canine fossa after raising a mucoperiosteal flap. This is called Caldwell-Luc approach.
25 B Most often it follows the use of an air driven dental handpiece or a compressed air spray bottle for irrigation. It leads to swelling where air can be felt to crakle under the palpating fingers. No active treatment is required. The air is absorbed within 1–2 weeks time.
26 C It usually occurs due to infection of the wound resulting in loss of clot or erosion of vessels in the granulation tissue. 'A' is primary haemorrhage and 'B' is reactionary haemorrhage.
27 D Birn has suggested that trauma and infection cause inflammation of the bone marrow resulting in the release of tissue activators which convert the plasminogen present in the clot to plasmin (fibrinolytic agent). This plasmin then dissolves the blood clot and releases Kinins from the kininogen (present in the clot itself) leading to pain.
28 A 'B', 'C' and 'D' refer to the 1st, 2nd and 4th stages of extraction wound healing respectively.
29 B
30 C All other positions will result in a larger chunk of the lingual bone being removed which might sometimes extend upto the coronoid process.
31 B
32 B This flap is scalloped to follow the gingival architecture and avoids elevation of attached gingiva to prevent shrinkage and exposure of margin of restorations.
33 B 'C' and 'D' are known as cellulitis and absceses respectively.
34 A The boundaries of 'Buccal Space' determine the shape of the abscesses. The 'Buccal Space' is bounded medially by buccinator muscle and buccopharyngeal fascia, laterally by skin and subcutaneous tissues, anteriorly by posterior border of zygomaticus major above and depressor anguli oris below; superiorly by zygomatic arch and inferiorly by the lower border of mandible.
35 B 'A' and 'C' are subsequent (intermediate) stages whereas 'D' represents the terminal stage.
36 C 'Hyperbaric oxygen' therapy uses 100%. Oxygen at a greater alveolar partial pressure than which occurs at normal atmospheric pressure. This results in increase in oxygen tension in the tissues leading to improved vascular supply and increased oxygen level also has bacteriostatic and bacteriocidal effects and fascilitate fibroblast proliferation and new capillary formation. All these above factors then aid in healing.
37 D
38 C 'D' is initial stage of cyst expansion where only the centre of the cyst is covered by a thin bone and can be indented without fracturing the thin bone.

'A' is when there is no bone between the cyst lining and the overlying mucosa i.e. the cyst lining is in direct contact with the mucosa.

39 A Whenever it is required to put a contrast medium into the cyst, the removal of the fluid content is mandatory. The Toller's double lumen needle prevents any negative pressure during aspiration and painful positive pressure during the injection of contrast medium.
40 C
41 D
42 B The Giant cell lesion of Hyperparathyroidism is 'Brown tumour'; where serum calcium level is raised and phosphorus level is lowered. The treatment for such lesion is parathyroidectomy and the Giant cell lesion most often subsides on its own following parathyroidectomy.
43 C

44 A All of these lesions reveal a multilocular radio lucency of varying diameter on radiographs. When the multiple radiolucencies are small, the radiographic picture is described as that of soap bubble appearance. 'B' is seen is osteomyelitis and 'C' is characteristic of osteosarcoma.

45 A Is otherwise known as 'marginal resection'. This procedure is advocated for the treatment of aggressive odontogenic tumors when the lesion does not extend closer than 1 cm to the inferior border of mandible.

46 B Here the incision is started subpalpebrally continuing upto just below medial canthus of eye. Then it turns along the lateral nasal crease, turning down and below the external nares of the same side then bisecting the upper lip at the philtrum. The incision is completed by extending it along the mucobuccal fold intra-orally upto the tuberosity.

47 A When the lingual frenum is short and attached high on the alveolar process, the tongue assumes a relatively flat position in the floor of the mouth which may produce abnormal pressure against mandibular incisors during speech and deglutition resulting in excessive labial tipping of mandibular teeth. This might also result in the palatal vault and maxillary arch being narrow and difficulty in tongue movement and speech.

48 B Cell mass constitutes about 55% of body weight 'A' and energy reserves in adipose tissues constitute about 15% 'C'.

49 C

50 B

51 A It is a benign inflammatory process that usually affects minor salivary glands of the palate and in other areas like nasal cavity etc. and is thought to be secondary to vascular infarction of salivary gland lobules. They appear as large painless or painful deeply ulcerated areas lateral to mid palatal raphe and near the junction of hard and soft palate. These lesions usually heal spontaneously within 6–10 weeks.

52 C Le Forte III fracture involves the cribriform plate of the ethmoid bone and when this structure is fractured, cerebrospinal fluid can leak and present as CSF rhinorrhoea.

53 A In mandibular body fracture, the periosteum is stripped most often. Blood then escapes into the sub-mucosal plane and presents as sublingual haematoma.

54 B When there is trauma to the extra occular muscles leading to their paralysis, the Hess chart is maintained to see whether there is any improvement in the acitivity of individual muscles over a period of few days.

55 D Dislocated en bloc fractures of zygomatic complex means there is detachment of the zygoma from all its 4 attachments i.e. maxilla, Temporal, frontal- and sphenoidal bones resulting in a inferior, medial or posterolateral rotation. These type of fractures usually require fixation following reduction at least at 2 points.

56 A Bilateral pre-auricular incisions are extended across the scalp within the hairline and reflected over the forehead by degloving. Then the dissection is carried down overnasal bridge, Frontozygomatic (FZ) sutures and medial canthi. 'B' This incision is for exposing the TMJ and sometimes the zygomatic arch. 'C' is to treat Nasal fractures and 'D' is to treat orbital rim, floor and zygomatic complex fracture with separation at zygomatico maxillary suture.

57 C The use of allogenic freezedried bone chips eliminates the need for host donor bone and is replaced by new host bone and the process is known as 'creeping substitution'.

58 A This technique demonstrates the site of a post traumatic CSF leak from the basal cisterns of the brain by injecting a non-ionic contrast medium into the lumbar subarachnoid space and seen on the CT scan as opacified CSF passing from the opacified basal cisterns into the nasal cavity or sphenoid sinus.

59 A If the displaced zygomatic arch fracture is not reduced immediately or within 1–2 weeks of trauma, the scar tissue might bind down the fracture segments with ensuing fibrosis and it becomes diffcult to maintain the stability of the reduced zygomatic arch fracture which might then require open reduction and fixation.

60 B The Gunning splint is fixed to the mandible by means of circummandibular wires and to the maxilla by peralveolar wires and fixed together with wires. In the anterior region there is a gap between the maxillary and mandibular splints to fascititate feeding during the fixation period.

61 C

62 A The early use of thrombolytic drugs can decrease the extent of necrosis and myocardial damage and dramatically improves the outcome and prognosis.

63 C

64 D

65 C

66 B This is the safest position. If kept in a Trendlenberg position or right lateral position, the fetus will compress on the inferior vena cava (Caval compression) also in a supine position. The fetus can cause respiratory distress (10° head down). 'C' Will be too unconfrontable for the patient and will put pressure on the fetus.

67 A Capryl hydrocuprienotoxin is a preservative that can be used in place of methylparaben and can cause less allergy as compared to methyl paraben and 'B' is a fungicide, 'C' is vasoconstrictor and 'D' is a local anaesthetic agent itself.

68 B The typical appearance of a B/L TMJ ankylosis is the vogelgeschit or 'Andygump' appearance due to retruded chin and decrease in B/L ramus heights.

69 B As it might precipitate cardiac arrhythmia.

70 C Via a stab incision in the cheek, the skin hook is inserted and positioned just beneath the body of the zygoma and pulled to elevate the fractured zygomatic complex.

71 A

72 B

73 A It lies just medial to the condylar neck and supplies the TMJ. So during surgeries of TMJ, it should be protected by a blunt instrument in order to prevent bleeding which is very difficult to control otherwise.

74 B

75 C The incision in the duct is not sutured as it will lead to narrowing of the ductal lumen.

76 A

77 C

78 D During parotid gland surgery, there might be damage to auriculotemporal nerve or to communicating branches to facial nerve resulting in gustatory sweating of skin of upper cheek, temporal region and forehead during eating. Facial paralysis can also occur due to physical damage to the facial nerve during parotid surgery.

79 A

80 C Rib grafts in girls are usually taken from the 5th and 6th ribs well below the breast to prevent damage to the mammary glands and ducts.

81 B

82 D

83 C

84 B (A) and (C) are systemic antihistaminics, and (D) is used as a decongestant in nasal drops.

85 B

86 A With one rescuer, the cardiopulmonary resuscitation should be performed at a ratio of 15: 2 with two very quick lung inflations after each 15 chest compressions.

87 C These are imaginary lines to describe fracture lines through various landmarks of mid face and mandible on an occipetomental view of skull. In total there are 4 lines described by McGregor and Campbell and the 5th line which runs along the lower border of mandible has been added by Trapnell.

88 A This view is primarily used to observe the occipital area of skull and sometimes the necks of the condylar processes.

89 C 'A' uses hematocrit and red cell count to estimate the volume of average red cell; 'B' uses the haemoglobin content and red cell count to estimate the haemoglobin content of individual red cell. 'D' The normal value of PCV is 45:55 (Red cell: Serum).

90 A

91 B

92 B A is 'Cloacae'.

93 D It forms chelate with compounds containing calcium and this chelate is taken up by growing bones and developing teeth, resulting in retardation of bone growth and permanent staining of teeth respectively in children. So the administration of this drug should be avoided during pregnancy and in children upto around 7 years of age.

94 A

95 C If the patient is hypoglycaemic, the recovery will be fairly rapid; but if the patient is hyperglycaemic then no harm will be done with the above injection. So any kind of diabetic coma (either hypo- or hyperglycaemic) should be treated as hypoglycemic as the adverse effects of hypoglycaemia are more dangerous.

96 A

97 B The apex of the upper lateral incisor is curved apically in around 50% of cases hence the common palatal infection.

98 A

99 D 'A' is used to retract soft tissues away from chin during osteotomies of chin, 'B' is used to retract temporalis muscle attachment from anterior border of ramus of mandible during osteotomies in this area; 'C' is used for circummandibular or circumzygomatic suspension wiring. All these instruments are Obwegeser's instruments.

100 B

Syllabus

1. Definition, scope, aim and objectives of periodontology.
2. Gingiva.
3. Periodontal ligament.
4. Cementum.
5. Alveolar bone.
6. Changes in periodontium and defence mechanism of gingiva.
7. Gingivitis and gingival bleeding.
8. Changes in colour, consistency, surface texture and position of gingiva.
9. Etiology of periodontal disease, dental plaque—its role in periodontal disease.
10. Materia alba, food debris, dental calculus and stains.
11. Plaque control and oral hygiene methods in India.
12. Instruments used in periodontal procedures.
13. Principles of instrumentation.
14. Extension of inflammation from gingiva to the deeper periodontal tissues.
15. Periodontal pockets—definition, histopathology classification, etc.
16. Classification of periodontal disease.
17. Acute gingival infection and teatment.
18. Gingival enlargement and treatment.
19. Chronic desquamative gingivitis and treatment.
20. Gingival changes in puberty, menstruation, pregnancy, Menopause and other periodontal changes associated with endocrine disorders.
21. Diagnosis of periodontal disease.
22. Food impaction.
23. Halitosis.
24. Bruxism and other parafunctional habits.
25. Nutritional influences in the etiology of periodontal diseases.
26. Hematological disorders in the etiology of periodontal disease.
27. Periodontal abscess and treatment.
28. Immune reactions in periodontal diseases.
29. Trauma from occlusion in the etiology of periodontal disease.
30. Mobility and migration of teeth.
31. Determination of prognosis.
32. Treatment plan, rationale for periodontal treatment oral physiotherapy.
33. Juvenile periodontitis and treatment.
34. Pocket eradication procedures in general and healing.
35. Root planning and curettage.
36. Flap surgery and modifications.
37. Gingivectomy and gingivoplasty.
38. Osseous defects and osseous surgery including bone graft.
39. Furcation involvement and treatment.
40. Periodontal-endodontic therapy.
41. Mucogingival problems and treatment.
42. Occlusal adjustments.
43. Periodontal splints.
44. Hypersensitivity of teeth, drugs used in periodontal therapy.
45. Prosthetic and restorative procedures in the management of periodontal disease.
46. Maintenance phase of periodontal therapy.

Chapter 15

Periodontics

BASIC TISSUES

1. **The free gingival groove is present in about**
   - **A.** Less than 25 percent
   - **B.** 50 percent
   - **C.** 70 percent
   - **D.** More than 95 percent of all cases
2. **The gingival sulcus is the shallow crevice around the tooth bounded by**
   - **A.** The junctional epithelium and the marginal gingiva
   - **B.** The cementum and the epithelium of gingival margin
   - **C.** The epithelial attachment and crest of gingival margin
   - **D.** The tooth surface and the epithelial lining of the free margin of gingiva
3. **The principle cell type of gingival epithelium is**
   - **A.** Melanocytes
   - **B.** Non keratinocytes
   - **C.** Keratinocytes
   - **D.** Merkel cells
4. **The protective function of gingival epithelium is dependant on**
   - **A.** The proliferation and differentiation of keratinocytes
   - **B.** Only proliferation of keratinocytes
   - **C.** Only differentiation of keratinocytes
   - **D.** None of the above
5. **As the basal cells of gingival epithelium migrate towards the superficial surface the molecular weight of the keratin in each layer**
   - **A.** Increases
   - **B.** First increase and then decreases
   - **C.** First decrease and then increases
   - **D.** Decreases
6. **The most differentiated cell of the gingival epithelium is**
   - **A.** Langerhan cells
   - **B.** Keratinocyte
   - **C.** Merkel cells
   - **D.** Corneocyte
7. **The most common mechanism of energy production in gingival epithelium is**
   - **A.** Tricarboxylic cycle in basal and parabasal cells and pentose shunt in superficial layer
   - **B.** Pentose shunt in basal and parabasal layer and tricarboxylic cycle in superficial layer
   - **C.** Tricarboxylic cycle and pentose shunt in the basal layer only
   - **D.** Independent of cell layer type
8. **The oxytalan fibres of periodontal ligament are thought to**
   - **A.** Give elasticity to periodontal ligament
   - **B.** Provide noci-ception
   - **C.** Give support to the principal fibres
   - **D.** Regulate blood flow

9. The collagen turn over in the periodontal ligament is regulated by
A. Collagenase activity
B. Functional stimulus/demand
C. Fibroblastic intracellular degradation
D. Fibrinolysis

10. Epithelial rests in periodontal ligament are distributed mostly
A. Close to the cementum, in the apical area only
B. Close to the alveolar bone in the cervical area only
C. Close to the cementum in the apical and cervical area only
D. Close to the alveolar bone in the cervical area only

11. When tipping forces are applied to a tooth
A. The apical portion of root moves in the same direction as coronal portion
B. The coronal portion moves at 90° angle to the root portion
C. The coronal portion moves at an angle of 180° to that of root portion
D. The coronal and apical portions move independent to each other

12. In a single rooted healthy tooth the axis of rotation is located
A. At the junction of the apical third and the middle third of the root
B. At the junction of the apical third and middle third of the tooth
C. In an area between the apical third and middle third of the root
D. In an area between the apical third and middle third of the tooth

13. Ruffini-like mechano-receptors are located in
A. Alveolar periosteum
B. Periodontal ligament
C. Cementum
D. Pulp

14. The mineral content of cementum
A. Increases with age
B. Decreases with age
C. First increases and than decreases
D. Not related to aging

15. A true periodontal pocket will not form
A. Around a deciduous tooth
B. Around a nonfunctional tooth
C. Around an implant
D. Around a tooth with increased functional demand

16. Multinucleated osteoclasts are formed under the influence of
A. Parathyroid hormone (PTH)
B. Leukaemia inhibiting factor (LIF)
C. Interleukin
D. None of the above

17. During bone resorption the acidic environment on bony surface can be produced by
A. Bone tumors
B. Proton pump of osteoclasts
C. Local pressure
D. All of the above

18. In maxillary molars interdental fenestrations are present in
A. 66.6% of cases
B. 12.5% of cases
C. 20.8% of cases
D. 70% of cases

19. The least stable of the all the periodontal tissues is
A. Gingiva
B. Periodontal ligament
C. Cementum
D. Alveolar bone

20. Gingival stippling is a form of
A. Specialized reinforcement
B. Adaptive specialization
C. Functional modification
D. Esthetic adaptation

21. In 'early lesion' stage gingivitis the main collagen fibre groups destroyed are
- A. Transeptal fibre
- B. Circular and dentogingival fibre
- C. Semicircular and transgingival
- D. All of the above

22. The most advantageous method of diagnosing early gingival inflammation is
- A. Change in color
- B. Pocket formation
- C. Change in consistency
- D. Bleeding on gentle probing

23. The "Cell rich, collagen poor tissue denotes
- A. Areas of proliferation
- B. Areas of tissue maturation
- C. Areas of inflamed tissues
- D. Areas of tissues repair

24. Current accepted terminology for increase in size of gingiva is
- A. Gingival hypertrophy
- B. Gingival hyperplasia
- C. Gingival enlargement/over growth
- D. Elephantiasis gingivale gingivae

25. Drug induced gingival enlargement characteristically
- A. Always involves attached gingiva
- B. Appears to project from beneath the gingival margin
- C. Have minutely pebbled surface
- D. Appears like a mushroom

26. The occurrence and severity of phenytoin induced gingival enlargement is related to
- A. Drug dosage
- B. Levels of drug in saliva
- C. Level of plaque control
- D. None of the above

27. Experimentally phenytoin induced gingival enlargement has been successful in
- A. Beagal dogs and guinea pigs
- B. White mice and sheep
- C. Cat and ferrel
- D. None of the above

28. In cyclosporin induced gingival enlargement
- A. The magnitude is related to plasma concentration
- B. Is more vascularized
- C. Has abundant plasma cell and amorphous intracellular substances
- D. All of the above

29. Gingival enlargement in pregnancy is called
- A. Pyogenic granuloma
- B. Angio granuloma
- C. Fibrous granuloma
- D. Giant cell granuloma

30. Clinically plasma cell gingivitis is
- A. Similar to plaque induced gingivitis
- B. Located in the IDP
- C. Located in the oral aspect of attached gingiva
- D. Confirmed to marginal gingiva on lingual aspects only

31. Other than gingival CT the source of fibroma in gingiva is
- A. CT of periodontal ligament
- B. Bone
- C. CT of alveolar mucosa
- D. None of the above

32. Malignant melanoma tends to occur in
- A. Soft palate and mandibular gingiva
- B. Hard palate and maxillary gingiva
- C. Buccal mucosa and mandibular gingiva
- D. Alveolar mucosa and maxillary gingiva

33. Periodontal pocket formation in NUG does not occur because
- A. Necrotic changes do not involve J. epithelium
- B. Necrotic changes involve J. epithelium
- C. The lesion does not destroy the underlying periodontal tissue
- D. Punched out depression of the crest of IDP

34. The microscopic appearance of NUG is comparable to changes resulting from
- A. Trauma
- B. Chemical irritation
- C. Application of caustic medication
- D. All of the above

35. Clinical diagnosis of NUG is based on
- A. Bacterial smear and history
- B. Histopath and bacterial smear
- C. Presence of gingival pain, ulceration and bleeding
- D. None of the above

36. Streptococcal gingivostomatitis can be differentiated from NUG by
- A. The presence of diffuse erythema of gingiva
- B. Presence of marginal hemorrhage
- C. Absence of streptococcus form of bacteria
- D. Absence of necrosis and fetid odour

37. Gingival findings in agranulocytosis is characterized by
- A. Absence of necrosis
- B. Presence of diffuse erythema
- C. Absence of severe inflammatory reaction
- D. Presence of more of plaque

38. Vincent's angina is
- A. Fusospirochetal infection of the oropharynx and throat
- B. Fusospirochetal infection of marginal gingiva (NUG)
- C. NUG in leukemia
- D. Streptococcal gingivostomatitis

39. NUG prone personality is associated with
- A. Depression
- B. Schizophrenia
- C. Dominance and abasement
- D. Psychopathic deviance

40. Eruption gingivitis is caused by
- A. Tooth eruption per se
- B. Tissue remodelling associated with eruption
- C. Plaque accumulation around erupting tooth
- D. Calculus formation around erupting tooth

41. The source of matrix metalloproteinases in the gingiva is
- A. Fibroblasts
- B. PMNLs
- C. Macrophages
- D. All of the above

42. In the pathogensis of periodontal pocket intra-epithelial cleavage occurs in
- A. The sulcular epithelium
- B. The junctional epithelium
- C. The periodontal ligament fibres
- D. Epithelial attachment

43. Most severe degenerative changes in periodontitis is usually seen in
- A. Junctional epithelium at the base of the pocket
- B. Cemental surfaces
- C. Lateral pocket wall
- D. Gingival epithelium at the crest of periodontal pocket

44. The rationale for pocket reduction is based on
- A. The need to eliminate areas of plaque accumulation
- B. The need to regenerate periodontal tissue
- C. The need to form long junctional epithelium
- D. The need to form new attachment apparatus

45. The junctional epithelium at the base of periodontal pocket is usually
- A. Longer than that of normal sulcus
- B. Shorter than that of normal sulcus
- C. Equal to that of normal sulcus
- D. Not present

46. The presence of bacteria in gingival tissue has been interpreted as
A. Bacterial invasion
B. Passive translocation
C. Both of the above
D. None of the above

47. The presence of pus in the pocket reflects
A. The depth of the pocket
B. Severity of destruction of the periodontal tissues
C. The amount of alveolar bone support present
D. The nature of inflammatory changes in the pocket wall

48. Diseased root surfaces when reimplanted in the oral mucosa of patient will
A. Not induce an inflammatory response
B. Not induce an inflammatory response if autoclaved
C. Induce an inflammatory response even if autoclaved
D. Induce diseased cementum formation

49. The mineral content of the cementum that is exposed to oral cavity is likely to
A. Increase
B. Decrease
C. Remain static
D. Decrease and then increase

50. The so-called plaque free zone is
A. Narrower in deeper pockets
B. Broader in deeper pockets
C. Wide in incisors than in molar
D. Narrower in molars than in incisors

51. The severity of attachment loss is
A. Always correlated with the depth of pocket
B. Independent of pocket depth
C. Generally, but not always correlated to pocket depth
D. Inversely proportional to pocket depth

52. Which of the following statement is true?
A. The pockets of same depth are always associated with same degree of attachment loss
B. The pockets of different depths are always associated with different amount of attachment loss
C. The pockets of same depth may be associated with different degree of attachment loss
D. The depth of pocket is always inversely proportional to the attachment loss

53. The distance from attached palque to bone is
A. Never less than 0.5 nm and never more than 2.7 nm
B. Never less than 0.5 cm and never more than 2.7 cm
C. Never less than 0.5 mm and never more than 2.7 mm
D. Never less than 0.7 mm and never more than 0.37 mm

54. Which of the following distance is most constant?
A. The distance between the apical end of JE and the alveolar bone
B. The distance between the CEJ and JE
C. The distance between the crest of the gingiva and alveolar bone
D. The distance between the apical extent of calculus and the alveolar crest

55. The "walling off" of the advancing lesion is effected by
A. Fibrin-fibrinolytic system
B. The encapsulation
C. The basement membrane protein
D. The inflammatory cascade

56. Interproximal angular defect can appear only in spaces that are
A. Narrower than 2.5 mm
B. Wider than 2.5 mm
C. Narrower than 0.25 mm
D. Wider than 0.25 mm

57. **"Refractory periodontitis**
   - A. Is unresponsive to any treatment provided
   - B. Responds to treatment intially
   - C. Reccurs soon after the treatment
   - D. Is characterized by refraction of alveolar bone

58. **Generalized aggressive periodontitis patient**
   - A. Will always have, very mild gingival inflammatory response clinically
   - B. Exhibit poor production of antibody response to pathogens
   - C. Will always have very severe gingival inflammatory response clinically
   - D. Exhibit normal production of antibody response

59. **The monocytes in cases of localized aggresive periodontits are**
   - A. Hypo responsive
   - B. Hyper responsive
   - C. Non-responsive
   - D. Legs in number

60. **The most important environmental factor influencing the extent of periodontal destruction in periodontal disease is**
   - A. Nutrition
   - B. Tobacco chewing
   - C. Smoking
   - D. Tongue thrusting

61. **The microflora of linear gingival erythema may mimic that of**
   - A. Gingivitis
   - B. Periodontitis
   - C. Herpetic gingivostomatitis
   - D. Candidiasis

62. **Necrotizing ulcerative stomatitis in HIV +ve patients appears to be identical to**
   - A. Allergic stomatitis
   - B. Herpetic stomatitis
   - C. Cancrum oris
   - D. Oral lichen planus

63. **The majority of HIV +ve patients experience periodontal disease**
   - A. Similar to general population
   - B. Greater to general population
   - C. Similar to RPP
   - D. Similar to NUP

64. **Gingiva must be dried before observation to**
   - A. Prevent infection
   - B. Prevent slipping of examining fingers
   - C. Remove surface debris
   - D. Prevent light reflection

65. **The only accurate method of detecting periodontal pocket is**
   - A. Radiographic examination
   - B. GP points used along with X-rays
   - C. Careful exploration with a periodontal probe
   - D. Careful exploration with an explorer

66. **The periodontal pocket depth**
   - A. Can change even in untreated patients
   - B. Can only change due to gain or loss of attachment
   - C. Can only change after surgical intervention
   - D. Can only change after periodontal regenerative procedures

67. **The level of attachment when compared to periodontal pocket**
   - A. Is poor indicator of periodontal destruction
   - B. Is a better indicator of periodontal destruction
   - C. Is not an indicator of periodontal destruction
   - D. Is as good an indicator of periodontal destruction

68. **If the distance from CEJ to gingival margin and depth of pocket is same then the loss of attachment is**
   - A. Is the sum of the two
   - B. Is twice the sum of the two
   - C. Is sum of the two divided by two
   - D. Is zero or the sum of the two

69. **The loss of attachment equals the pocket depth when**
   A. Gingival margin is on crown
   B. Gingival margin is on CEJ
   C. Gingival margin is on cementum
   D. None of the above

70. **The loss of attachment is greater than pocket depth when**
   A. The gingival margin is on CEJ
   B. The gingival margin is coronal to CEJ
   C. The gingival margin is apical to CEJ
   D. The gingival margin is in the apical third

71. **The absence of gingival bleeding as a single test is**
   A. Not a good predictor of periodontal stability
   B. Good predictor of disease progression
   C. Excellent predictor of periodontal stability
   D. Good predictor of periodontal stability

72. **The most common micro-organism implicated in association with puberty gingivitis is**
   A. Capnocytophaga
   B. A actinomycetam comitans
   C. Eikenalla corodlus
   D. P. intermedia

73. **Increased susceptibility to gingival inflammation in pregnancy is thought to be due to**
   A. Heightened maternal immune response
   B. Suppressed maternal immune response
   C. Decreased PGE_1 production
   D. Decreased PGE_2 production

74. **Scaling, polishing and root planning**
   A. Should not be performed during pregnancy
   B. Should be performed only during the 2nd trimester
   C. Should be performed only during the 3rd trimester
   D. Can be performed whenever required throughout the pregnancy

75. **In hypertensive patients small doses of epinephrine should not be injected**
   A. Submucosally
   B. Intra mucosally
   C. Subdermally
   D. Intra ligamentory

76. **Whenever possible, in patients at high risk of developing infective endocarditis undergoing periodontal surgical procedures**
   A. Non resorbable sutures should be used
   B. Resorbable sutures that resorb in a long time should be used
   C. Resorbable sutures that resorb in a short time should be used
   D. Non resorbable sutures should be used but should be removed after a longer time post surgically

77. **The most common dental office complication seen in diabetic patient taking insulin is**
   A. Hyperglycemia
   B. Hypoglycemia
   C. Diabetic ketoacidoses
   D. Diabetic coma

78. **Prophylactic systemic steroid supplementation in patients undergoing periodontal procedures is generally not warranted in**
   A. Patients taking > 20 mg cortisol equivalent/day
   B. Patients taking > 40 mg cortisol equivalent/day
   C. Patients taking < 5 mg cortisol equivalent/day of < 1 month
   D. Patients taking > 60 mg cortisol equivalent/day for > 1 month

79. **To prevent hypotension in pregnant females**
   A. The patient should be made to lie in a supine position
   B. Placing the patient on her right side
   C. Elevating the right hip 5-6 inches
   D. Elevating the left hip 5-6 inches

80. The difference between after five and minimum five curette is
A. In the length of the shank
B. The width of the blade
C. The length of the blade
D. The design of the blade

81. In gracey curettes
A. The blade length is 50% longer than conventional gracey curette
B. The blade length is same as conventional gracey curette
C. The blade length is 25% shorter than conventional gracey curette
D. The blade length is 50% shorter than conventional gracey curette

82. Gingival curettage should always be
A. Preceded by scaling and root planning
B. Followed by scaling and root planning
C. Preceded by use of antiplaque agents
D. Preceded by systemic antibiotic therapy

83. Gingivectomy should be performed in
A. Shallow infrabony pockets
B. Deep infrabony pockets
C. Shallow suprabony pockets
D. Suprabony pockets regardless of depth

84. Electrocautery should not be used in
A. Incising periodontal abscess
B. Relocation of frenum attachments
C. Pericoronal flap removal
D. Periodontal flap surgery

85. In gingival enlargement patients with limited keratinized tissue, the treatment of choice is
A. Periodontal flaps
B. Gingivectomy
C. Gingivoplasty
D. Plaque control only

86. The amount of keratinized tissue that should remain after gingivectomy is at least
A. 6 mm B. 3 mm
C. 2 mm D. 1 mm

87. "Holding suture" is a type of
A. Sling suture
B. Figure "8" suture
C. Interdental suture
D. Horizontal mattress suture

88. The main purpose of modified widman flap is
A. Pocket elimination
B. Pocket reduction
C. Periodontal regeneration
D. Instrumentation facilitation

89. The undisplaced flap may be considered as
A. Modified widman flap
B. Slightly coronally placed flap
C. Papilla preservation flap
D. Internal bevel gingivectomy

90. The flap design of choice for regenerative surgery is
A. Modified widman flap
B. Apically displaced flap
C. Undisplaced flap
D. Papilla preservation flap

91. Non-graft associated new attachment is most likely to be attained in
A. One walled defects
B. Gingival abscess
C. Endodont and periodontal abscess
D. Two walled defects

92. In combined endo perio lesion the prognosis depends upon the
A. The amount of endo lesion
B. The amount of periodontal lesion
C. The type of microorganism
D. The amount of crown material remaining

93. The aim of crown lengthening is to expose the clinical crown to
A. Prevent the placement of crown margin into the area of biologic width
B. Facilitate the placement of crown margin into the area of biologic width
C. Reduce the length of biologic width
D. To facilitate the placement of crown margin beyond the biologic width

94. **The distance between the most apical extension of restoration margin and alveolar bone crest should be**
A. At least 6 mm
B. At least 3 mm
C. At least 2 mm
D. More than 2 mm

95. **The management of interdental papilla during restoration fabrication is best approached by viewing the papilla as a**
A. A 3 D triangle
B. A 3 D tent
C. Balloon
D. A 3 D rectangle

96. **Females taking oral contraceptives when compared with controls, exhibit**
A. Lower periodontal index and higher Gingival index scores
B. Higher periodontal index and lower Gingival index scores
C. Higher periodontal as well as Gingival index scores
D. Similar periodontal index and Gingival index scores

97. **Smokers suffer from more progressive periodontal disease because of**
A. Reduced phagocytosis
B. Reduced local blood supply
C. Decreased levels of circulating Ig G_2
D. All of the above

98. **"Modern periodontal epidemiology" concentrates on**
A. Determinants at community level
B. Determinants at society level
C. Determinants at organ, tissue or cell level
D. All of the above

99. **Which of the following micro-organism is considered to be a "bona fide" pathogen influencing periodontal disease initiation and progression?**
A. Fusobacterium nucleatum
B. Eikenella corrodens
C. P. Gingivalis
D. Capno cytophaga

100. **Gingipains are**
A. Micro-organisms causing pain in the gingiva
B. Host Matrix Metalloprotienases
C. Bacterial cystiene proteinases
D. Painful gingivae

Answers

1 B Free gingival groove is a linear depression present at the junction of marginal gingiva and attached gingiva but is not always present.

2 D Gingival sulcus is formed around the tooth neck and so is bounded by the marginal gingiva and the tooth surface.

3 C

4 A The rapid cell turnover (proliferation) prevents the bacteria from entering the deeper cell layer and also as the cells mature (differentiate) the inter cellular spaces are obliterated.

5 A

6 D The end cell of the differentiation process of the gingival epithelium is the corneocyte present on the most superficial layer (stratum corneum).

7 A In the basal layer the oxygen tension is high due to close proximity to blood vessel so the energy production is by tricarboxylic cycle.

8 D Oxytalan fibres are present around the blood vessels and as such help in regulating the blood flow.

9 C

10 C

11 C The opposing parts of the tooth well move in opposite directions when tipping forces are applied on the tooth.

12 C

13 B

14 D The mineral content of the cementum remain fairly constant in healthy individual.

15 C

16 B

17 D

18 B

19 D Out of all the periodontal tissues the alveolar bone is the most plastic tissues that keeps on remodelling, resorbing and forming under the influence of various factors.

20 B Gingival stipplings are adaptive specialisation as gingiva is masticatory mucosa. The stipplings increase the surface area of contact between epithelium the surface area of contact between epithelium and connective tissue, helping gingiva to withstand masticatory forces.

21 B The early lesion of gingivitis involve the circular and dento gingival fibers as they are the most superficial of the gingival fibres.

22 D Gingival bleeding is most objective criteria, better than color change and consistency.

23 C Inflammation by itself increase the number of cellular elements in the area and inprocess, degrades the collagen, thus giving rise to cell rich, collagen poor tissue picture.

24 C Most of the gingival enlargement do not strictly fall into hypertrophy or hyperplasia in the true sense, so the term enlargement is most accepted.

25 B

26 D

27 C

28 D

29 B

30 C

31 A Fibromas of gingiva can arise from the connective tissue of periodontal ligament also.

32 B

33 B For periodontal pocket to form, the marginal gingival shift should be lesser than the apical shift of JE as in NUG, the marginal gingiva is necrosed hence pocket do not form.

34 D The microscopic picture of NUG is non-specific hence is comparable to trauma and chemical irritation.

35 C Presence of gingival pain, ulceration and bleeding are the most reliable signs for the clinical diagnosis of NUG.

36 D Strep to coccal gingivo stomatites does not cause necrosis and fetid odour whereas NUG does.

37 C As granulocytes are one of the major cell types involved in inflammation, their absence would also result in an attenuated inflammatory host response.

38 A Vincents angina typically involves the oropharynx as well as the throat. Where as NUG does not.

39 C

40 C Eruption gingivitis is not caused by tooth eruption per se but due to plaque accumulation around an erupting tooth, where plaque control becomes difficult due to eruption.

41 D

42 B

43 C The lateral pocket wall is the most reactive and dynamic area in the periodontal pocket, hence the most of the degenerative changes occur in this area only.

44 A As periodontal pocket is a healing lesion, the rationale of pocket reduction lies in the elimination of areas of plaque accumulation and thus helping in regeneration.

45 B

46 B

47 D The presence of pus in the pocket reflects more on the nature of destructive changes rather than the severity of disease.

48 C

49 A

50 A

51 C Severe attachment loss can occur along with gingival recession and as such a shallow or no pocket formation thus the severity of CAL is not always related to depth of pocket.

52 C Pocket depth is the distance between marginal gingiva and base of the pocket. Whereas attachment loss is the distance between CEJ and level of JE. Hence the pockets of some depth may be associated with different degree of attachment loss.

53 C

54 D

55 A

56 B For angular defects to occur the bone should atleast be wider than 2.5 mm which is the dia of destruction of dental plaque. In spaces narrower than 2.5 mm whole of the bone is destroyed giving rise to horizontal defects.

57 A A truly refractory periodontitis is nonresponsive to any treatment provided whereas the recurrent periodontitis recurs soon due to inadequate treatment.

58 B Aggressive periodontitis has two clinical presentations (inflammatory and non inflammatory type). But will always exhibit poor antibody production.

59 B

60 C Smoking has been documented as the most important factors ahead of all the other environmental factors viz nutrition habits etc.

61 B

62 C

63 A

64 D

65 C As radiographs show only the amount of bone present, they are not accurate for detecting pockets which is a soft tissue lesion as well.

66 A Pocket depth keep on varying in untreated patients due to reduction or increase in the inflammation.

67 B As periodontal destruction is determined by the level of attachment, it is a better indicator of periodontal destruction than periodontal pocket which is the distance between marginal gingiva and the base of the pocket.

68 D

69 B

70 C The gingival margin is apical to CEJ
A = Attachment loss
B = Depth of the pocket

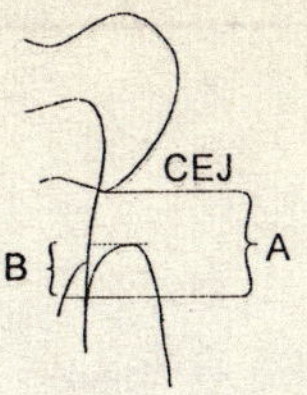

So, A > B

71 C Presence of bleeding does not predict disease progression. But its absence is an indicator of periodontal health.

72 D

73 B Suppresed maternal response which is important for the well being of foetus is responsible for the increased gingival inflammation.

74 D With proper precautions, pregnancy is not a contraindication for scaling polishing and root planing.

75 D

76 C Sutures are a source of bacteremia, hence, resorbable sutures resorbing in a very short time should be used.

77 B

78 C

79 C Elevating the right hip decreases the pressure on vena cava thus increasing venous return to heart.

80 C

81 D

82 A

83 D

84 D

85 A

86 B

87 D

88 D

89 D

90 D

91 C

92 B

93 A

94 B

95 C

96 A

97 D

98 C

99 C

100 C

Notes

Syllabus

- Introduction, definition, historic background, aims and objectives of Orthodontics and the need for Orthodontic care.
- Growth and development in general
  a. Definition of growth and development.
  b. Differential growth and growth spurts.
  c. Factors influencing growth and development.
  d. Methods of measuring growth.
- Morphologic development of craniofacial structures
  a. Osteology and myology of bones and muscles of cranium and face.
  b. Methods of bone growth.
  c. Prenatal growth of craniofacial structures.
- Post natal growth and development of:
  a. Cranium – vault.
  – base of skull.
  b. Maxilla.
  c. Mandible.
  d. Dental arches and occlusion.
- Theories of growth control and genetics as applied to Orthodontics.
- Functional development of dental arches and occlusion:
  a. Factors influencing development of dental arches and occlusion.
  b. Forces of occlusion.
  c. Wolff's law of transformation of bone.
  d. Trajectories of forces.
- Clinical applications of growth, development and occlusion:
- Malocclusion in general:
  a. The concept of normal occlusion, its characteristics and factors responsible for establishment and maintenance and normal occlusion.
  b. Definition of malocclusion.
  c. Description of different types viz., dental, skeletal, dentoskeletal and functional malocclusion.
- Classification of malocclusion:
  a. Definition and importance of classification of malocclusion.
  b. Principles, description, advantages and disadvantages of classification systems by Angle, Dewey, Simon, Lischer, Health and Ackermann and Profit.
- Normal and abnormal functions of the stomatognathic system.
- Etiology of malocclusion:
  a. Definition, importance, classification of etiology of malocclusion.
  b. Role of each factor in the causation of malocclusion.
  c. Etiology of different types of malocclusion:
  – midline diastema.
  – crowding.
  – cross bites.
  – deep bite.
  – class III malocclusion.
- Diagnosis and diagnostic aids and their interpretation:
  a. Definition, importance and classification of diagnostic aids and differential diagnosis.
  b. Importance of case history and clinical examination in Orthodontics.
  c. Study models:
  – Importance and uses.
  – Preparation and preservation of study models.
  d. Importance of intra oral X-rays and photographic analysis in Orthodontics.
  e. Panoramic radiographs.

f. Cephalometrics:
   - Different methods of study of the relation of skeletal bases.
   - Definition of cephalometrics.
   - Roentgenographic cephalometrics.
   - Description and uses of cephalostat.
   - Description and uses of anatomical landmarks, lines and angles used in cephalometric analysis.
   - Uses of cephalometrics.

g. Electromyography and its use in Orthodontics.

h. Wrist X-rays and its importance in Orthodontics.

- General principles in Orthodontics theory and treatment planning.
- Anchorage in Orthodontics:
  - Definition, classfication, different types and stability of anchorage.
- Biomechanical principles in Orthodontic tooth movement:
  a. Tissue response to Orthodontic force application.
  b. Histological changes during different types of tooth movement.
  c. Optimum force for different types of tooth movement.
- Preventive Orthodontics:
  a. Definition.
  b. Different procedures that are undertaken in preventive Orthodontics.
  c. The approach to preventive Orthodontics.
  d. Limitations of preventive Orthodontics.
- Interceptive Orthodontics:
  a. Definition.
  b. Procedures undertaken.
  c. Serial extraction as an interceptive procedure, principles, definition, indications, techniques, advantages, disadvantages and summary.
  d. Role of muscle exercise as an interceptive procedure.
- Corrective Orthodontics:
  a. Definition, factors to be taken into consideration in treatment planning.
  b. Model analysis.
  c. Methods of gaining space in the arch, indications, relative merits and demerits of proximal stripping, arch expansion and extractions.
  d. Extractions in Orthodontics:
     - Factors to be taken into consideration.
     - Indications and choice of teeth for extraction.
- General principles in selection, designing and construction of various appliances, and materials used in Orthodontics.
- Orthodontics appliances–general:
  a. Definition.
  b. Requisites for Orthodontics appliances.
  c. Classification.
  d. Indications, advantages, disadvantages of removable and fixed appliances.
  e. Methods of force application.
  f. Technical considerations–curing acrylic.
  g. Principles of welding, soldering, different methods of welding and soldering, solders, fluxes and antifluxes principles of spot welding.
- Orthodontic appliances–removable:
  a. Component parts of removable, mechanical appliances.
  b. Different types of clasps and their uses.
  c. Different types of active components.
  d. Appliances used to bring about palatal, labial, mesial, distal movement and rotation correction.
  e. Expansion appliances used in Orthodontics:
     - Principles of arch expansion.
     - Indications for arch expansion.
     - Description of expansion devices.
     - Different types of expansion devices.
     - Different uses of expansion devices.
  f. Habit breaking appliances.

- Orthodontic appliances–fixed:
  a. Definition.
  b. Indications.
  c. Component parts of fixed appliances and their uses.
  d. Basic principles of different fixed appliance techniques.
    – Edgewise, Begg light wire, Twin-arch wire, Labio–lingual, straight wire etc.
- Orthodontic appliances–Myofunctional therapy:
  a. Definition and principles of myofunctional therapy.
  b. Muscle exercises and their uses in Orthodontics.
  c. Functional appliances:
    – Definition, indications, uses, mode of action and construction of different functional appliances–activator, oral screen, bite planes inclined plane, Frankel's appliance.
- Orthodontic management of cleft lip and palate.
- Surgical Orthodontics:
  – Definition, indications and procedures undertaken to correct mandibular prognathism, maxillary prognathism, anterior open bite.
- Principles and methods of treatment of some common malocclusions:
  a. Midline distema.
  b. Cross bites.
  c. Open bites.
  d. Deep bites.
  e. Class II division 1.
  f. Class II division 2.
  g. Class III.
- Retention:
  a. Definition.
  b. Need for retention–causes of relapse.
  c. Methods of retention.
  d. Different types of retention appliances.
  e. Duration of retention.
- Age factor in Orthodontics.

Chapter 16

Orthodontics and Dentofacial Orthopedics

1. **Baker's anchorage is a type of**
   A. Intermaxillary anchorage
   B. Intramaxillary anchorage
   C. Extraoral anchorage
   D. Muscular anchorage

2. **Which of the following is not a tooth borne myofunctional appliance?**
   A. Activator
   B. Bionator
   C. Herbst's appliance
   D. Frankl

3. **Which of the following functions of the bone is the most prominent?**
   A. Calcium reservoir
   B. Sodium reservoir
   C. Phosphate reservoir
   D. Buffering

4. **Which of the following movements are performed by a non-working condyle?**
   A. Straight forward
   B. Downwards, forwards, lateral
   C. Downwards, forwards medial
   D. Downwards, backward medial

5. **Tooth in the mandibular arch which is most likely to be displaced due to arch size discrepancy is**
   A. First molar
   B. Second molar
   C. First premolar
   D. Second premolar

6. **Which of the following enzymes decreases the rate of orthodontic tooth movement?**
   A. Cyclooxygenase
   B. Metalloprotein
   C. Alkaline phosphatase
   D. Protein kinase

7. **Which of the following appliances is not used for slow maxillary expansion?**
   A. Jack screw B. Coffin spring
   C. Quad helix D. Hyrex appliance

8. **Maxillary marrow contains**
   A. All fatty marrow
   B. Red marrow
   C. Fibrous marrow
   D. Fatty and fibrous marrow

9. **The setting time of zinc phosphate cement may be retarded by**
   A. Increase in the ratio of powder to liquid
   B. Diluting the liquid with powder
   C. Increase the addition of powder to liquid
   D. Decrease the addition of powder to liquid

10. **Which of the following head gear is preferred while treating a Class 11 div. 2 malocclusion with a horizontal growth pattern?**
    A. High pull headgear
    B. Medium pull headgear
    C. Cervical headgear
    D. Reverse pull headgear

11. Increased amount of residual monomer in an acrylic denture will result in
- A. Increased expansion
- B. Increased shrinkage
- C. Low impact strength
- D. Increased brittleness

12. Which of the following is an adhesive?
- A. Composite
- B. Direct filling resins
- C. Polycaroxylate cement
- D. BIS-GMA resins in pit and fissure sealants

13. In intramembranous bone formation
- A. Osteoblasts are converted to osteocytes
- B. Osteoblasts are converted to obsteoclasts
- C. Replacement of cartilage by bone
- D. Mesenchymal membrane is converted to bone

14. Mesiodens can cause
- A. Maxillary incisor protrusion
- B. Delayed eruption of maxillary incisors
- C. Canine impaction
- D. Maxillary retrusion

15. Hypercementoses of root apex is seen in
- A. Ankylosis
- B. Orthodontic tooth movement
- C. Periapical pathology
- D. All of the above

16. Lingual cusp of a maxillary first premolar occludes with
- A. The mesial marginal ridge of lower first premolar
- B. The lingual embrassure between the lower canine and first premolar
- C. The lingual embrassure between the lower first premolar and second premolar
- D. None of the above

17. The term superior protrusion was given by
- A. Angle
- B. Tweed
- C. Dr R Ahmed
- D. Simon

18. Supernumerary teeth are not associated with
- A. Ectodermal dysplasia
- B. Cleidocranial dysostosis
- C. Teeth
- D. Cleft and palate

19. Acromegaly results in
- A. Class I malocculsion
- B. Class II malocculsion
- C. Class III malocculsion
- D. Deep bite

20. Apertognathia is
- A. Open bite
- B. Deep bite
- C. Cross bite
- D. Scissor bite

21. Visible light in a light cured composite resin causes
- A. Conjunctivitis
- B. Retinitis
- C. Cataract
- D. Iritis

22. Swallowing threshold is controlled by
- A. Taste
- B. Olfaction
- C. Gustation
- D. Salivary flow

23. Anterior posterior skeletal discrepancy is best visualized in a cephalogram by
- A. Facial angle
- B. ANB angle
- C. SN-FHP angle
- D. SN-mandibular plane angle

24. In maxillary impression, coronoid process influences
- A. Maxillary buccal flange thickness
- B. Posterior palatal seal
- C. Labial flange thickness
- D. None of the above

25. Heavy orthodontic forces leads to
- A. Hyalinization
- B. Osteblastic activity all around
- C. Odontoblastic activity all around the tooth
- D. Loss of alveolar crest

26. Cervical cross section of which tooth is roughly triangular
- A. Mandibular 2nd premolar
- B. Mandibular 1st premolar
- C. Mandibular 1st molar
- D. Maxillary 2nd molar

27. The most common lesion due to local irritating factor is
- A. Pyogenic granuloma
- B. Irritation fibroma
- C. Epulis
- D. None of the above

28. Torsiversion is
- A. Rotation of tooth around its axis
- B. Transposition
- C. Bodily movement
- D. Tipping

29. A successful orthodontic treatment completed at 12 years of age, patient developed crowding at 20 years of age, could be attributed to
- A. Restarting the treatment
- B. Is physiological/maturation
- C. Retention period was overlooked by orthodontist
- D. This does not occur

30. Peck-n-Peck analysis, which is not correct?
- A. Is usually for anterior teeth
- B. Has been incorporated nowadays in Ponts analysis
- C. Ratio of mesiodistal to labiolingual measurements
- D. Is usually included in the history sheet of orthodontic treatment

31. Canine placed much buccally in the dental arch is aligned preferably by
- A. Palatal canine retractor
- B. Buccal canine retractors
- C. Finger springs
- D. Split labial low

32. Which orthodontic tooth movement is most difficult to achieve?
- A. Intrusion
- B. Mesial movement
- C. Retraction
- D. Distal movement

33. Bodily tooth movement could be attributed to
- A. Reciprocal anchorage
- B. Stationary anchorage
- C. Cervical headgear
- D. Bent in tie back loops

34. In the correction of anterior cross bite which clinical condition is most advantageous
- A. Deep bite
- B. Edge to edge bite
- C. Tongue thrusting
- D. Hawley's retainer

35. In light forces usually the centre of rotation tends to be more towards
- A. Apex of the root
- B. Beyond apex of the root
- C. Centre of resistance
- D. Cervical region

36. Which orthodontic tooth movement is most difficult to retain?
- A. Intrusion
- B. Extrusion
- C. Rotation
- D. Migration

37. In orthodontic treatment, appliances when initially instituted leads to pain, this phenomonen is
- A. Normal, usual settles without medication
- B. Orthodontist should ensure there is no pain and discomfort to the patient
- C. Initial pain should be foreseen and antibiotics cover should short prior to placement of multifaceted appliances
- D. All of the above are correct

38. Class III skeletal growth pattern is characterized by all *except*
- A. Acute cranial base angle
- B. Anteriorly positioned articular
- C. Middle cranial fossa align posteriorly and superiorly
- D. Makes having more proclaimed maxillary incisors than females

39. In a bonded palatal expansion (hyrex) appliance the wire framework is made of
- A. 0.040 inch stainless steel
- B. 0.040 inch elgiloy
- C. 0.032 inch stainless steel
- D. 0.036 inch stainless steel

40. All these appliances are fixed functional appliances *except*
- A. Jasper jumper
- B. Mandibular protraction appliance (MPA)
- C. Pendulum appliance
- D. Herbst's appliance

41. Infantile swallowing pattern is
- A. Visceral
- B. Somatic
- C. Pleomorphic
- D. Combination of all

42. Which of the following cephalometric parameter is used to diagnose a long face syndrome patient?
- A. Angle ANB B. Angle SNA
- C. Jarabak ratio D. Saddle angle

43. Which of the following is rapid palatal expansion device?
- A. Quad helix B. Coffin's spring
- C. W-arch D. Jackson screw

44. Which of the following contemporary orthodontic arch wire has maximum surface friction?
- A. Stainless steel B. AJW wire
- C. TMA wire D. NiTi wire

45. The movement of bone in response to its own growth is termed as
- A. Rotation
- B. Secondary displacement
- C. Primary displacement
- D. Differentiation

46. The copper NiTi wires are not available in the temperature ranges of
- A. 15° B. 29°
- C. 35° D. 40°

47. The 7th key to normal occlusion is
- A. Molar relation
- B. Occlusal plane
- C. Crown angulations and inclinations
- D. Bolton ratio

48. Bjork used the implants for predicting facial growth changes. This approach is
- A. Longitudinal approach
- B. Metric approach
- C. Structural approach
- D. Computerized prediction

49. The functional matrix concept as revisited by Moss does not include
- A. Connected cellular network (CCN)
- B. Mechano transduction
- C. Epigenetic—Epithesis
- D. Septo maxillary ligament development

50. What is the normal average distance between the crest of the alveolar bone and the cemento enamel junction in young adult
- A. 1.0 mm B. 1.08 mm
- C. 2.08 mm D. 2.80 mm

51. If the grading of malocclusion is classified as "mild", "moderate" and "severe" the scale of measurement used is
- A. Interval B. Nominal
- C. Ordinal D. Ratio

52. The articular cartilage is characterized by all of the following features *except*
- A. It is devoid of perichondrium
- B. It has a rich nerve supply
- C. It is avascular
- D. It lacks the capacity to regenerate

53. In a disease free temporomandibular joint, posterior end of the articular disc remains at
- **A.** 9 O'clock position
- **B.** 10 O'clock position
- **C.** 12 O'clock position
- **D.** 2 O'clock position

54. Which of the teeth has maximum sensory receptors?
- **A.** Maxillary permanent 1st molar
- **B.** Mandibular permanent 1st molar
- **C.** Mandibular permanent canine
- **D.** Maxillary permanent canine

55. Resorption of cementum as compared to bone occurs
- **A.** Less readily
- **B.** More readily
- **C.** Almost similar
- **D.** Undermining resorption

56. Enamel etched by a tooth conditions but not covered with a fissure sealant will
- **A.** Remineralize within a month
- **B.** Remineralize within 3 months
- **C.** Absorb stain and discolor the tooth
- **D.** Leave the tooth more susceptible to caries attack

57. Reduction genioplasty in mild class III malocclusion cases is performed when
- **A.** Crossbite is present in the anterior teeth
- **B.** Anterior crossbite is not present
- **C.** Posterior crossbite
- **D.** Maxillary contraction is present

58. Which of the following procedures is used to prevent relapse after correction of a rotated permanent maxillary canine
- **A.** Recontour of the crown
- **B.** Supracrestal fibrotomy
- **C.** Establishment of cuspid protected occlusion
- **D.** Removal of all functional contacts with the canine in lateral and protrusive excursion

59. Growth of the maxilla in the vertical direction is due to
- **A.** Growth of the alveolus
- **B.** Growth at sutures
- **C.** Growth of the cranial base
- **D.** Growth of synchondroses

60. Muscle determining the buccal frenum is:
- **A.** Levator angulii oris
- **B.** Zygomaticus major
- **C.** Triangularis
- **D.** Orbicularis oris

61. A child with thumb sucking habit shows
- **A.** Unilateral expansion of the maxilla
- **B.** Bilateral expansion of the maxilla
- **C.** Bilateral expansion of maxilla with deviation of mandible
- **D.** Unilateral posterior crossbite

62. Extraction of maxillary first molar is indicated
- **A.** To facilitate the eruption of second molars
- **B.** When extraction of premolars provide insuffcent space
- **C.** Poor prognosis of first molars
- **D.** Rotation of first molar

63. Tipping of a tooth results in the fibres of the periodontal ligament to be
- **A.** All compressed
- **B.** All stretched
- **C.** Half compressed half stretched
- **D.** No effect

64. Ashley-Howe model analysis is used in
- **A.** Tooth material excess
- **B.** Maxillomandibular relationship
- **C.** Basal bone relationships
- **D.** Growth prediction

65. In a skeletal class II, the value of ANB will be
- **A.** 10 degree
- **B.** + 2 degree
- **C.** 0 degree
- **D.** + 6 degree

66. All of the following about the temporomandibular joint are true *except*
A. It is a condylar joint
B. It has a meniscus
C. It is supplied by auriculotemporal nerve
D. Fibrous capsule is deficient at the neck of condyle

67. The fibre group of the periodontal ligament which provides the maximum resistance to masticatory forces is
A. Transeptal B. Oblique
C. Apical D. Horizontal

68. Achondroplasia is associated with
A. Maxillary retrusion
B. Mandibular retrusion
C. Maxillary protrusion
D. None of the above

69. Gas used for soldering torch is
A. Acetylene B. Propane
C. Oxygen D. Oxyacetylene

70. Hypoplastic enamel radiographically appears as
A. Radioopaque B. Radiolucent
C. Normal D. Sclerotic

71. Radiographic appearance of lamina dura is seen as
A. Continuous radioopaque line
B. Continuous radiolucent line
C. Interrupted opaque line
D. Uninterrupted line

72. Which property has maximum effect on chemical strength of zinc phospahte cement?
A. Liquid powder ratio
B. Spatulation time
C. Particle size
D. Increment addition

73. Generalised recession of gingiva is related to
A. Tooth brushing
B. Occlusal trauma
C. Alveolar dehiscence
D. Chronic gingival inflammation

74. Hypercementosis is associated with
A. Pulp necrosis B. Hyperfunction
C. Hypofunction D. Hypoplasia

75. If length of wire is doubled, the deflection becomes
A. Two times B. Four times
C. Six times D. Eight times

76. Translation occurs when the centre of rotation is
A. Apex of root
B. Infinity
C. Between apex and middle third of root
D. Middle of root

77. Primary stress bearing area in maxilla is
A. Alveolar ridge B. Incisive papilla
C. Rugae D. Hamular notch

78. The most common curvature of the palatal root of the maxillary first molar is to the
A. Facial B. Mesial
C. Distal D. Lingual

79. Activator in self curing resin is
A. Benzoin methyl ether
B. Peroxide
C. Amine
D. EDTA

80. Which of the following has high irritant property to pulp?
A. Zinc phosphate
B. Silicate
C. Glass ionomer
D. Polycarboxylate

81. Taurodontism is usually seen in
A. Incisors B. Canines
C. Premolars D. Molars

82. Siamese brackets are used in
A. Beggs technique
B. Edgewise
C. Twin wire
D. All of the above

83. Facial photographs will not predict
- A. Profile
- B. Lip competency
- C. Chin prominence
- D. Anterior crossbite

84. Odontodysplasia is most common in
- A. Mandibular premolar
- B. Mandibular canine
- C. Mandibular third molar
- D. Maxillary central incisor

85. Anterior openbite is most common in
- A. Guerin fracture
- B. Mandibular condylar fracture
- C. Symphysis fracture
- D. Angle fracture

86. Most common morphological variation is seen in
- A. A maxillary lateral incisor
- B. Mandibular lateral incisor
- C. Maxillary canine
- D. Mandibular canine

87. Mandible is formed by
- A. Endochondral ossification of Meckels cartilage
- B. Endochondral ossification of Reichters cartilage
- C. Is an offshoot of maxillary process
- D. Combination of all of above

88. Trisodium phosphate in alginate acts as
- A. Retarder
- B. Reactor
- C. Accelerator
- D. Plasticizer

89. All of the following are true for light cure composite *except*
- A. Held at a distance of 1 cm from tooth
- B. Curing cycle of 40-60 secs
- C. Use of orange glass shield for eye protection
- D. Adding increments of 1-2 mm

90. Rate of abrasion by polishing agent is increased by all *except*
- A. Pressure
- B. High speed
- C. Lubricant
- D. Size of particle

91. Which of the following feature is not seen with cleft palate?
- A. Supernumerary tooth at site of cleft
- B. High vault palate
- C. Bilateral maxillary constriction
- D. Missing lateral incisor

92. Cu-Ni-Ti wires used in orthodontics, could be attributed
- A. High tensile strength
- B. Low creep
- C. High corrosion
- D. None of the above

93. Proprioceptors are absent in
- A. Skeletal muscle
- B. TMJ
- C. Pulp
- D. All of the above

94. In trauma from occlusion, no change is seen in
- A. Alvoelar bone
- B. Lamina dura
- C. Periodontal ligament
- D. Epithelial attachment

95. Eruption is mostly influenced by
- A. Cell proliferation in crypt
- B. Osteoblastic activity in primary tooth
- C. Hormonal changes
- D. Shedding of primary teeth

96. "Infraclusion" is given by
- A. Angle
- B. Lischer
- C. Dewey
- D. Pierre Fauchard

97. The percentage of maxillary growth remaining after 10 years of age is
- A. 45%
- B. 10%
- C. 25%
- D. 35%

98. Which of the following terms refer to a type of fusion in which of formed teeth are joined only along the line of cementum?

A. Gemination

B. Fusion

C. Concrescence

D. Dilaceration

99. Into how many segments is the infant gum pad divided?

A. Two in each quadrant

B. Three in each quadrant

C. Two in each jaw

D. Five in each quadrant

100. What will satisfy the prevalence of Angle's class II malocclusion?

A. 67%

B. 20%

C. 75%

D. 2%

Answers

1 A
2 D Frankel appliances are tissue borne passive appliance system.
3 A Normal bone contains between 32 and 36 percent of organic matter and 47 to 51 percent of ash. The mineral constituents of bone are mainly tricalcium phosphate, $Ca_3 (PO_4)_2$, which forms about 85 percent, and calcium carbonate ($CaCO_3$) about 10 percent. The skeletal system holds about 99 percent of the calcium in the body.
4 C
5 D
6 C
7 D Hyrex expansion screw is used for rapid maxillary expansion.
8 B
9 D
10 C
11 B
12 C
13 D In intra membranous ossification, a group of undifferentiated cells in a connective tissue form a cluster. Osteoblasts arise from this concentration and subsequently produce an osteoid matrix which becomes calcified. As the process spreads mesh work of bony trabecular is formed. As the osteoblasts continue to form an osteoid they become "entrapped" in their own matrix and become osteocytes.
14 A Mesiodens is a super numerary tooth in region of incisors. It may be erupted or lie in the bone and accordingly may protrude the teeth.
15 D Is a sequale of orthodontic tooth movement. Generally this condition develops when orthodontic tooth movement and treatment is either prolonged or excessive forces are employed.
16 D
17 B
18 D
19 C
20 A
21 B
22 C
23 B
24 A
25 A Heavy orthodontic forces acting on the tooth causes a severe compression of the membrane. Closing of the blood vessels and cellular necrosis result, and the growth capacity of the membrane destroyed. Remodelling changes on the periodontal alveolar surface are precluded. This is presumed to trigger undermining resorption. In this process the resorptive changes then proceed from the endosteal cancellous spaces deep to the alveolar surface, since the alveolar surface itself is closed off owing to vascular occlusion.
26 A
27 C
28 A
29 B Often successful orthodontic treatment completed in early teens, it is observed crowding in the lower dental arch in the teens, when third molars erupt. Many attribute this phenomenon to the mesial thrust of the erupting third molars. Belief of mesial thrust of molars has not been proved. Conclusively. Still physiological maturation of the dentition is described as the best reason as this phenomenon is observed in those patients in whom third molars are congenitally missing or extracted much earlier.
30 C
31 A
32 A Intrusion is believed to be most difficult tooth movement to be achieved in orthodontics. In meeting the objective compression of pulpal nerves, vessels and surrounding alveolar bone. Condition is of paramount concern. While attempting intrusion alignment of adjoining teeth gets disturbed, which again is a paramount consideration.
33 B Stationary anchorage is defined as such.
34 A See question 46.
35 C
36 C
37 A
38 C
39 B
40 B
41 A Infantile swallowing is visceral in nature by definition and persists upto 4-5 years of age.
42 B
43 D
44 B
45 C
46 B
47 D
48 A
49 D
50 A
51 C
52 A
53 D
54 A
55 A

56 A
57 B
58 B
59 A
60 A
61 D
62 C
63 C
64 A
65 B
66 D
67 B
68 C
69 A
70 B
71 A
72 D
73 A
74 C
75 D
76 B
77 A
78 D
79 C
80 B
81 D
82 B
83 D
84 D
85 B
86 A
87 A
88 B
89 B
90 C
91 D
92 B
93 C
94 C
95 A
96 B Infraclusion by definition is given by Lischer's classification. Also includes other terms as supraclusion and so on.
97 C
98 C
99 B
100 B

Syllabus

I. Oral Medicine and Diagnosis:

1. Terminology in Oral Medicine.
2. Laboratory investigations in Oral Medicine.
3. Developmental disorders affecting jaws, tongue and oral mucosa.
4. Disorders of blood and blood forming organs.
5. Lymphatic drainage; anatomy of head and neck lymph nodes, D/D of cervicofacial lymphadenopathy.
6. Salivary gland disorders.
7. Acute and chronic infections of jaws.
8. Nutritional deficiencies.
9. Halitosis.
10. Metabolic and endocrine disorders.
11. Systemic review in oral medicine.
12. Red and white lesions of oral cavity.
13. Ulcerative, vesicular and bullous lesions.
14. Facial pain.
15. Pigmented lesions of oral cavity.
16. Gingival enlargement.
17. Benign tumors of oral cavity.
18. Malignant tumors.
19. Oral Cancer.
20. TMJ anatomy and disorders.
21. Immunologic disorders.

II. Radiology:

1. Construction and working of X-ray tube.
2. Collimation, filteration, quality and quantity, properties of X-rays, electromagnetic spectrum.
3. Films used in Dental Radiography.
4. Intensifying screens, grid, cassettes.
5. Intraoral radiographic techniques. Bisecting, Paralleling, Comparison.
6. Hazards of X-rays radiation.
7. Radiation protection.
8. Ideal Radiograph, criteria to evaluate periapical radiograph and factors controlling the diagnostic quality of dental radiograph.
9. Processing of radiographs.
10. Causes of faulty radiographs.
11. Localization techniques.
12. Anatomic landmarks in intraoral radiographs.
13. Extraoral views.
14. Radiographic features of dental caries.
15. Radiographic features of periodontal disease.
16. Diseases and disorders of dentition.
17. Fractures of jaws and teeth.
18. Diseases, disorders of soft tissue.
19. Periapical radiolucencies.
20. Pericoronal radiolucencies.
21. Solitary cyst like radiolucencies.
22. Multilocular radiolucencies.
23. Solitary radiolucencies with ragged and poorly defined borders.
24. Multiple, separate well defined radiolucencies.
25. Generalised radiolucencies.
26. Mixed radioluscent-radiopaque lesion.

27. **Radiopacities of jaws.**
28. **Radiographic features of diseases of maxillary antrum-TMJ.**
29. **Sialography.**
30. **Principles of interpretation of radiograph.**

Chapter 17

Oral Medicine, Diagnosis and Radiology

1. **EBV has been demonstrated to be having a cause-and-effect relationship with:**
   A. Oral hairy leukoplakia
   B. African Burkitts lymphoma
   C. Naso pharyngeal carcinoma
   D. None of the above
2. **In adults (> 40 yrs) suffering from (EBV) infectious mononucleus the predominant findings are**
   A. Fever and pharyngitis
   B. Lymphadenopathy
   C. Hepatomegaly
   D. Splenomegaly
3. **Cases of NUG that are refractory to conventional therapy should be evaluated to rule out**
   A. HSV
   B. VZV
   C. EBV
   D. None of the above
4. **Corticosteroid therapy in infectious mono nucleosis should be restricted to patients having**
   A. Pharyngitis
   B. Splenomegaly
   C. Massive tonsillar enlargement
   D. None of the above
5. **Cytomegalovirus (HHV-5) can reside latently in**
   A. Salivary gland cells
   B. Endothelium
   C. Macrophages and lymphocytes
   D. All of the above
6. **Developmental tooth defects can be produced by neonatal**
   A. CMV
   B. HSV
   C. VZV
   D. None of the above
7. **"Owl eye" cell is histological diagnostic feature of**
   A. Kissing disease
   B. Herpes zoster
   C. Cytomegalovirus
   D. Varicella zoster
8. **Infection with enterovirus encompasses**
   A. Herpangina
   B. Hand-foot and mouth disease
   C. Acute lymphonodular pharyngitis
   D. All of the above
9. **The least significant source for the transmission of AIDS is**
   A. Blood
   B. Oral fluids
   C. Breast milk
   D. Vaginal secretion
10. **Kaposi's sarcoma is associated with**
    A. HSV-2 B. VZV
    C. HSV-8 D. HSV-1

11. The presence of candidiasis in a patient infected with HIV is
A. Diagnostic of development of AIDS
B. Pathognomonic of development of AIDS
C. Predictive for development of AIDS
D. None of the above

12. HIV associated linear gingival erythema
A. Does not respond to improved plaque control
B. Resolves after professional plaque removal
C. Respond to systemic antifungal medication
D. All of the above

13. NUP is characterized by all of the following *except*
A. Gingival necrosis
B. Rapidly progressing bone loss
C. Deep pocketing
D. Spontaneous hemorrhage

14. The most common EBV related lesion in patients with AIDS is
A. Lymphoma
B. Kaposi sarcoma
C. Oral hairy leukoplakia
D. NUP

15. Lesions of aphthous ulcers in HIV patient that are unresponsive to topical steroids should be treated with
A. Antifungals (azoles)
B. Cyclosporin
C. Thalidomide
D. None of the above

16. The most common site for lesions caused by Human Papilloma virus in HIV patients is
A. Intra oral
B. Peri oral
C. Anogenital area
D. Oral mucosa tightly bound to underlying structures

17. HPV related lesions in patients with AIDS mandate
A. No treatment
B. Close observation
C. Palliative treatment
D. Use of corticosteroids

18. The most common oral presentation of histoplasmosis in AIDS patient is
A. Intrabony lesion invading the deeper structures
B. A shallow ulcer at the vermillion border
C. Indurated mucosal ulceration with raised borders
D. Deep ulcers (punched out) in the interdental gingiva

19. The most common site for HIV associated salivary gland disease is
A. Parotid glands
B. Submandibular gland
C. Sublingual salivary gland
D. Mucous salivary glands of the palate

20. Hyperpigmentation in HIV patient is microscopically similar to
A. Kaposi sarcoma
B. Melanoma
C. Focal melanosis
D. Cafe-au-lait spots

21. The most common site for lymphoma in AIDS patient is
A. Gingiva B. Palate
C. CNS D. Maxilla

22. The antiretroviral therapy in AIDS has dramatically reduced the prevalance of
A. Opportunistic infections
B. Kaposi sarcoma
C. Non Hodgkins lymphoma
D. None of the above

23. Acquired double lip may be
A. A component of Ascher syndrome
B. Result of trauma or sucking on the lip
C. All of the above
D. None of the above

24. Fordyce's granules are closely similar to sebaceous glands found in the skin *except*
A. Sebaceous cells are polygonal in shape
B. The nuclei are centrally placed
C. Absence of hair follicles
D. Abundant foamy cytoplasm

25. The preliminary test for differentiating leukodema from leukoplakia is
A. Biopsy
B. Stretching of mucosa
C. FNAC
D. Exfoliative cytology

26. The most common cause for macroglossia is
A. Vascular malformations
B. Benign tumors
C. Cretinism
D. Neurofibromatosis

27. Which of the following factor(s) is/are associated with Hairy Tongue?
A. Radiation therapy
B. Use of antacid
C. Poor oral hygiene
D. All of the above

28. Hairy tongue most commonly spares
A. The midline of the tongue
B. Lateral and anterior borders of the tongue
C. Posterior half of the tongue
D. Area anterior to the circumvallate papillae

29. The most common type of oral varicosity is
A. Varices of the lip
B. Varices of the buccal mucosa
C. Sublingual varix
D. Submandibular varix

30. The most common site for caliber persistent artery is
A. Lip mucosa
B. Floor of the mouth
C. Ventral surface of the tongue
D. Buccal mucosa

31. Caliber persistent artery is
A. A vascular malformation
B. A varice
C. A local extravasation of blood
D. None of the above

32. Most of the Bifid condyles have
A. Antero medial and postero-lateral heads
B. Medial and lateral heads
C. Anterior and posterior heads
D. Antero lateral and postero medial heads

33. The most positive laboratory method of identification of HSV1 is
A. Cytology
B. HSV Isolation
C. Antibody Titre
D. None of the above

34. Paralysis of bladder; the extremeties and diaphragm can be caused by
A. HSV1 infection
B. Shingels
C. Hand foot and mouth disease
D. Herpangina

35. Dental anamolies can result because of infection during tooth development by
A. HSV1 infection
B. Coxsackie virus
C. Herpes zoster (Varicella zoster)
D. HSV2 infection

36. Toxic epidermal necrolysis (TEN) is
A. Severe form of EM
B. Chronic form of EM
C. Milder form of EM
D. Not related to EM

37. Triggers for erythema multiforme (EM) include
A. Benign and Malignant Tumors
B. Progesterone
C. Histoplasmosis
D. All of the above

38. A. Old age
B. UV light exposure
C. Emotional stress
D. Respiratory illness
___ Has been demonstrated unequivocally to induce HSV lesion, experimentally.

39. **In reccurrent attacks of erythema multiforme which of the following is warranted**
A. Antibiotic prophylaxsis
B. Antihistamin prophylaxsis
C. Antiviral prophylaxsis
D. None of the above

40. **People exposed to HSV–1, later in life often demonstrate**
A. Gingivostomatitis
B. Mumps
C. Pharyngo tonsilitis
D. Genital lesions

41. **The most common site for recurrent HSV1 infection is**
A. Gingiva
B. Tongue
C. Pharyngo tonsillar region
D. Vermilion border and adjacent skin

42. **Scrumpox is**
A. Smallpox in children
B. Lesions of herpes zoster in children who are in immuno compromised
C. Lesions of primary HSV–1 infection in areas of abrasion
D. Lesions of HSV–1 on the digits

43. **The most important factor in usage of antivirals in the treatment of HSV–1 infection is**
A. Dosage of the antivirals
B. Generation of the antivirals
C. Duration of antiviral therapy
D. Time of initiation of antiviral therapy

44. **Acyclovir in the treatment of HSV–1 has been shown to work synergistically with**
A. Betadine
B. Essential oils
C. Chlorhexidine
D. Triclosan

45. **Acyclovir resistant HSV–1 recurrent episode patient can be treated in future episodes by**
A. Acyclovir
B. Steroids
C. Antibiotics
D. None of the above

46. **The most common and serious complication of varicella is**
A. Reyes syndrome
B. Sickle cell crisis
C. Encephalitis
D. Varicella pneumonitis

47. **Zoster sine herpete is a term used to denote**
A. HSV–1 with rash
B. Varicella zoster with rash
C. Varicella zoster without rash
D. Zoster without rash

48. **Herpes zoster involving trigeminal nerve may be associated with**
A. Devitalization of teeth in the affected area
B. Bone necrosis with loss of teeth in the affected area
C. All of the above
D. None of the above

49. **Ophthalmic referral is mandatory in cases of herpes zoster when the lesion involve**
A. Skin of the upper lip
B. Intra oral tissues
C. Skin of the cheeks
D. Tip of the nose

50. **Which is the only malignant neoplasm of jaws that invades the pulp of the tooth?**
A. Osteosarcoma
B. Chondrosarcoma
C. Burkitts lymphoma
D. Hodgkins disease

51. In causation of Burkitts lymphoma which of the following can act as a co-factor?
A. Malarial parasites
B. Cytomegalo virus infecton
C. HSV infection
D. Ascaris infestation

52. The only reservoirs for mumps virus is
A. Rabbit B. Sheep
C. Man D. Cat

53. Infantile cortical hyper osteosis may be clinically confused with
A. Pagets disease
B. Fibrous dysplasia
C. Cherubism
D. Osteopetrosis

54. Blue sclera is seen in patients with
A. Rickets
B. Marphan's syndrome
C. Cleidocranial dysostosis
D. Peirre Robins syndrome

55. Parrot beak like face is characteristic
A. Mandibulo-facial dysostosis
B. Pierre-Robins syndrome
C. Cleidocranial dysostosis
D. None of the above

56. Oral lympho epithelial cyst is microscopically similar to
A. Thyroglossal cyst
B. Branchial cleft cyst
C. Sebaceous cyst
D. Dentigerous cyst

57. Extra osseous counterpart of lateral periodontal cyst is
A. Inflammatory periapical cyst
B. Residual cyst
C. Gingival cyst of adult
D. Cyst of new born

58. The only white lesion that can be scrapped of is
A. White sponge nevous
B. Slaked lime lesion and candidasis
C. Candidiasis only
D. None of the above

59. The malignant neoplasm that invades pulp tissue
A. Ameloblastoma
B. CEOT
C. Squamous cell carcinoma
D. Burkitt's lymphoma

60. The functions of tongue are reduced in
A. Mysthenia gravis
B. Scleroderma
C. Oral submucous fibrosis
D. Muscle dystrophy

61. The presence of multiple uninterrupted super-numerary teeth is usually seen in
A. Cowden's syndrome
B. Gardner's syndrome
C. Cleidocranial dysostosis
D. PL syndrome

62. The rudimentary teeth showing dysplastic dentin are a feature of skin disease
A. Pemphigus vulgaris
B. Acanthosis Nigricans
C. Epidermolysis bullosa complex
D. Systemic sclerosis

63. Bumpy lips are feature of
A. Traumatic neuroma
B. Schwanoma
C. MENS syndrome
D. None of the above

64. For a lesion to be considered as dentigerous cyst the surrounding radiolucent space should be at least
A. 1 to 2 mm
B. 3 to 4 mm
C. 5 to 6 mm
D. 1 to 2 mm

65. Lateral periodontal cyst arise from
A. Periodontal ligament fibres
B. Reduced enamel epithelium
C. Rests of Malassez
D. Rests of Dental lamina

66. Lateral periodontal cysts occur more commonly in
A. Males in mandibular premolar and cuspid region
B. Females in maxillary molar region
C. Males in mandibular molar region
D. Females in mandibular molar region

67. Botryoid odontogenic cyst is
A. Multiloculated dentigerous cyst
B. Uniloculated periodontal cyst
C. Multiloculated odontogenic keratocyst
D. Multiloculated lateral periodontal cyst

68. Patients with multiple odontogenic keratocyst show
A. No recurrence
B. Same recurrence as seen in solitary OKC
C. More recurrence than solitary OKC
D. Less recurrence than solitary OKC

69. COC may mimic in its late phase (Radiographically)
A. OKC
B. Dentigerous cyst
C. Only AOT
D. AOT, partially mineralized odontoma, CEOT and ameloblastic fibro-odontoma

70. Aneurysmal bone cyst is a
A. Neoplastic lesion
B. Cystic lesion
C. Reactive pseudo-cystic lesion
D. Hamartoma

71. The psuedo cystic lesion of maxilla containing salivary gland tissue may be a
A. Static bone cyst
B. Nasopalatine duct cyst
C. Traumatic bone cyst
D. Salivary gland inclusion cyst

72. Intra oral counterpart of branchial cyst is
A. Lympho epithelial cyst
B. Dermoid cyst
C. Median palatine cyst
D. None of above

73. Multicystic ameloblastoma when treated with curettage
A. May not reoccur
B. May show a recurrence rate from 50–90%
C. May show a recurrence rate 10–20%
D. None of the above

74. Sentinel tubercles are the features of
A. Tuberculosis
B. Syphilis
C. Sarcoidosis
D. Candidiasis

75. Viral etiology of oral cancer comprises
A. 15% of human malignancies
B. 30% of human malignancies
C. 50% of human malignancy
D. None of the above

76. The father of Dental Radiology is
A. Wilhelm C Roentgen
B. Pierre Fauchard
C. Otto Wolkhoff
D. Edmund C Kells

77. Size of an adult periapical radiograph film is
A. 22 × 35 mm
B. 24 × 40 mm
C. 32 × 41 mm
D. 35 × 45 mm

78. Most sensitive IOPA film is
A. Intermediate speed
B. Ekta speed
C. Fast speed
D. Ultra speed

79. All of the following dental restorative materials are radiolucent *except*
A. Calcium hydroxide cement
B. Silicate cement
C. BISGMA resin
D. Poly-methyl-methacrylate

80. Another name for 'Jug-handle view' is
A. Occipito-menton view
B. Lateral oblique view
C. Submento-vertex view
D. Water's view

81. An elderly individual presents with expansion of alveolar ridge and migration of teeth. Investigations reveal that serum calcium level is normal and generalised cotton wool appearance is seen on extra-oral radiograph. The likely diagnosis is
- A. Osteopetrosis
- B. Ameloblastoma
- C. Odontogenic myxoma
- D. Paget's disease

82. A routine extra-oral radiograph reveals unusual, multiple elongated radiopaque areas in orofacial region. The patient is a butcher by profession and he does not illicit any relevant medical or dental history. A likely differential diagnosis could be
- A. Bone marrow space
- B. Cysticercosis
- C. Basal cell carcinoma
- D. All of the above

83. Basic composition of an X–ray film consists of
- A. Base and emulsion
- B. Base and activator
- C. Filler and matrix
- D. Filler and activator

84. X–rays belong to the group of
- A. Electromagnetic radiation
- B. Photon radiation
- C. Ionizing radiation
- D. All of the above

85. Unit of measurement for radiation absorbed by the body is
- A. Roentgen
- B. RAD
- C. Coulomb per kilogram
- D. All of the above

86. Least radiosensitive body organ among the following is
- A. Salivary glands
- B. Intestines
- C. Growing bone
- D. Growing cartilage

87. Somatic effects of radiation exposure do not include
- A. Mucositis
- B. Xerostomia
- C. Chromosome mutations
- D. None of the above

88. Sharpness of a radiographic image can be enhanced by
- A. Increasing the distance between the object and radiograph
- B. Increasing the distance between the focal spot and object
- C. Using a large focal spot at all times
- D. All of the above

89. Taking a posterior IOPA as compared to an anterior IOPA is controlled by a dentist in terms of
- A. Higher KVP
- B. Greater Ma
- C. Larger duration
- D. All of the above

90. Main use of hydroquinone in processing of radiographs is as
- A. Developing agent
- B. Preservative
- C. Activator
- D. Retarder

91. Sodium sulfite is a constituent of radiograph fixing solution that is used as
- A. Acidifier
- B. Hardner
- C. Solvent
- D. Preservative

92. Time temperature method of processing an intra-oral radiograph manually consists of immersing the film in a developing solution for
- A. 4 minutes at 65°F
- B. 5 minutes at 68°F
- C. 6 minutes at 72°F
- D. Any of the above

93. A middle-aged patient reports to dental O.P.D. with complaint of xerostomia. Her sialogram reveals a cherry blossom like appearance of parotid gland. The likely diagnosis is
A. Pleomorphic adenoma
B. Parotitis
C. Sjögren's syndrome
D. Atresia

94. X-rays and ultraviolet rays are different from each other in the following ways, *except*
A. Perception to human sense
B. Fluorescence
C. Wavelength
D. None of the above

95. Size of an X-ray beam is reduced by
A. Filteration
B. Collimation
C. Grid
D. All of the above

96. A faulty radiograph shows herring bone pattern as a result of
A. Film exposed from wrong side
B. Excessive bending of film
C. Increased vertical angulation
D. Double exposure

97. Following is/are true periapical radiolucency(ies) in contact with tooth apex
A. Surgical defects
B. Bone marrow spaces
C. Naris
D. All of the above

98. Following is/are advantage(s) of bisecting angle technique over paralleling technique for recording intraoral radiographs
A. Distortion
B. Less exposure to radiation
C. Use in edentulous mouth
D. All of the above

99. Tube shift principle states that
A. If an object is placed buccal to a reference structure, it appears to move distally when X-ray tube is moved mesially
B. If an object is placed lingual to a reference structure, it appears to move distally when X-ray tube is moved mesially
C. If an object is placed buccal to a reference structure, it does not appear to move irrespective of whether X-ray tube is moved mesially or distally
D. None of the above

100. Following is not an indication for localization
A. Tracking a broken endodontic file
B. Determining position of root canals in maxillary first premolar
C. Identifying spatial position of anatomic radiolucency
D. Determining mesio-distal position of impacted tooth.

Answers

1 D
2 A B, C, D are predominant finding in children younger than 4 years.
3 C Because NUG is fairly common in infectious mononucleosis.
4 C Massive tonsillar enlargement may cause airway obstruction warranting steroid therapy.
5 D
6 A
7 C
8 D
9 B Saliva appears to reduce the ability of HIV to infect lymphocytes.
10 C
11 C
12 D
13 A Gingival necrosis does not let pocket formation to occur.
14 C
15 C But must be used with caution as thalidomide can enhance the production of HIV.
16 C
17 B Because many HIV patients exhibit dysplasia within HPV-related lesion.
18 C
19 A
20 C
21 C
22 C
23 C
24 C
25 B
26 A
27 D
28 B
29 C
30 A
31 A Caliber persistent artery is a vascular anomaly in which a main arterial branch extends upto superficial submucosal tissues without reduction in its diameter.
32 B
33 B
34 B
35 C
36 A
37 D
38 B A cause and effect relationship has not been demonstrated though EBV is associated with Burkitt's lymphoma.
39 C Antivirals are recommended in chronic recurrent EM because more than 15% of such cases are preceded by symptomatic recurrence of HSV.
40 C
41 D
42 C
43 D
44 C
45 A Because only the peripheral viruses mutate and become resistant to drugs whereas the resident virus remain sensitive.
46 D
47 D
48 C
49 D Involvement of the tip of the nose suggest the involvement of naso-cilliary branch of the fifth crainal nerve, suggesting potential for ocular infection that may lead to permanent blindness.
50 C
51 A
52 C
53 C
54 A
55 C
56 B
57 C
58 D
59 D
60 A
61 C
62 C
63 C
64 B
65 D
66 A
67 D
68 C
69 D
70 C
71 B
72 A
73 B
74 A
75 A
76 D 'A' discovered X-rays, 'B' is the father of modern dentistry.
77 C
78 B
79 A
80 C
81 D
82 B Tapeworm infestation in oro-facial region generally manifests without any clinical symptoms. Occupation (Butcher) is a predisposing factor.
83 A

84 D X-rays are positively charged particles of the electromagnetic spectrum.

85 B 'A' is the unit of exposure and 'C' measures the degree of potential danger to health.

86 A 'B' has high sensitivity and 'C' and 'D' have intermediate sensitivity.

87 C Chromosome mutations are result of genetic effects from radiation exposure.

88 B A shall blur the radiographic image and C is inappropriate.

89 C Voltage and current are constant, while exposure time varies:

	Vertical Angulations (°)	
	Maxillary	*Mandibular*
Incisiors	+ 50	– 20
Caninex	+ 45	– 15
Premolars	+ 30	– 10
Molars	+ 25	– 5 (For III molar)

90 A

91 D

92 B

93 C Age, gender and radiographic appearance indicate that patient is having Sjögren's syndrome.

94 B Both X-rays and ultra-violet rays can emit fluorescence.

95 D

96 A 'B' causes elongation of few teeth 'C' causes shortening of image, 'D' causes double image formation.

97 A 'B' and 'C' are false periapical shadows cast over teeth that can be shifted by taking additional radiographs with different angulation.

98 C

99 A SLOB-Same lingual, opposite buccal.

100 D Localization can measure bucco-lingual position of impacted tooth.

Chapter 18

All India Postgraduate Entrance Examination-2004

1. **In a disease free temporomandibular joint, posterior end of the articular disc remains at**
   A. 9 O'clock position
   B. 10 O'clock position
   C. 12 O'clock position
   D. 2 O'clock position
2. **Which of the following teeth has maximum sensory receptors?**
   A. Maxillary permanent 1st molar
   B. Mandibular permanent 1st molar
   C. Mandibular permanent canine
   D. Maxillary permanent canine
3. **In a healthy gingival, the distance between gingival margin and free gingiva groove is**
   A. 0.1-0.5 mm **B.** 1.5-1 mm
   C. 0.5-1.5 mm **D.** 1-2 mm
4. **Which of the following structures is not present on the internal surface of mandible?**
   A. Genial tubercle **B.** Mylohyoid ridge
   C. Lingula **D.** Mental foramen
5. **Among all of the following foramens in the base of skull which is the most posteriorly present**
   A. Foramen spinosum
   B. Foramen rotundum
   C. Foramen lacerum
   D. Foramen ovale
6. **Enamel etched by a tooth conditioner but not covered with a fissure sealant will**
   A. Remineralize within a month
   B. Remineralize within 3 months
   C. Absorb stain and discolor the tooth
   D. Leave the tooth more susceptible to caries attack
7. **The strength of dental investment for gold alloy is dependent on the amount of**
   A. Silica **B.** Carbon
   C. Copper **D.** Gypsum
8. **In Erythema migrans, which papilla of tongue are absent?**
   A. Fungiform **B.** Foliate
   C. Filliform **D.** Circumvallate
9. **Thistle-tube appearance of pulp chamber is a feature of**
   A. Coronal dentin dysplasia
   B. Regional odontodysplasia
   C. Dentigenesis imperfecta
   D. Amelogenesis imperfecta
10. **On clinical examination a 60-year-old female had a tumor in the right Buccal mucosa. The size of the tumor was about 2 cm in diameter. There was no involvement of regional lymph nodes and also had no distant metastasis. The TNM of the tumor is**
    A. $T_1 N_0 M_o$ **B.** $T_1 N_1 M_o$
    C. $T_1 N_2 M_o$ **D.** $T_2 N_0 M_o$

11. **Which of the following is not a feature of torus mandibularis?**
   A. Common in mongoloids
   B. Present on the lingual surface of mandible below the mylohyoid line
   C. Usually bilateral
   D. May or may not be associated with torus palatinus

12. **The time gap between appearance of Kopilk's spot and cutaneous rash in measles is**
   A. 24 hrs B. 3-4 days
   C. 2 weeks D. 10 days

13. **The drug that causes intrinsic staining of teeth due to calcium chelation is**
   A. Alizarin B. Ampicillin
   C. Tetracycline D. Erythromycin

14. **Which of the following medications shortens the recovery period of primary herpetic gingivostomatitis?**
   A. Acyclovir
   B. Ziduvidine
   C. Kenalog in orachase
   D. All of the above

15. **The occurrence of dental caries in the population at a given point of time may be termed as**
   A. Incidence
   B. Point prevalence
   C. Period prevalence
   D. None of the above

16. **The CPITN probe has a ball end of which diameter and marking at what level?**
   A. 0.5 mm diameter ball and marking at 3, 5, 8 and 11 mm
   B. 1.0 mm diameter ball and marking at 3.5, 5.5, 8.5 and 11 mm
   C. 0.5 mm diameter ball and marking at 3.5, 5.5, 8.5 and 11 mm
   D. 1.0 mm diameter ball and marking at 3, 5, 8 and 11 mm

17. **The WHO index for fluorosis is based on**
   A. Dean's index
   B. McKay's index
   C. Community fluorosis index
   D. Public health fluorosis index

18. **While planning for a clinical trial for finding out the effect of a particular mouthwash on human subjects, which kind of study design will be able to give best results?**
   A. Randomized controlled trial with double blind planning
   B. Clinical trial with single blind plan and cross-over
   C. Randomized controlled trial with no blinding and cross-over
   D. Randomized controlled trial with double blind plan and cross-over

19. **DMFT index is a**
   A. Simple reversible index
   B. Cumulative irreversible index
   C. Cumulative reversible index
   D. Simple irreversible index

20. **Recommended average daily intake of fluoride from all sources combined for adults and children is**
   A. 2.0 to 2.2 mg and 1.2 mg
   B. 1.2 to 2.0 mg and 1.2 mg
   C. 2.2 to 2.4 mg and 1.5 mg
   D. 2.6 to 2.8 mg and 1.4 mg

21. **Mineral trioxide aggregate used in apexification**
   A. Forms an integral part of the root canal filling
   B. Dissolves as the apical barrier formation progresses
   C. Has not yielded good results
   D. Is available in a paste form

22. **Which of the following is the most recommended endodontic obturating material for deciduous teeth?**
   A. Kri paste B. ZOE
   C. $Ca(OH)_2$ paste D. Maisto's paste

23. Which of the following is the best indication for propofol as an intravenous induction agent?
A. Neurosurgery
B. Day care surgery
C. Patients with coronary artery disease
D. In neonates

24. Which of the following volatile anaesthetic agents should be preferred for induction of anaesthesia in children?
A. Enflurane B. Isoflurane
C. Sevoflurane D. Desflurane

25. When a patient develops supraventricular tachycardia with hypotension under general anaesthesia, all of the following treatments may be instituted *except*
A. Carotid sinus massage
B. Adenosine 3-12 mg IV
C. Direct current cardioversion
D. Varapamil 5 mg IV

26. A 25-year-old male with roadside accident underwent debridement and reduction of fractured both bones right forearm under axillary block. On the second post-operative day the patient complained of persistent numbness and paresthesia in the right forearm and the hand. The most common cause of this neurological dysfunction could be all of the following *except*
A. Crush injury to the hand and lacerated nerves
B. A tight cast or dressing
C. Systemic toxicity of local anaesthetics
D. Tourniquet pressure

27. The first costochondral joint is a
A. Fibrous joint B. Synovial joint
C. Syndesmosis D. Syncendrosis

28. Which of the following is the feature of Y chromosome?
A. Acrocentric B. Telocentric
C. Submetacentric D. Metacentric

29. Shine-Dalgarno sequence in bacterial mRNA is near
A. AUG condon B. UAA condon
C. UAG condon D. UGA condon

30. Which of the following is a membrane-bound enzyme that catalyzes the formation of cyclic AMP from ATP?
A. Tyrosine kinase
B. Polymerase
C. ATP synthase
D. Adenylate cyclase

31. A small Ca^{2+} binding protein that modifies the activity of many enzymes and other proteins in response to changes of Ca^{2+} concentration is known as
A. Cycline B. Calmodulin
C. Collagen D. Kinesin

32. An enzyme that makes a double stranded DNA copy from a single stranded RNA template molecule is known as
A. DNA polymerase
B. RNA polymerase
C. Reverse transcriptase
D. Phosphokinase

33. A segment of an eucaryotic gene that is not represented in the mature mRNA is known as
A. Intron B. Exon
C. Plasmid D. TATA box

34. The articular cartilage is characterized by all of the following features *except*
A. It is devoid of perichondrium
B. It has a rich nerve supply
C. It is a vascular
D. It lacks the capacity to regenerate

35. All of the following are categorised as secondary lymphoid organs *except*
A. Lymph nodes
B. Spleen
C. Thymus
D. Subepithelial collections of lymphocytes

36. An inhaled foreign body is likely to lodge in the right lung due to all of the following features *except*

A. Right lung is shorter and wider than left lung
B. Right principal bronchus is more vertical than the left bronchus
C. Tracheal bifurcation directs the foreign body to the right lung
D. Right inferior lobar bronchus is in continuation with the principal bronchus

37. A person on a fat free carbohydrate rich diet continues to grow obese. Which of the following lipoproteins is likely to be elevated in his blood?

A. Chylomicrons B. VLDL
C. LDL D. HDL

38. The transmembrane region of a protein is likely to have

A. A stretch of hydrophilic amino acids
B. A stretch of hydrophobic amino acids
C. A disulphide loop
D. Alternating hydrophilic and hydrophobic amino acids

39. Radio isotopes are used in the following techniques *except*

A. Mass spectroscopy
B. RIA
C. ELISA
D. Sequencing of nucleic acid

40. Which of the following substances acts to increase the release of Ca^{++} from endoplasmic reticulum?

A. Inositol triphosphate
B. Parathyroid hormone
C. 1.25-dihydroxy cholecalciferol
D. Diacyl glycerol

41. Which of the following elements is known to influence the body's ability to handle oxidative stress?

A. Calcium B. Iron
C. Potassium D. Selenium

42. Which of the following groups of proteins assist in the folding of other proteins?

A. Proteases B. Proteosomes
C. Templates D. Chaperones

43. A highly ionized drug

A. Is excreted mainly by the kidneys
B. Crosses the placental barrier easily
C. Is well absorbed from the intestine
D. Is highly protein bound

44. All of the following are used as proxy measures for incubation period *except*

A. Latent period
B. Period of communicability
C. Serial interval
D. Generation time

45. The current recommendation for breast-feeding is that

A. Exclusive breast-feeding should be continued till 6 months of age followed by supplementation with additional foods
B. Exclusive breast-feeding should be continued till 4 months of age followed by supplementation with additional foods
C. Colostrum is the most suitable food for a new born baby but it is best avoided in first 2 days
D. The baby should be allowed to breast-feed till one year of age

46. The following statements about breast milk are true *except*

A. The maximum milk output is seen at 12 months
B. The coefficient of uptake of iron in breast milk is 70%
C. Calcium absorption of human milk is better than that of cow's milk
D. It provides about 65 K cals per 100 ml

47. Multi-purpose worker scheme in India was introduced following the recommendation of

A. Srivastava Committee
B. Bhore Committee
C. Kartar Singh Committee
D. Mudaliar Committee

48. The usefulness of a 'screening test' in a community depends on its

A. Sensitivity B. Specificity
C. Reliability D. Predictive value

49. If the grading of malocclusion is classified as "mild", "moderate" and "severe" the scale of measurement used is

A. Interval B. Nominal
C. Ordinal D. Ratio

50. If prevalence of dental caries is 10%, the probability that three people selected at random from the population will have diabetes is

A. 0.01 B. 0.03
C. 0.001 D. 0.003

51. A study began in 1970 with a group of 5000 adults in Delhi who were asked about their 'Gutka' consumption. The occurrence of cancer was studied in this group between 1990-1995. This is an example of

A. Cross-sectional study
B. Retrospective cohort study
C. Concurrent cohort study
D. Case-control study

52. Hair and nails are usually preserved in poisoning from

A. Arsenic B. Phosphorous
C. Barbiturates D. Carbon monoxide

53. The occurrence of hyperthyroidism following administration of supplemental iodine to subjects with endemic iodine deficiency goiter is known as

A. Jod-Basedow effect
B. Wolff-Chaikoff effect
C. Thyrotoxicosis factitia
D. de Quervain's thyroiditis

54. A 39-year-old female presents with fever. The blood culture from the patient grows Gram-positive small to medium coccobacilli that are pleomorphic, occurring in short chains. Direct wet mount from the culture shows tumbling motility. The most likely organism is

A. *Listeria monocytogenes*
B. *Corynebacterium sp*
C. *Enterococcus sp*
D. *Erysipelothrix rhusiopathiae*

55. In all of the following bacterial diarrhoeas toxins are implicated as a major pathogenetic mechanism *except*

A. *Vibrio cholerae*
B. *Shigella sp*
C. *Vibrio parahaemolyticus*
D. *Staphylococcus aureus*

56. All of the following clinical features are associated with Enteroviruses *except*

A. Myocarditis
B. Pleurodynia
C. Herpangina
D. Hemorrhagic fever

57. A post-operative patient developed septicemia and was empirically started on combination chemotherapy by a new resident doctor. However, when the patient did not respond even after 10 days of antibiotics treatment, the review of the charts was done. It was found that the resident doctor had started the combination of antibiotics which was mutually antagonistic in action. Which one of the following is the most likely combination that was given?

A. Vancomycin and Amikacin
B. Cephelexin and Gentamicin
C. Ampicillin and Chloramphenicol
D. Ciprofloxacin and Piperacillin

58. In some old fractures, cartilaginous tissue forms over the fractured bone ends with a cavity in between containing clear fluid. This condition is called as

A. Delayed union
B. Slow union
C. Non union
D. Pseudarthrosis

59. A police recruit, smoker and 6 months into training started complaining of pain at posterior medial aspect of both legs. There was acute point tenderness and the pain was aggravated on physical activity. The most likely diagnosis is
A. Burger's disease
B. Gout
C. Lumbar canal stenosis
D. Stress fracture

60. In which of the following locations there is collection of pus in the quinsy?
A. Peritonsillar space
B. Parapharyngeal space
C. Retropharyngeal space
D. Within the tonsil

61. Fordyce's (Spots) Granules in Oral Cavity arise from
A. Mucous glands
B. Sebaceous glands
C. Taste buds
D. Minor salivary glands

62. Which of the following statements best represents Bell's paralysis?
A. Hemiparesis and contralateral facial nerve paralysis
B. Combined paralysis of the facial trigeminal, and abducens nerves
C. Idiopathic ipsilateral paralysis of the facial nerve
D. Facial nerve paralysis with a dry eye

63. Retardation of skeletal maturity can be caused by all *except*
A. Chronic renal failure
B. Hypothyroidism
C. Protein energy malnutrition (PEM)
D. Congenital adrenal-hyperplasia

64. Bone marrow transplantation can be used as a treatment for all *except*
A. Osteopetrosis
B. Adrenoleukodystrophy
C. Huler's syndrome
D. Hemochromatosis

65. HBA1$_C$ level in blood explains
A. Acute rise of sugar
B. Long term status of blood sugar
C. Hepatorenal syndrome
D. Chronic pancreatitis

66. To which of the following family of chemical mediators of inflammation, the Lipoxins belong?
A. Kinin system
B. Cytokines
C. Chemokines
D. Arachidonic acid metabolites

67. The most abundant glycoprotein present in basement membrane is
A. Laminin
B. Fibronectin
C. Collagen type 4
D. Hepman sulphate

68. Which of the following is a precognition protein?
A. Thrombomodulin
B. Protein C
C. Protein S
D. Thrombin

69. Which of the following is an antiapoptotic gene?
A. C-myc
B. P53
C. bcl-2
D. bax

70. The most common site of oral cancer among Indian population is
A. Tongue
B. Floor of mouth
C. Alveobuccal complex
D. Lip

71. Persistent vomiting most likely causes
A. Hyperkalaemia
B. Acidic urine excretion
C. Hypochloraemia
D. Hyperventilation

72. Ram Kumar, a 70-year-old male who has been chewing tobacco for the past 50 years presents with a six months history of a large, fungating, soft papillary lesions in the oral cavity. The lesion has

penetrated into the mandible. Lymph nodes are not palpable. Two biopsies taken from the lesion proper show benign appearing papillomatosis with hyperkeratosis and acanthosis infiltrating the subjacent tissues. The most likely diagnosis is

A. Squamous cell papilloma
B. Squamous cell carcinoma
C. Verrucous carcinoma
D. Malignant mixed tumour

73. All of the following anticancer agents cause bone marrow depression *except*

A. Chlorambucil
B. Daunorubicin
C. Doxorubicin
D. Flutamide

74. Clinically significant drug interaction occurs between pyridoxine and all the following drugs *except*

A. Isoniazid B. Cyclosporine
C. Levodopa D. Hydralazine

75. In which of the following phases of clinical trial of drugs ethical clearance is not required?

A. Phase I B. Phase II
C. Phase III D. Phase IV

76. Which of the following is not a nucleoside reverse transcriptase inhibitor?

A. Zalcitabine
B. Lamivudine
C. Nevirapine
D. Didanosine

77. Which of the following antimicrobials has antipseudomonal action?

A. Cefpodoxime proxetil
B. Ceforanide
C. Cefotetan
D. Cefoperazone

78. Which of the following statements is not true regarding sulfonamides?

A. Sulfasalazine is absorbed well from gastrointestinal tract
B. Crystalluria can occur with sulfonamide administration
C. Sulfonamide administration to newborn may cause kernicterus
D. Sulfonamides are of value in treatment of infections due to Nocardia species

79. Epoxy resin is not compatible with

A. Polysulfide
B. Polyether
C. Addition silicone
D. Condensation silicone

80. Which of the following actions is ascribed to delta type of opioid receptors?

A. Ciprofloxacin
B. Trovafloxacin
C. Lomefloxacin
D. Sparfloxacin

81. Which of the following actions is ascribed to delta type of opioid receptors?

A. Supraspinal analgesic
B. Respiratory depression
C. Euphoria
D. Reduced intestinal motility

82. Which cement base has the highest elastic modulous?

A. Zinc phosphate
B. Polymer-reinforced ZOE
C. Zinc polycarboxylate
D. Glass-ionomer cement

83. The main excitatory neurotransmitter in the CNS is

A. Glycine B. Acetylcholine
C. Aspartate D. Glutamate

84. The blood in the vessels normally does not clot because

A. Vitamin K antagonists are present in plasma
B. Thrombin has a positive feedback on plasminogen
C. Sodium citrate in plasma chelates calcium ions
D. Vascular endothelium is smooth and coated with glycocalyx

85. The force of muscle contraction can be increased by all of the following *except*

A. Increasing the frequency of activation of motor units
B. Increasing the number of motor units activated
C. Increasing the amplitude of action potentials in the motor neurons
D. Recruiting larger motor units

86. A 37-year-old multipara construction labourer has a blood picture showing hypochromic anisocytosis. This is most likely indicative of

A. Iron deficiency
B. Folic deficiency
C. Malnutrition
D. Combined iron and folic acid deficiency

87. Maximum permissible setting expansion of high strength stone is

A. 0.1% B. 0.05%
C. 0.3% D. 0.2%

88. The Non-REM (NREM) sleep is commonly associated with

A. Frequent dreaming
B. Frequent penile erections
C. Increased blood pressure
D. Night terrors

89. Coefficient of thermal expansion currently available porcelain is

A. $6 \times 10^{-6}/°C$
B. $8 \times 10^{-6}/°C$
C. $10 \times 10^{-6}/°C$
D. $14 \times 10^{-6}/°C$

90. Which of the following brain tumors does not spread via CSF?

A. Germ cell tumors
B. Medulloblastoma
C. CNS Lymphoma
D. Craniopharyngoma

91. Which of the following is the most penetration beam?

A. Electron beam
B. 8 MV photons
C. 18 MV photons
D. Proton beam

92. Which of the following does not bind to GABA receptor chloride channels?

A. Ethanol B. Alphaxolone
C. Zolpidem D. Buspirone

93. Jai Pratap, a 20-year-old male presented with chronic constipation, headache and palpitations. On examination he had marfanoid habitus, neuromas of tongue, medullated corneal nerve fibers and a nodule of 2 × 2 cm size in the left lobe of thyroid gland. This patient is a case of

A. Sporadic medullary carcinoma of thyroid
B. Familial medullary carcinoma of thyroid
C. MEN II A
D. MEN II B

94. The most common condition of inherited blindness due to mitochondrial chromosomal anomaly is

A. Retinopathy of prematurity
B. Leber's herediatry optic neuropathy
C. Retinitis pigmentosa
D. Retinal detachment

95. The movement at the following joint permits a person to look towards right or left

A. Atlanto-occipital joint
B. Atlanto-axial joint
C. C2-C3 joint
D. C3-C4 joint

96. Which one of the following preservatives is used while packing catgut suture?

A. Isopropyl alcohol
B. Colloidal iodine
C. Glutaraldehyde
D. Hydrogen peroxide

97. Which one of the following preservatives is used while packing catgut suture?

A. Isopropyl alcohol
B. Colloidal iodine
C. Glutaraldehyde
D. Hydrogen peroxide

98. Which of the following is the earliest manifestation of Cushing's syndrome?
A. Loss of diurnal variation
B. Increased ACTH
C. Increased plasma cortisol
D. Increased urinary metabolites of cortisol

99. Thoracic extension of cervical goiter is usually approached through
A. Neck
B. Chest
C. Combined cervico-thoracic route
D. Thoracoscopic

100. The most common malignant tumor of adult males in India is
A. Oropharyngeal carcinoma
B. Gastric carcinoma
C. Colo-rectal carcinoma
D. Lung cancer

101. In complete denture construction labio-dental sound F and V are used to determine the
A. Vertical placement of upper anterior teeth
B. Labio-lingual position of anterior teeth
C. Anterio posterior position of anterior teeth
D. Space between tongue and anterior part of hard palate

102. If a edentulous patient has torus palatinus, what is the most preferred treatment while constructing a denture
A. Relief in denture before insertion
B. Relief at the impression stage
C. Relief on master cast before packing
D. Scraping of torus on master cast

103. In maxillary denture thickness of flange in distobuccal area is determined by
A. The bucinator and masseter muscle
B. The ramus, buccinator and masseter muscle
C. Coronoid process, buccinator and masseter muscle
D. The ramus, coronoid process and masseter muscle

104. Material of choice for final impression in a patient with submucous fibrosis is
A. Zinc-oxide eugenol impression paste
B. Light body silicon
C. Regular body silicon
D. Irreversible hydrocolloide

105. Palatal cusp of upper posterior teeth in complete denture patients should fall on
A. Crest of mandibular ridge
B. Lingual to crest of mandibular ridge
C. Buccal to crest of mandibular ridge
D. Buccal vestibule

106. If a complete denture patient has genial tubercle at the level of the crest of mandibular ridge, then denture base
A. Can cover them
B. Should not cover them
C. Should cover them but relief is not necessary
D. Should cover them and relief is must

107. Posterior palatal seal is recorded when the head is bent at
A. 30°
B. 150°
C. 60°
D. 45°

108. A complete denture patient complains that he has pain in his throat during swallowing. This indicates
A. Over extended PPS
B. Over extended lingual flange
C. Over extended lingual flange in retromyelohyoid region
D. His tonsils are inflamed

109. The sprue in wax pattern should be placed
A. At right angle
B. At acute angle
C. At obtuse angle
D. It depend upon type of wax pattern

110. Fovea palatine are situated in
A. Hard palate
B. Soft palate
C. At the junction of hard and soft palate
D. Their position is not fixed

111. Extension of distolingual flange in retromylohyoid area is determined by
- **A.** Superior constructor and mylohyoid muscle
- **B.** Tongue movement with mylohyoid muscle
- **C.** Superior constructor, medial ptergoid and tongue
- **D.** Superior constructor muscle and tongue musculature

112. The gagging reflex indicates
- **A.** Making and breaking content of the posterior palatal seal
- **B.** Under extended upper denture
- **C.** Too deep posterior palatal seal
- **D.** Under extended disto lingual flange of lower denture

113. How long prior to taking an impression should the retraction cord be left in place?
- **A.** 1 min **B.** 2 min
- **C.** 5 min **D.** 8 min

114. Coefficient of thermal expansion ot metalceramic alloy is
- **A.** Same as porcelain
- **B.** More than porcelain
- **C.** Less than porcelain
- **D.** More than or equal to porcelain but not less the porcelain

115. Titanium casting is done
- **A.** Under vacuum in argon atmosphere
- **B.** Under air pressure, in nitrogen atmosphere
- **C.** In specially fabricated aluminum vanadium crucibles
- **D.** Using CAD-CAM technique

116. The following is the list of elastomeric impression material which is the most biocompatible?
- **A.** Polysulfide
- **B.** Polyether
- **C.** Addition silicone
- **D.** Condensation silicone

117. Monophase elastomeric impression materials are based on
- **A.** Putty **B.** Heavy body
- **C.** Regular body **D.** Light body

118. Passivating alloys are
- **A.** Cr, Al, Ti **B.** Cr, Mo, Ti
- **C.** Cr, Fe, Mo **D.** Cr, Gold, Ti

119. Crucible indicated for casting base metal alloys is
- **A.** Carbon crucible
- **B.** Clay crucible
- **C.** Quartz crucible
- **D.** High melting plastic crucible

120. Which of the following wax coating is present on dental floss?
- **A.** Bess wax
- **B.** Spermaceti wax
- **C.** Japan wax
- **D.** Carnauba wax

121. Which of the following materials acts as an anti expansion agent in impression plaster?
- **A.** NaCl **B.** Potassium sulfate
- **C.** Calcium sulfate **D.** Silica quartz

122. Which of the following is not a mouth temperature waxes?
- **A.** Adaptol
- **B.** Korrecta type I
- **C.** HL physiologic paste
- **D.** IOWA wax

123. The mode of curing in microwave cured dentures is by
- **A.** Heat conduction
- **B.** Energy conversion
- **C.** Electrical resistance
- **D.** Magnetic field creation

124. All are consequences of odontulism *except*
- **A.** Prognathic appearance
- **B.** Thinning of lips
- **C.** Decreased length of lip
- **D.** Increase in columella-philtrum angle

125. Minimum criteria for success of an implant is

A. Success rate of 95% at end of 5 year observation period and 85% at end of 10 year

B. Success rate of 90% at end of 5 year and 80% at end of 10 year

C. Success rate of 85% at end of 5 year and 80% at end of 10 year

D. Success rate of 90% at end of 5 year and 87% at end of 10 year

126. RPI stands for

A. Occlusal rest, proximal plate, I bar

B. Cingulum rest, proximal plate, I bar

C. Rest, proximal guide plane, I bar

D. Rest, proximal plate, indirect retainer

127. Into how many segments the infant's gum pad is divided?

A. Two in each quadrant

B. Three in each quadrant

C. Two in each jaw

D. Five in each quadrant

128. Which statement best describes tooth development during eruption?

A. The crown pierces the alveolar crest when 2/3 root is complete

B. The crown reaches the occlusal plane when 2/3 root is complete

C. The crown pierces the alveolar crest when 3/4 of root is complete

D. The crown does not emerge in the oral cavity until root formation is complete

129. The presence of higher amounts of proline-rich proteins (PRP) can have what kind of effect on caries causation?

A. Caries promoting since they help in bacterial adherence

B. Make tooth surface resistant to caries since it enhance fluoride action

C. It has role during tooth mineralization only therefore no effect on caries

D. Aid in super saturation of saliva therefore make tooth resistant to caries

130. Snyder test

A. Is a method to detect acid formation in saliva

B. Is a method to find out pH of crevicular fluid

C. Is a method to identify caries causing microorganisms

D. Is a method to detect fungal growth on skin

131. Fiber-optic trans-illumination (FOTI) method of caries diagnosis is based on the principle of

A. When laser beam falls on carious enamel, it gives a bluish hue

B. A fluorescent dye is taken up by carious dentine which can be viewed easily

C. There is a different index of light transmission for decayed of sound enamel

D. The conductance of normal and decayed tooth tissue is different

132. Among the common food items, fluoride is found in higher PPM in

A. Pineapple	B. Tea

C. Sea fish	D. Coconut water

133. Fluoride is carried in the blood via

A. Plasma

B. RBC's

C. Both plasma and RBC's

D. WBC's

134. Enamel of primary and permanent teeth differ in

A. Enamel prism arrangement

B. Mineral content

C. Enamel is same in primary and permanent dentition, only dentin is different

D. None of the above

135. Patients with Down's Syndrome normally have

A. IQ score above 80

B. Brachycephalic skull

C. Stiff muscles

D. All of the above

136. Mulberry molars are characteristic features of
A. Severe fluorosis
B. Trauma at the time of birth
C. Congenital syphilis
D. Due to chronic suppurative abscess in overlying gingival tissue

137. What is the latest name of multiple caries in children involving most of the teeth?
A. Rampant caries
B. Maternally derived *Strepotoccus Mutans* disease
C. Early childhood caries
D. Early childhood syndrome

138. Famous Vipcholm study was conducted to
A. To find out role of sticky and non-sticky form of sugars on dental caries
B. To find out the role of water fluoridation on dental caries
C. To find out role of xylitol on dental caries
D. All of the above

139. Aspartane is a
A. Non-caloric sweetener
B. Caloric sweetener
C. Sugar complex
D. None of the above

140. Dry socket following extraction of a tooth is caused due to
A. Staph aureus infection
B. Distintegration of blood clot
C. Prolonged antibiotic cover
D. Unsutured socket

141. In Winter's WAR line, Amber line represents the
A. Relative depth of the III molar
B. Point of application of the elevator
C. Bone level covering the impacted tooth
D. Axial inclination of the impacted tooth relative to II molar

142. Multiple odontogenic keratocyst are associated with
A. Gardner's syndrome
B. Gortin-Goltz syndrome
C. Goldenhar's syndrome
D. Grinspan syndrome

143. The fascial spaces involved in Ludwig's Angina are
A. Unilateral-submandibular and sublingual spaces
B. Bilateral-submandibular and sublingual spaces
C. Unilateral-submandibular, sublingual and submental spaces
D. Bilateral-submandibular, sublingual and submental spaces

144. Unilateral TMJ ankylosis is associated with the following features, *except*
A. Multiple carious teeth
B. Facial asymmetry with fullness on the normal side of mandible
C. Chin deviated towards the affected side
D. Prominent ante gonial notch on the affected side

145. In dislocated condylar fractures, the condyle is dislocated
A. Medially due to the attachment of medial pterygoid
B. Laterally due to the attachment of lateral pterygoid
C. Laterally due to the attachment medial pterygoid
D. Medially due to the attachment of lateral pterygoid

146. Battle's sign is
A. Sub-conjunctival ecchymosis
B. Sublingual ecchymosis
C. Palatal ecchymosis
D. Ecchymosis is the mastoid region

147. The safe dose of adrenaline in a patient with compromised cardiac condition is
A. 0.2 mg
B. 0.02 mg
C. 0.4 mg
D. 0.04 mg

148. Rumpel-Lede test measures the
- **A.** Bleeding time
- **B.** Platelet count
- **C.** Capillary fragility
- **D.** ESR

149. Etiology of mucocele is related to
- **A.** Mechanical trauma to the minor salivary gland excretory duct
- **B.** Salivary calculi in the excretory duct major salivary gland
- **C.** Acute infections
- **D.** Smoking tobacco

150. Which of the following is the first drug of choice in anaphylactic reaction?
- **A.** Epinephrine 1:1000
- **B.** Dexamethasone 8 mg
- **C.** Hydrocortisone 100 mg
- **D.** Epinephrine 1:1,00,000

151. The role of sodium metabisulfite in local anaesthetic agent is
- **A.** Preservative
- **B.** Fungicide
- **C.** Reducing agent
- **D.** Vasoconstrictior

152. Which of the following features is not associated with acute osteomyelitis of mandible?
- **A.** Severe pain
- **B.** Purulent exudate
- **C.** Parasthesis of lower lip
- **D.** Radiographic evidence of bone destruction

153. Ostectomy procedure is indicated in
- **A.** Physiologial architecture of alveolar bone
- **B.** Correction of Tori
- **C.** Reverse architecture bony defects
- **D.** Correction of bone ledges

154. Which of the following antibiotic prescribed in case of juvenile periodontitis?
- **A.** Tetracycline
- **B.** Erythromycine
- **C.** Sulfadiazine
- **D.** Cephalexin

155. Which of the following is true is case of AIDS patient?
- **A.** Acute pain
- **B.** Diffuse red lesion of the attached gingival
- **C.** Gingiva covered with pseudomembrane
- **D.** Gingival itching

156. What is the difference between gingivitis and periodontitis?
- **A.** Gingival sulcus
- **B.** Periodontal pocket
- **C.** Loss of epithelial attachment
- **D.** Mobility of tooth

157. Which of the following step should be most preferably taken in root planning procedure?
- **A.** Removal of root caries
- **B.** Removal of necrosed cementum and calculus
- **C.** Removal of calculus
- **D.** Removal of dentine

158. If periodontal surgery is necessary in case of horizontal bone loss in upper anterior region. Which of the following procedure is the most appropriate?
- **A.** Papilla preservation flap
- **B.** Widman flap
- **C.** Coronary displaced flap
- **D.** Gingivectomy

159. A young adult shows non-fluctuant, tender and redness swelling in the marginal gingival lesion. This is most likely
- **A.** Periodontal abscess
- **B.** Periapical abscess
- **C.** Gingival abscess
- **D.** Periapical sinus

160. Which of the following periodontal disease does not have calculus?
- **A.** ANUG
- **B.** Chronic adult periodontitis
- **C.** Juvenile periodontitis
- **D.** Periodontal abscess

161. Which of the following conditions gingivectomy is contraindicated?
A. Gingival sulcus beyond mucogingival junction
B. Enlargement of the gingival
C. Papillary enlargement
D. Enlargement due to acute systemic disease

162. What is the normal average distance between the crest of the alveolar bone and the cementoenamel junction in young adult?
A. 1.0 mm B. 1.08 mm
C. 2.08 mm D. 2.80 mm

163. In which percentage chlorhexidine is used as a mouthwash?
A. 2 percent B. 0.02 percent
C. 0.2 percent D. 1.0 percent

164. Which of the following dental material shows most tear resistance?
A. Polysulfide
B. Condensation silicone
C. Addition silicone
D. Polyether

165. Which probe is used to detect the furcation involvement?
A. Periodontal probe
B. Nabers probe
C. Florida probe
D. Probe No.11

166. The percentage of maxillary growth remaining after 10 years of age is
A. 45% B. 10%
C. 25% D. 35%

167. The functional Matrix concept as revisited by Moss does not include
A. Connected cellular network (CCN)
B. Mechanotransduction
C. Epigenetic-Epithesis
D. Septopremaxillary ligament development

168. Björk used the implants for predicting facial growth changes. This approach is called as
A. Longitudinal approach
B. Metric approach
C. Structural approach
D. Computerized prediction

169. The 7th key to normal occlusion is
A. Molar relation
B. Occlusal plane
C. Crown angulations and inclination
D. Bolton ratio

170. The copper NiTi wires are not available in the temperature range of
A. 15° B. 29°
C. 35° D. 40°

171. Which of the following has the highest modulus of elasticity?
A. Dentin B. Enamel
C. Amalgum D. Composite resin

172. The two blocks in the Twin Block functional appliance are angulated at
A. 75° B. 70°
C. 65° D. 80°

173. Class III skeletal growth pattern is characterized by all except
A. Acute cranial base angle
B. Anteriorly positioned articular
C. Middle cranial fossa align posteriorly and superiorly
D. Males having more proclined maxillary incisors than females

174. In a bonded palatal expansion (Hyrax) appliance the wire framework is made of
A. 0.040 inch stainless steel
B. 0.040 inch elgiloy
C. 0.032 inch stainless steel
D. 0.036 inch stainless steel

175. All these appliances are fixed functional appliances except
A. Churio jumper
B. Mandibular protraction appliance (MPA)
C. Pendulum appliance
D. Herbst

176. All of the following weights of different components of the PAR Index are correct *except*

A. Overjet (Score × 6)
B. Overbite (Score × 2)
C. Midline (Score × 4)
D. Buccal segment (Score × 2)

177. Which of the following index is primarily used to measure the success of orthodontics treatment?

A. IOTN
B. ICON
C. PAR index
D. Goslon index

178. Which of the following condition is an absolute contraindication for orthodontic treatment?

A. Patient having history of subacute bacterial endocarditis
B. Patient receiving insulin for juvenile diabetes mellitus
C. Recently diagnosed case of acute leukemia
D. An treated case of juvenile periodontitis

179. Negative growth is a characteristic of

A. Testis
B. Brain
C. Mandible
D. Thymus

180. Which of the following cephalometric parameter is used to diagnose a long face syndrome patient?

A. Angle ANB
B. Angle SNA
C. Jaraback ratio
D. Saddle angle

181. Normal facial index

A. 65-75%
B. 75-80%
C. 80-90%
D. 100%

182. Which of the following is rapid palatal expansion device?

A. Quad helix
B. Coffin's spring
C. W-arch
D. Jackson screw

183. Which of the following contemporary orthodontic arch wire has maximum surface friction?

A. Stainless wire
B. AJW wire
C. TMA wire
D. NiTi wire

184. The movement of bone in response to its own growth is termed as

A. Rotation
B. Secondary displacement
C. Primary displacement
D. Differentiation

185. The body tissue that grows rapidly but shows minimal growth after the age of 6-7 years is

A. Neural tissue
B. Lymphoid tissue
C. Skeletal tissue
D. Genital tissue

186. The implant method of studying growth was proposed by

A. Scammon
B. Borg
C. Belchier
D. Björk

187. Maxilla is "primarily" formed by

A. Intramembranous bone formation
B. From cartilage
C. Endochondral bone formation
D. Equally by intramembranous and endochondral bone formation

188. Which of the following areas of the oral cavity are affected by inflammatory papillary hyperplasia affects?

A. Lips
B. Tongue
C. Palate
D. Gingival

189. The main causative organism in Ludwig Angina is

A. Streptococcus viridans
B. Staphylococcus albus
C. Staphylococcus aureus
D. Streptococcus haemolyticus

190. Which of the following terms refers to a type of fusion in which the formed teeth are joined only along the line of cementum?

A. Gemination
B. Fusion
C. Concrescence
D. Dilaceration

191. Which is degeneration disorder characterized by atrophic changes of the deeper structures (e.g. fat, muscle, cartilage and bone) involving one side of the face?
- A. Scleroderma
- B. Parry Romberg syndrome
- C. Miescher's syndrome
- D. Peutz-Jeghers syndrome

192. Virus responsible for infectious mononucleosis is
- A. RNA Paramyxo virus
- B. Varicella zoster virus
- C. Epstein Barr virus
- D. Coxsackie virus A 16

193. Microabrasion involves the use of
- A. Sulphuric acid
- B. Acetic acid
- C. Phosphoric acid
- D. Hydrochloric acid

194. Name of lesion which is not a radiolucent lesion of the jaws
- A. Ameloblastoma
- B. Cherubism
- C. Focal periapical osteopetrosis
- D. Odontogenic cyst

195. Name the lesion where cotton wool, multifocal radiodense conglomerates is not seen usually
- A. Gardner's syndrome
- B. Cemento-osseous dysplasia
- C. Paget's disease
- D. Fibrous dysplasia

196. The syndrome of geographic tongue should be treated by
- A. Excision of the lesion
- B. Penicillin therapy
- C. Topical application of Nystatin
- D. Routine observation at recall time

197. Radiographically latent period of an acute periapical abscess is
- A. 7-10 days
- B. 10-15 days
- C. 2-5 days
- D. 3-7 days

198. What is not characteristic of Eagle's syndrome?
- A. Excessive lacrimation
- B. Pain during mandibular movement
- C. Stabbing type pain originate in the tonsillar regions
- D. When the jaws are closed the pain subsided

199. What is not included in the contents of the sublingual space?
- A. Sublingual gland
- B. Facial artery
- C. Hypoglossal nerve
- D. Lingual nerve

200. The clinical picture of hair in black hairy tongue is caused by hyperkeratinized hyperplastic
- A. Filiform papillae
- B. Fungiform papillae
- C. Vallate papillae
- D. Filiform and fungiform papillae

Answers

1 D
2 D
3 C
4 D
5 C
6 B
7 D The essential ingredients of investment material are gypsum and allotropic forms of silica. Most investment materials contain α–hemihydrate of gypsum because it provides greater strength. The gypsum serves as binder to hold the other ingredients together and to provide rigidity. The strength of the investment is dependent on the amount of binder present.
8 C
9 A
10 A
11 B
12 B
13 C
14 A
15 B Prevalence is the total number of cases in a given population at a **point** or over a **period** of time.
Incidence is the number of new cases in a given population occurring within a defined time period.
16 C
17 A
18 D **Double blind** plan is preferable over single blind plan. Similarly **cross-over design** is more advantageous.
19 B DMFT is both **cumulative** and **irreversible** index. Cumulative indices measure past as well as present condition. Irreversible indices measure conditions which, once manifested, cannot be reverted back to normal.
20 A
21 D
22 B
23 B Propofol has a faster recovery period which is advantageous in day care surgery.
24 C
25 D
26 C
27 D
28 A
29 B
30 D The cyclic phosphodiester cAMP is formed from ATP in a reaction catalyzed by adenyl cyclase. Adenyl cyclase activity is regulated by complex interactions, many of which involve hormone receptors. The second messenger camp participates in diverse regulatory functions in the cell. As a regulatory molecule comparatively little camp is required. Consequently the intracellular camp concentration is about 1 nmol/L, which is three orders of magnitude below that of ATP.
31 B In place of troponin, smooth muscle cells contain large amount of another regulatory protein called as calmodulin. This protein is similar to troponin in that it reacts with four calcium ions; it is different in the manner that it initiates contraction. Calmodulin does that by activating the myosin cross-bridges.
32 C Certain types of viruses can cause some kind of cancers. This usually results by either two ways. In the case of DNA virus, the DNA strand of the virus can insert itself directly into one of the chromosomes and cause mutation that leads to cancer. In the case of RNA virus some of these carry with them an enzyme called as reverse transcriptase that causes DNA to be transcribed from the RNA. Then the transcribed DNA inserts itself into the animal cell genome.
33 A The coding regions of DNA, the transcripts of which ultimately appear in the cytoplasm as single mRNA molecules, are usually interrupted in the eukaryotic genome by large intervening sequence of noncoding DNA. Most coding sequences for a single mRNA are interrupted in the genome by atleast one–and as many as 50 in some cases–noncoding intervening sequences called as interons. In most cases the interons are much longer than the continuous coding regions (exons).
34 B
35 C The lymphatic system represents an accessory route by which fluid can flow from the interstitial spaces into the blood. The system consists of peripheral lymphatics, lymph nodes, thoracic duct, and spleen. Thymus is not a part of lymphatic system.
36 A There is no disparity in size of the lungs on the right and left side. It is only the right bronchus, which is more vertical, which leads to foreign body lodgment to the right lung.
37 B Adipose tissue triacylglycerol is the main fuel reserve of the body. Subsequent to its hydrolysis fatty acids are released into the circulation as free fatty acids. These are taken up by most tissue and esterified to acyl-glycerol or oxidized as major fuel to CO_2. Surplus triacylglycerol arising from lipogenesis and free fatty acids is secreted into the circulation as VLDL (very low

density lipoprotein). They undergo the fate similar to that of chylomicrons.

38 C In addition to peptide bonds, covalent disulfide loops conform between transmembrane regions of protein. These disulfide loops confer additional stability to specific conformation of protein such as enzymes and structural protein (keratin).

39 A Isotopes are used to tag bio-molecules so that their metabolic fate could be monitored. Radio isotopes are never used in mass spectroscopy, which is used to determine the structure of biomolecules.

40 A Some hormones activate transmembrane receptors that inactivate the enzyme phospholipase C attached to the inside projections of the receptors. This enzyme catalyses the breakdown of some phospholipids in the cell membrane, especially phosphatidylinositol biphosphate into two different second messenger products, inositol triphosphate and diacylglycerol. The inositol triphosphate mobilizes calcium ions from the mitochondria and the endoplasmic reticulum, and the calcium ions than have their own second messenger effects.

41 D Selenium is the only antioxidant among the mentioned elements. Selenium is a constituent of glutathione peroxidase. It is an antioxidant with vitamin E. Its deficiency is seen when the soil content is low or secondary to parenteral nutrition and during protein–energy–malnutrition. Symptoms of its toxicity are hair loss, dermatitis and irritability.

42 D Exit from the endoplasmic reticulum may be rate-limiting step in the secretary pathway. In this context it has been found that certain proteins play a role in the assembly or proper folding of other proteins without themselves being components of later. Such proteins are called as molecular chaperones.

43 A

44 B **Latent period** is a term used in non-infections disease epidemiology as equivalent of incubation period in infectious diseases. **Serial interval** is a practical way of estimating incubation period based on the gap between primary and secondary cases. **Generation time** is roughly equal to incubation period.

45 B

46 A Maximum milk output is seen during first year after child birth but not necessarily at 12 months.

47 C

48 A Screening of community is done to identify those who have the disease or condition of interest. **Sensitivity** of a test satisfies this requirement.

49 C Ordinal scales grade qualitative conditions (codes) in a logical order when quantitative data (scores) is not available (or for convenience).

50 C If prevalence is 10% or 1/10 then the probability that one person selected at random would have the disease is 0.1. Hence the probability that three people would have the disease is $0.1 \times 0.1 \times 0.1 = 0.001$.

51 C Since the investigation proceeds from cause to effect it is a **cohort** study. Furthermore the study group was followed up from 1970 to 1995 hence it is also **prospective or concurrent.**

52 A

53 A

54 A

55 C

56 D

57 C

58 D

59 A

60 A

61 B

62 C

63 D

64 D

65 B

66 B

67 A

68 D

69 C

70 C

71 C

72 C

73 D

74 B

75 D

76 C

77 D

78 A

79 B Polyether is not compatible with epoxy resins because a separator must be used to prevent the epoxy resin from bonding to the impression.

80 B

81 A

82 A The modulus of elasticity reflects the stiffness of the material. Amongst the given material zinc phosphate has the maximum modulus of elasticity.

Zinc phosphate	9.3-13.4 Gpa
Polymer reinforced ZOE	2.7 Gpa
Zinc polycarboxylate	6.7 Gpa
Glass ionomer	3.5-6.5 Gpa

83 D Glutamate is secreted by the presynaptic terminals in many of the sensory pathways entering the central nervous system, as well as in many areas of cerebral cortex. It probably always causes excitation.

84 D Probably the most important factors for preventing clotting in the normal vascular system are (1) the smoothness of the endothelial surface which prevents contact activation of the intrinsic clotting system, (2) a layer of glycocalyx on the endothelium which repels clotting factors and platelets, (3) a protein called thrombomodulin which binds thrombin.

85 C The force of contraction of muscle can be increased by (1) increasing the number of motor units contracting simultaneously which is called multiple fibre summation and (2) by increasing the frequency of contraction which is called frequency summation and which can lead to tetanization.

86 A Classical iron deficiency anemia shows red cells, which are produced, that are much smaller than normal and have too little hemoglobin inside them giving rise to microcytic, hypochromic anemia. In extreme conditions the blood picture becomes that of hypochromic and anisocytosis.

87 A All gypsum products expand externally upon setting.
Plaster expands the most—0.2 to 0.3%;
Stone expands—0.08 to 0.10%;
And high-strength stone expands the least— 0.05 to 0.07%.

Theoretically, a contraction on setting can be calculated; however, the growing crystals of the gypsum cause an outward crystal thrust. This thrust results in an external expansion with resulting internal porosities in the set mass. A minimal setting expansion is desirable for accurate dimensional reproduction for most casts and dies.

88 C During night a person goes through two types of sleep that alternate with each other. (1) Slow wave sleep, non-REM sleep and (2) Rapid eye movement sleep.

During REM the muscle tone through out the body is exceedingly depressed and the heart rate and the respiratory rate becomes irregular. Therefore the blood pressure is reduced. On the contrary during the non-REM sleep the blood pressure is increased.

89 D The coefficient of thermal expansion of most of the ceramics now a day is in the range of 12-16 ppm/°C (25°– 500°C).
For example:

Duceram LFC	12.2	ppm/°C (25°–500° C)
Finesse	11	ppm/°C (25°–500° C)
Duceram plus	14.2	ppm/°C (25°–500° C)
Duceram	14.2	ppm/°C (25°–500° C)
Duceram gold	15.8	ppm/°C (25°–500° C)

90 D
91 C
92 D
93 D
94 B
95 B
96 A
97 D
98 A
99 A
100 A

101 A The labio-dental or fricative sounds are used in the anterior tooth positioning. This technique was developed by Pound and Murell in which the position of the artificial maxillary anterior is determined by the position of the maxillae when the patient says words beginning with "f" or "v". The incisal edges of upper anteriors should touch the vermilion border of the lower lip.

102 B During fabrication of a denture of a patient with torus palatinus most preferred method is giving relief on master cast before packing. By doing so the impressions are recorded as exactly as possible without any alteration and relief can be determined by using the surveyor in the lab to determine the degree of undercut. Hence this method is accurate, saves patient's time and is not arbitrary like relief in the denture before insertion.

103 D In maxillary denture thickness of flange in disto-buccal area is determined when the jaws are separated and the patient moves the mandible to right and left lateral positions. The thickness distal to alveolar tubercle area is being contacted by anterior border of the ramus of mandible, coronoid process and masseter.

104 B Amongst the given impression materials zinc oxide eugenol impression material will not be used because it may cause some tissue irritation. Alginate will not be a material of choice as for alginate the size of the tray should be as big as possible which is not going to be comfortable for a patient with limited mouth opening. Between the light body and regular body light body is preferred, as it will have better flow and therefore accurate recording of the tissues.

105 A The palatal cusp of the upper posterior teeth in complete denture should fall on the crest of the mandibular ridge. By doing so it is ensured that the palatal cusp of upper teeth will fall in the central groove of the lower, which are placed over the center of the ridge. Therefore most of the occlusal forces will fall on the center of the ridge.

106 D If the genial tubercle are at the level of the crest of the ridge then definitely the muscle attached to them also become superficial (1) genioglossal and (2) geniohyoid.

There is no way the denture can be made without covering the tubercles otherwise the denture will be too narrow and fracture plus it will not develop the peripheral seal. If it has to be covered then relief is a must so that when the muscles get activated during movement the denture is not lifted.

107 A The position of the head and tongue during the fluid wax procedure is of particular importance. According to nelson the effective posterior seal is to be established without inducing tissue irritation, the soft palate should be impressioned in its most functionally depressed position. The maximum depression of the soft palate will be recorded when the Frankfurt plane (porion-orbitale) is 300 below the horizontal and the tongue is firmly positioned against the mandibular teeth.

108 C Overextended PPS will lead to gagging of the patient. Overextended lingual flange leads to ulceration and lifting of the lower denture as the floor of the mouth is raised during any movement. Overextended lingual flange in retromylohyoid region causes pain in the throat sensation.

109 C The sprue should be attached to the bulkiest part of the wax pattern away from the margins and occlusal contacts. It is always attached at an obtuse angle so that the molten metal is directed to all parts of the mold without having to flow opposite the direction of the casting force. The sprue must also allow proper positioning of the pattern in the ring.

110 A There are two glandular openings within the tissue of the posterior portion of the hard palate, usually lying on either side of the midline. They are known as fovea palatini. They are the ductal openings into which the ducts of other palatal mucous glands drain.

111 C The retromylohyoid space lies at the distal end of the Alveolingual sulcus. It is bounded medially by the anterior tonsillar pillar, posteriorly by the retromylohyoid curtain which is formed posteriorly by the superior constrictor muscle, laterally by the mandible and pterygomandibular raphe, anteriorly by the lingual tuberosity and inferiorly by the mylohyoid muscle.

112 A Major causes of gagging are:
- Hypersensitive patients
- Insertion and removal of dentures may induce gagging (making and breaking of the posterior palatal seal)
- Overextended upper dentures
- Bulky posterior margins of the upper denture.

113 D The retraction cord must be placed in the sulcus for a period of 5-15 minutes (on an average of 10 minutes). Cord should be around 2 inches long and packed nicely in the sulcus except the last 2-3 mm of the cord. After 10 minutes the cord is removed slowly to avoid bleeding. Remember the impression material should be injected only if the sulcus remains dry.

114 D The coefficient of thermal expansion of porcelain is about $12 \times 10^{-6}/°C$. The coefficient of thermal expansion is important when porcelain is bonded to metal. The expansion of the metal and porcelain must be properly matched or the alloy must be more than porcelain otherwise porcelain will fracture when the crown cools from the temperature of the porcelain oven to room temperature.

115 A Titanium has a high melting point (1668°C), a special casting machine with arc–melting capability and an argon atmosphere under vacuum is used, along with a compatible casting investment, to ensure acceptable castability.

116 A Comparing the cell cytotoxicity for different impression materials reveal that polysulfide results in the lowest cell death count and set polyether impression material produces the highest cell cytotoxicity.

117 C Medium (regular) viscosities of polyether and addition silicone impression materials are used for the monophase or single viscosity technique. The procedure is similar to that of the multiple-mix technique, except that only one mix is made; part of the material is placed in the tray and another part in the syringe for injection in the cavity preparation, on prepared teeth or on the soft tissue. The success of this technique depends on the pseudo plastic properties of the material.

118 A Corrosion resistance is derived from the material components being either too noble to react in the oral environment (gold or palladium) or by the ability of one or more of the metallic elements to form an adherent passivating surface film, which inhibits any surface reaction (chromium in Ni-Cr and Co–Cr alloys and titanium in commercially pure titanium and in Ti-6Al-4V alloy.

119 C Four types of casting crucibles are available, clay, carbon, quartz and zirconia-alumina.
- Clay crucibles are used for many crown and bridge alloys such as high noble and noble types.
- Carbon crucibles are used higher fusing gold based alloys.
- Quartz crucibles are used high fusing alloys of any type, mainly alloys which are sensitive to carbon contamination. Crown and bridge alloys with high palladium content for metal-ceramic copings and any of the nickel based or cobalt based alloys are included in this category.

120 B

121 B The most effective method of controlling the setting expansion is through the addition of chemicals by the manufacturer. The setting expansion can be reduced by adding either potassium sulfate or borax.

122 B IOWA wax, developed by Dr. Smith.
- Korecta wax No. 4 developed by Dr. Applegate.
- Physiologic paste developed by Dr. Harkins.
- Adaptol developed by Nathan Kaye, are the waxes which flow at room temperature.
- Korecta No. 1 is not a mouth temperature wax.

123 A Polymethyl methacrylate resin can also be polymerized using microwave energy. A conventional microwave oven is used to supply the thermal energy required for polymerization. This mode of curing is done via conduction of heat.

124 C

125 C

126 A The current concept of bar clasp design is the RPI system (rest, proximal plate, I-bar). This assembly consists of a mesiocclusal rest with the minor connector placed into mesiolingual embrasure, a distal guiding plane, extending from the marginal ridge to the junction of middle and gingival third of the abutment. The I–bar is placed in the gingival one third of the buccal or labial surface of the abutment in 0.01 inch-undercut.

127 B

128 A

129 D

130 A

131 C

132 C

133 A

134 A

135 B

136 C

137 B

138 A

139 A

140 B

141 C

142 B

143 D

144 B

145 D

146 D

147 D

148 C

149 A

150 A

151 C

152 D

153 A

154 A

155 B

156 C

157 B Removal of calculus and altered cementum is the primary objective of root planning procedure.

158 A Papilla preservation flap is indicated as esthetics is of prime importance in the upper anterior region.

159 C

160 C Agressive form of periodontal diseases are usually associated with very less amount of calculus.

161 A As atleast 2-3 mm of attached gingiva should be left after gingivectomy.

162 B

163 C

164 A The tear resistance of
Polysulfide is 2500-7000 N/m
Condensation silicone–2300-2600 N/m
Addition silicone–1500-4300 N/m
Polyether–1800-4800 N/m

Therefore polysulfide has the highest tear resistance.

165 B

166 C

167 D

168 A

169 D

170 B

171 B Modulus of elasticity of few important dental materials is given below:

Dentin	18600 MPa
Enamel	83000 MPa
Amalgam	27600 MPa
Composite	16600 MPa
Zinc phosphate	13800 MPa
Glass ionomer	5520 MPa
Polysulfide rubber	1-3 MPa

Therefore enamel has the highest modulus of elasticity.

172 C

173 D

174 B

175 B

176 C PAR Index or PEER Assessment Rating was proposed by Richmond S et al. In 1992 to measure malocclusion and assess the outcome of orthodontic treatment. Overjet, overbite, midline, buccal segment and buccal occlusion are components of PAR Index. Weights of these components can be as follows: overjet (Score 0-8), Overbite (Score 0-8), Midline (Score 0-2), Buccal segment (0-5). Hence a midline score of 4 is a misnomer.

177 C
178 C
179 D
180 C
181 A
182 D
183 C
184 C
185 A
186 D
187 A
188 C
189 C
190 C
191 B
192 C
193 D
194 C
195 A
196 D
197 B Osteoclast cells take at least 10-15 days to resorbe the bone and they arrive much after neutrophils.
198 A
199 B
200 A